Tumors
of the
Central Nervous System

Atlas
of
Tumor Pathology

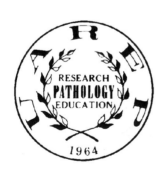

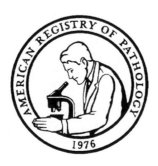

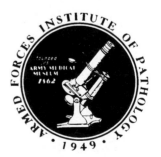

ATLAS OF TUMOR PATHOLOGY

Third Series
Fascicle 10

TUMORS OF THE CENTRAL NERVOUS SYSTEM

by

PETER C. BURGER, M.D.
Professor of Pathology, Oncology, and Neurosurgery
The Johns Hopkins University
School of Medicine
Baltimore, Maryland

and

BERND W. SCHEITHAUER, M.D.
Consultant and Professor of Pathology
Mayo Clinic and Mayo Graduate School of Medicine
Rochester, Minnesota

Published by the
ARMED FORCES INSTITUTE OF PATHOLOGY
Washington, D.C.

Under the Auspices of
UNIVERSITIES ASSOCIATED FOR RESEARCH AND EDUCATION IN PATHOLOGY, INC.
Bethesda, Maryland
1994

Accepted for Publication
1993

Available from the American Registry of Pathology
Armed Forces Institute of Pathology
Washington, D.C. 20306-6000
ISSN 0160-6344
ISBN 1-881041-10-7

ATLAS OF TUMOR PATHOLOGY

EDITOR
JUAN ROSAI, M.D.
Department of Pathology
Memorial Sloan-Kettering Cancer Center
New York, New York 10021-6007

ASSOCIATE EDITOR
LESLIE H. SOBIN, M.D.
Armed Forces Institute of Pathology
Washington, D.C. 20306-6000

EDITORS' NOTE

The Atlas of Tumor Pathology has a long and distinguished history. It was first conceived at a Cancer Research Meeting held in St. Louis in September 1947 as an attempt to standardize the nomenclature of neoplastic diseases. The first series was sponsored by the National Academy of Sciences-National Research Council. The organization of this Sisyphean effort was entrusted to the Subcommittee on Oncology of the Committee on Pathology, and Dr. Arthur Purdy Stout was the first editor-in-chief. Many of the illustrations were provided by the Medical Illustration Service of the Armed Forces Institute of Pathology, the type was set by the Government Printing Office, and the final printing was done at the Armed Forces Institute of Pathology (hence the colloquial appellation "AFIP Fascicles"). The American Registry of Pathology purchased the Fascicles from the Government Printing Office and sold them virtually at cost. Over a period of 20 years, approximately 15,000 copies each of nearly 40 Fascicles were produced. The worldwide impact that these publications have had over the years has largely surpassed the original goal. They quickly became among the most influential publications on tumor pathology ever written, primarily because of their overall high quality but also because their low cost made them easily accessible to pathologists and other students of oncology the world over.

Upon completion of the first series, the National Academy of Sciences-National Research Council handed further pursuit of the project over to the newly created Universities Associated for Research and Education in Pathology (UAREP). A second series was started, generously supported by grants from the AFIP, the National Cancer Institute, and the American Cancer Society. Dr. Harlan I. Firminger became the editor-in-chief and was succeeded by Dr. William H. Hartmann. The second series Fascicles were produced as bound volumes instead of loose leaflets. They featured a more comprehensive coverage of the subjects, to the extent that the Fascicles could no longer be regarded as "atlases" but rather as monographs describing and illustrating in detail the tumors and tumor-like conditions of the various organs and systems.

Once the second series was completed, with a success that matched that of the first, UAREP and AFIP decided to embark on a third series. A new editor-in-chief and an associate editor were selected, and a distinguished editorial board was appointed. The mandate for the third series remains the same as for the previous ones, i.e., to oversee the production of an eminently practical publication with surgical pathologists as its primary audience, but also aimed at other workers in oncology. The main purposes of this series are to promote a consistent, unified, and biologically sound nomenclature; to guide the surgical pathologist in the diagnosis of the various tumors and tumor-like lesions; and to provide relevant histogenetic, pathogenetic, and clinicopathologic information on these entities. Just as the second series included data obtained from ultrastructural (and, in the more recent Fascicles, immunohistochemical) examination, the third series will, in addition, incorporate pertinent information obtained with the newer molecular biology techniques. As in the past, a continuous attempt will be made to correlate, whenever possible, the nomenclature used in the Fascicles with that proposed by the World Health Organization's International Histological Classification of Tumors. The format of the third series has been changed in order to incorporate additional items and to ensure a consistency of style throughout. This includes the dropping of the 's possessive in eponymic terms, in accordance with the WHO and the International Nomenclature of Diseases. Close cooperation between the various authors and their respective liaisons from the editorial board will be emphasized to minimize unnecessary repetition and discrepancies in the text and illustrations.

To its everlasting credit, the participation and commitment of the AFIP to this venture is even more substantial and encompassing than in previous series. It now extends to virtually all scientific, technical, and financial aspects of the production.

The task confronting the organizations and individuals involved in the third series is even more daunting than in the preceding efforts because of the ever-increasing complexity of the matter at hand. It is hoped that this combined effort—of which, needless to say, that represented by the authors is first and foremost—will result in a series worthy of its two illustrious predecessors and will be a suitable introduction to the tumor pathology of the twenty-first century.

Juan Rosai, M.D.
Leslie H. Sobin, M.D.

ACKNOWLEDGMENTS

We are, first and foremost, honored to recognize Mrs. Bonnie Lynch as our secretarial collaborator who has contributed so much to this volume. Her dedication, equanimity, and sense of good humor are as constant as the high quality of her work. Similar praises need be extended also to Ms. Susan Reeves, the principal photographer for this project. Although increasingly curious as to when this long project would be finished, she never compromised her meticulous attention to detail which, we hope, is apparent in the photomicrographs. Mr. Steve Conlon was also a great help in preparing illustrations. Dr. Ian Sutherland deserves many thanks for his editorial assistance.

Able colleagues who assisted by reviewing the manuscript include Drs. Thomas Montine, Douglas Anthony, Gregory Fuller, James Goldman, Hannah Kinney, and Jacob Vandersteenhoven. Drs. Orest Boyko and Allan Friedman aided in the descriptions of radiographic and clinical features. For the illustrations, we owe much to the many generous contributors of case material who are credited in the figure legends.

Much of the work done by one of us (PCB) was carried out in the Department of Pathology of the Duke University Medical Center. We are grateful for the generous support of the Department in the preparation of this volume.

We recognize also unwitting, and perhaps unwilling, participants in this project, such as journal editors and co-workers, for their patience while our attention was diverted to this effort.

Finally, special thanks must be given to our understanding families as this large and complicated endeavor increasingly encroached on our already restricted precious time at home.

Peter C. Burger, M.D.
Bernd W. Scheithauer, M.D.

TUMORS OF THE CENTRAL NERVOUS SYSTEM

Contents

TUMORS OF THE CENTRAL NERVOUS SYSTEM

INTRODUCTION

Over 20 years have passed since the previous edition of the Fascicle, *Tumors of the Central Nervous System*. Although the pace at which major new entities are recognized has slowed somewhat, the process of discovery is ongoing and descriptions of new lesions or tumor subcategories continue to appear. Important diagnostic techniques such as immunohistochemistry and the determination of proliferating indices have become available. Molecular biologic methods are now being applied, but are just beginning to encroach upon the primacy of routine histologic diagnosis. Innovations and refinements in surgical procedures, such as the operating microscope and stereotactically directed needle biopsy, have had major impacts since the surgeon can sample freely lesions that previously were approached only with trepidation. Spectacular advances have been made in neuroimaging. When the second series Fascicle, *Tumors of the Central Nervous System,* was written such techniques were limited to skull radiographs, angiography, pneumoencephalography, ventriculography, myelography, and radioisotope scanning. The elegant in vivo delineation by radiography of the details of nervous system anatomy which we now take for granted was not available. Radiographs are now the same indispensable diagnostic aids for the study of central nervous system tumors that they have long been in the pathologic study of bone lesions.

As a consequence of these clinical and radiologic advances, neoplastic and non-neoplastic lesions are not only sampled at will, but are often detected early in the course of disease. Small, often fragmented specimens are commonplace. The pathologist's task is complicated by a larger list of potential diagnoses and smaller specimens. In addition, clinicians are increasingly attuned to the subtleties of tumor classification and grading. For example, there is a tendency to suggest or reject radiotherapy as a treatment option on the basis of small and subjective differences in tumor grade. Entities that were previously treated similarly, e.g., astrocytomas and oligodendrogliomas, must now be distinguished in view of the relative chemosensitivity of the latter. Equally important is the increasing need to recognize certain primary brain tumors that are not infiltrative biologically malignant lesions deserving aggressive postsurgical therapy.

For all of these reasons, the publication of a new Fascicle on Tumors of the Central Nervous System seems appropriate. This volume is intended to serve as a practical diagnostic aid in the context of surgical pathology, rather than as a review of such issues as etiology and molecular pathogenesis. The details of these latter rapidly evolving fields are better left to other sources. The discussions of most entities therefore include a summary of clinical features and, as is evident on even casual perusal of this book, descriptions of radiographic features. In the context of surgical neuropathology, these images in many respects constitute the "gross examination" of the day, with the added benefit of providing functional information about the lesion and surrounding tissue.

In the sections describing microscopic features, we have emphasized not only the stereotypic appearances expected in an atlas, but also the deviations from the classic presentations so commonly encountered in practice. Reactive and inflammatory processes are emphasized since they are finding their way to surgical pathologists with increasing frequency. The evaluation of needle biopsy specimens is described as well since these small, sometimes suboptimal fragments are now a fact of professional life. The perennial difficulties inherent in interpretation of frozen sections are addressed also. Finally, special attention is given throughout the text, figures, and appendices to better differentiated and hamartomatous lesions for which aggressive treatment may be administered inadvertently.

The authors hope that these modifications will in some measure advance the task begun so successfully by the authors of the central nervous system Fascicles of the first and second series.

1
CLASSIFICATION OF CENTRAL NERVOUS SYSTEM TUMORS

Like most other current classifications of central nervous system (CNS) tumors, the one adopted in this volume has its roots in the Bailey and Cushing system of 1929 (1). Viewed in the context of human ontogeny and cytogenesis, CNS tumors were related to a specific cell lineage and, when possible, were identified as primitive or "-blastic" or as differentiated or "-cytic." The common lesions now recognized as fibrillary or "diffuse" astrocytic neoplasms (astrocytoma, anaplastic astrocytoma, glioblastoma) were thus categorized as astrocytoma, astroblastoma, and spongioblastoma multiforme, respectively. Embryonal tumors, long viewed as malignant caricatures of embryogenesis, were categorized as medulloepithelioma, neuroepithelioma, and various "blastomas," of which medulloblastoma is the most common representative. By today's standards the classification was simple, but its concepts are deeply rooted and readily apparent in current classifications, including the one employed here.

In the first Fascicle, *Tumors of the Central Nervous System* (1951), Kernohan and Sayre largely respected the Bailey and Cushing system for embryonal tumors, but greatly modified the approach to gliomas (4). In a vigorous attempt at simplification, the authors presented these latter neoplasms as variable degrees of dedifferentiation, but not as stages of cytogenesis. The astrocytoma, astroblastoma, and spongioblastoma multiforme of Bailey and Cushing became the familiar astrocytomas grades 1 to 4. The Kernohan approach was popular because it dealt readily with the tendency of many gliomas to transform to higher grade and explained the regional heterogeneity so often encountered in practice. It also clearly established the inverse relation between tumor grade and duration of survival. Although recently there has been a retreat from strict application of the Kernohan system, its underlying concepts have been retained.

Grading continues to be important in the diagnosis of gliomas, both astrocytic and nonastrocytic. Whether descriptive terms or numbers are used, grading is applied de facto to the full spectrum of CNS neoplasms. Even neuronal neoplasms, such as pineal parenchymal tumors, are in effect graded with a recognition that, as in gliomas, variable and occasionally mixed degrees of differentiation are common.

Insights into CNS tumor biology found in both the Bailey and Cushing and the Kernohan and Sayre approaches were incorporated into the detailed second series Fascicle, *Tumors of the Central Nervous System* (1972) by Lucien Rubinstein (6), as well as in the classic and authoritative text, *Pathology of Tumours of the Nervous System* coauthored with Rubinstein's former mentor and lifelong collaborator, Professor Dorothy Russell (7). Both books presented a more detailed analysis of a field with an increasingly apparent complexity. In these volumes, the authors retained the Bailey and Cushing approach to embryonal tumors and added two entities, ependymoblastoma and primitive polar spongioblastoma. They expounded at length upon embryonal tumors as consequences of neoplastic transformation at certain, and often fleeting, stages of neurocytogenesis. Kernohan and Sayre's concept of progressive anaplasia in gliomas was accepted, but not the notion that all gliomas could be simply classified into four grades. The uniqueness of the pilocytic astrocytoma and the importance of its distinction from diffuse or fibrillary astrocytomas, were also emphasized. Manifold inflammatory lesions and non-neuroectodermal tumors were also included since they are "tumors" in the broad sense of the term. Recent additions to the Russell/Rubinstein text include descriptions of more recently recognized entities such as pleomorphic xanthoastrocytoma, central neurocytoma, and infantile desmoplastic ganglioglioma.

As a part of a wide-ranging attempt by the World Health Organization (WHO) to standardize nomenclature for most human tumors, an international committee of neuropathologists was convened to prepare the WHO "Blue Book" entitled *Histological Typing of Tumours of the Central Nervous System*, edited by Professor Klaus Zülch (8). The classification in this 1979 publication was to a certain extent similar to that of the second series CNS Fascicle, but had to accommodate the sometimes divergent views of the participants. The classification's origin as a committee project is apparent where, for example, glioblastoma and medulloblastoma are combined under "Poorly Differentiated and Embryonal

Tumors." By design, the book was not a comprehensive text but rather a brief outline seeking to provide a consensus classification rather than detailed descriptions of histopathologic features.

The initial WHO classification came to grips with the issue of predicting clinical behavior by assigning grades I to IV. These were based upon histologic factors and were intended to provide a general estimate of a lesion's anticipated biologic behavior. There was, however, little information about the prognostic significance of specific histologic variables and the grading system was, by today's standards, somewhat rigid. The diffuse or fibrillary astrocytic tumors noted above ranged from grade II (astrocytoma) through grade III (anaplastic astrocytoma) to grade IV (glioblastoma). Functionally, therefore, the WHO method of grading these tumors was a three-tiered system, similar to that of the second series CNS Fascicle and to the approach of Russell and Rubinstein. Pilocytic neoplasms were, appropriately, considered grade I. This standardized approach was obviously arbitrary and, with regard to gliomas, was readily confused with grades 1 to 4 of the Kernohan system. Particularly outside the United States, the WHO system was, nonetheless, highly influential. Its lack of precision in assigning grades only became a limitation in recent years when the decision to administer radiotherapy or chemotherapy often hinged upon the sometimes subtle distinction of tumors of grade II from those of grade III or above.

The Blue Book was recently revised by a second WHO committee that retained the general outline of the preceding volume but added newly described entities, including central neurocytoma, dysembryoplastic neuroepithelial tumor, infantile desmoplastic ganglioglioma, pleomorphic xanthoastrocytoma, and papillary craniopharyngioma (5). Upon general consensus, it also recognized that the glioblastoma is, in most instances, a high-grade diffuse or fibrillary astrocytic neoplasm which is not akin to the medulloblastoma except in its poorly differentiated state. Despite reluctance on the part of some, the group gave the meningeal hemangiopericytoma a nosologic niche independent of meningioma. As expected, considerable discussion surrounded the classification of embryonal tumors, particularly the place for the popular term "primitive neuroectodermal tumor." The book retained the general approach to grading

of the prior volume, but the grades of astrocytomas were more rigidly defined.

The classification employed in this Fascicle contains elements of all of the above systems. It is not identical to any of these, however, nor does it strictly comply with our previous text which is to a large extent organized along regional rather than strictly histogenetic lines (2). We have freely expressed our own preferences in several areas, adding comments where our approach differs significantly from the aforementioned classifications. We did not, for example, use the modified "PNET" concept advanced by the second WHO committee for reasons discussed in the chapter, Embryonal Tumors. In addition, the wide range of mesenchymal tumors now known to frequent the nervous system required an expanded classification. We modified the classification used for soft tissue tumors in the textbook of Enzinger and Weiss (3). In accord with the recent WHO deliberations, but at variance with the stance taken by the second series Fascicle, we placed the primitive polar spongioblastoma in a category of uncertain histogenesis, rather than among the embryonal tumors. In regard to grading, we have not attempted to numerically stratify gradations of malignancy within the tumor groups but retained categories defined by verbal designations. Where appropriate, comments are added to clarify the relationship of these divisions to synonymous numerical grading systems of proven utility.

In light of these problems in the classification of CNS tumors, the subjectivity of histologic interpretation and the difficulty inherent in classifying lesions on the basis of phenotypic features alone become apparent, as does the morphologic overlap between some CNS tumors, such as astrocytomas and oligodendrogliomas. Precise definitions, such as for mixed gliomas or certain embryonal tumors, thus become difficult to establish and apply. It is also clear that there are, as yet, many undefined subcategories of tumors or tissue patterns in which the nosologic and clinical significance remain to be defined. That practical, everyday tumor classification is not yet an exact science is a consequence of the incomplete understanding of histologic and clinical features, as well as an even more incomplete grasp of the ultimate details of molecular anatomy. We have made an effort to provide a clinically relevant classification, in full awareness that there will be further evolution in CNS tumor classification.

HISTOLOGIC CLASSIFICATION OF
TUMORS OF THE CENTRAL NERVOUS SYSTEM

1. Tumors of Neuroglia and Choroid Plexus Epithelium
    1.1   Astrocytic neoplasms
          1.1.1   Fibrillary or "diffuse" astrocytic tumors
                  1.1.1.1   Astrocytoma
                  1.1.1.2   Anaplastic astrocytoma
                  1.1.1.3   Glioblastoma multiforme
                  1.1.1.4   Gliosarcoma
                  1.1.1.5   Protoplasmic astrocytoma
                  1.1.1.6   Granular cell astrocytic neoplasms
                  1.1.1.7   Gliomatosis cerebri
                  1.1.1.8   Meningeal gliomatosis
          1.1.2   Other astrocytic tumors
                  1.1.2.1   Pilocytic astrocytoma
                  1.1.2.2   Pleomorphic xanthoastrocytoma
                  1.1.2.3   Subependymal giant cell astrocytoma (tuberous sclerosis)
                  1.1.2.4   Infantile desmoplastic astrocytoma
                  1.1.2.5   Gliofibroma
    1.2   Oligodendroglial neoplasms
          1.2.1   Oligodendroglioma and anaplastic oligodendroglioma
    1.3   Ependymal neoplasms
          1.3.1   Ependymoma and anaplastic ependymoma
          1.3.2   Subependymoma
    1.4   Choroid plexus neoplasms
          1.4.1   Choroid plexus papilloma
          1.4.2   Choroid plexus carcinoma
    1.5   Gliomas of mixed composition
          1.5.1   Mixed gliomas
    1.6   Other gliomas
          1.6.1   Astroblastoma
          1.6.2   Granular cell tumor of the infundibulum
2. Neuronal and Glio-Neuronal Tumors
    2.1   Gangliocytoma and ganglioglioma
    2.2   Desmoplastic infantile ganglioglioma
    2.3   Dysplastic cerebellar gangliocytoma (Lhermitte-Duclos disease)
    2.4   Central neurocytoma
    2.5   Dysembryoplastic neuroepithelial tumor
    2.6   Other glio-neuronal lesions
3. Embryonal Tumors
    3.1   Primitive neuroectodermal tumor
    3.2   Medulloepithelioma
    3.3   Neuroblastoma and ganglioneuroblastoma
    3.4   Olfactory neuroblastoma (esthesioneuroblastoma)
    3.5   Retinoblastoma
    3.6   Melanotic neuroectodermal tumor of infancy
    3.7   Ependymoblastoma
    3.8   Medulloblastoma
    3.9   Medullomyoblastoma and melanotic medulloblastoma
    3.10 Other embryonal tumors

4.   Tumors of the Pineal Gland
    4.1   Pineocytoma
    4.2   Pineoblastoma
    4.3   Mixed pineocytoma - pineoblastoma and pineal parenchymal neoplasms of intermediate differentiation
    4.4   Pineal cyst
    4.5   Gliomas

5.   Tumors of Uncertain Origin
    5.1   Hemangioblastoma
    5.2   Primitive polar spongioblastoma
    5.3   Atypical teratoid/rhabdoid tumor

6.   Germ Cell Tumors

7.   Tumors of Meningothelial Cells
    7.1   Meningioma
    7.2   Atypical meningioma
    7.3   Malignant meningioma

8.   Tumors of Mesenchymal Tissue
    8.1   Vascular tumors and tumor-like lesions
        8.1.1   Vascular malformations
            8.1.1.1   Arteriovenous malformation
            8.1.1.2   Cavernous angioma
            8.1.1.3   Venous malformation
            8.1.1.4   Capillary telangiectasis
            8.1.1.5   Other vascular lesions
        8.1.2   Vascular neoplasms
            8.1.2.1   Hemangiopericytoma
            8.1.2.2   Hemangioendothelioma
            8.1.2.3   Angiosarcoma
    8.2   Nonvascular mesenchymal tumors and tumor-like lesions
        8.2.1   Benign nonvascular tumors
            8.2.1.1   Lipoma
            8.2.1.2   Lipoma of the internal auditory canal
            8.2.1.3   Chondroma and osteochondroma
            8.2.1.4   Fibroma and fibromatosis
            8.2.1.5   Other benign mesenchymal lesions
        8.2.2   Malignant nonvascular tumors
            8.2.2.1   Chordoma
            8.2.2.2   Chondrosarcoma
            8.2.2.3   Mesenchymal chondrosarcoma
            8.2.2.4   Rhabdomyosarcoma
            8.2.2.5   Fibrosarcoma
            8.2.2.6   Malignant fibrous histiocytoma
            8.2.2.7   Other sarcomas

9.   Tumors of Paraganglionic Tissue
    9.1   Paraganglioma

10.   Primary Tumors of Hematopoietic Tissue
    10.1   Primary central nervous system lymphoma
    10.2   Plasmacytoma
    10.3   Microgliomatosis

18. Metastatic and Secondary Neoplasms
    18.1 Metastatic carcinoma and sarcoma
    18.2 Leukemia
    18.3 Secondary malignant lymphoma
    18.4 Spinal epidural lymphoma
    18.5 Intravascular lymphoma
    18.6 Lymphomatoid granulomatosis

REFERENCES

1. Bailey P, Cushing H. A classification of tumors of the glioma group. Philadelphia: JB Lippincott, 1926.
2. Burger PC, Scheithauer BW, Vogel FS. Surgical pathology of the nervous system and its coverings. 3rd ed. New York: Churchill Livingstone, 1991.
3. Enzinger FM, Weiss SW. Soft tissue tumors. 2nd ed. St. Louis: CV Mosby, 1988.
4. Kernohan JW, Sayre GP. Tumors of the central nervous system, Section X—Fascicles 35 and 37. Atlas of Tumor Pathology. Washington DC: Armed Forces Institute of Pathology, 1952.

5. Kleihues P, Burger PC, Scheithauer BW. Histological typing of tumours of the central nervous system. World Health Organization. Berlin: Springer-Verlag, 1993
6. Rubinstein LJ. Tumors of the central nervous system. Atlas of Tumor Pathology, 2nd Series, Fascicle 6. Washington DC: Armed Forces Institute of Pathology, 1972.
7. Russell DS, Rubinstein LJ. Pathology of tumours of the nervous system. 5th ed. Baltimore: Williams & Wilkins, 1989.
8. Zülch KJ. Histological typing of tumours of the central nervous system. Geneva: World Health Organization, 1979.

2
NORMAL EMBRYOLOGY AND ANATOMY

Embryology

The developing central nervous system (CNS) first emerges as a plate of embryonic epithelium which, when uplifted, delimits a midline longitudinal trench, the primitive neural groove (9,30). In tectonic fashion, by a process of uplifting and subvention, the opposing edges of the groove approach the midline, make contact in the mid-dorsal region, and undergo rostral to caudal fusion. The result is a cylinder which remains open at both ends until the time of closure of the anterior and posterior neuropores. Early in embryogenesis, the cylinder becomes constricted to form four segments: the prosencephalon, mesencephalon, rhombencephalon, and a caudal elongation which remains undivided as the forerunner of the spinal cord. In accordance with the C-shape of the early embryo, the neural tube is angulated or flexed in the cervical and cephalic regions. A subsequent posterior shift of the cerebrum necessitates an additional kink in the region of the future pons.

The crowning touch in the development of the human brain is the appearance and enlargement of the telencephalic vesicles. These aneurysmal expansions bud from the prosencephalon and expand dramatically as they begin to assert their role as the brain's dominant divisions, the cerebral hemispheres. Their lumina, the future lateral ventricles, retain their connection with the third ventricle via the foramina of Monro. Being narrow, these apertures are vulnerable to obstruction by regional tumors such as colloid cysts, neurocytomas, and a wide spectrum of gliomas.

The second prosencephalic division, the diencephalon, gives rise to the thalami and hypothalamus. The mesencephalon, or midbrain, retains a generally tubular profile and a short simple lumen, the aqueduct of Sylvius, which persists as a narrow but functionally important channel for the passage of cerebrospinal fluid into the fourth ventricle. In subsequent development, the rhombencephalon or hindbrain evolves into the metencephalon (pons and cerebellum) and myelencephalon (medulla).

As a primitive reflex and relay structure, the spinal cord lacks the complicated structure of the more rostral segments of the CNS which subserve cognition, intellect, and coordination. As a result, the cord retains the basic tubular architecture of the early developing nervous system as well as the dorsal/ventral segregation of sensory and motor functions, respectively. Motor functions initiated ventrally in the anterior gray columns are conducted to the periphery through the anterior roots, whereas sensory impulses are received dorsally through the posterior roots. Although at birth the central canal is patent along its length, it becomes discontinuous by puberty, leaving only clusters and small tubules of ependymal cells. The most common intramedullary cord tumor (ependymoma) is derived from these cells.

The choroid plexus projects into the ventricular system along both the embryonic choroidal fissure of the cerebrum and the rhombic lip of the cerebellum. In the mature brain, the plexus intrudes into the lateral, third, and fourth ventricles but not into the aqueduct of Sylvius. In the trigone or atrium of the lateral ventricles, at the juncture of the temporal horn, occipital horn, and body, the plexus forms an especially prominent mass, the glomus. As discussed in chapter 19, asymptomatic xanthogranulomatous degeneration occurs frequently in this region. In the fourth ventricle, the plexus follows the lateral recesses to emerge in the subarachnoid space of the cerebellopontine angle, thus explaining the occasional papilloma occurring lateral to the brain stem and ostensibly arising outside the ventricular system. Meningothelial cells, and therefore occasional meningiomas (see fig. 9-5), are found within the stroma of the choroid plexus.

Early in development, the neural tube evolves to form: 1) an internal ventricular zone which ultimately gives rise to choroid plexus epithelium and ependyma; 2) a subventricular zone which contains the mitotically active precursors of neurons and glia, both of which migrate from the ventricular region; 3) an intermediate zone which serves first as a transit area for migrating neurons only to later evolve into the white matter; and 4) a superficial cortical layer. The cell lineage of neurons and glia is a subject of great interest and relevant to the classification and biology of CNS tumors. Increasing use is being made of retroviral vectors which, by genetically marking cells, can be used to identify an "infected" cell's progeny (2,12). Various species have been used to study whether individual infected cells can produce neuronal or glial clones, or both. It is beyond the scope of this chapter to summarize the details of this rapidly evolving field, however, in concept, the transformation of pluripotential cells can produce neoplasms exhibiting divergent differentiation, as is discussed in the chapter, Embryonal Tumors.

The elongated radial glia, which are positive for the intermediate filament protein glial fibrillary acidic protein (GFAP), span the thickness of the neural tube's wall and serve as ropes up which the gymnastic neuroblasts "climb" into the developing cortex (3,19,29,36,40). The horizonal laminar organization of the cerebral cortex owes its existence to these neuronal precursors which ascend in coordinated flights, with subsequent waves climbing higher into the cortical zone than those of preceding generations. The columns of neurons seen in fortuitous sections are also a consequence of this radial migration. Once having served their function as neuronal guidewires, the radial glia lose their distal processes and evolve into astrocytes (29).

Although it is difficult to reconcile historic and current word usage, elongated radial glia seem to be the equivalent to what were once termed spongioblasts. The term spongioblastoma multiforme, later modified to glioblastoma multiforme, became synonymous with a highly malignant and presumably primitive glioma. The term spongioblastoma polare was used for pilocytic astrocytomas because of their cellular elongation. The primitive polar spongioblastoma, with a rare but highly distinctive pattern of disputed significance, has also been linked by some to the radial glia. The Bergmann glia of the cerebellum and cells with Rosenthal fiber–forming potential have also been attributed to these developmentally important cells. Thus, though the radial glia appear to play a role in neuronal migration and in the evolution of glia, particularly astrocytes, their place in oncogenesis remains highly speculative. Radial glia may not even be the only source of astrocytes, since studies using retroviral vectors suggest that astrocytes can also be generated from a pool of undifferentiated cells in the subventricular zone (21,22). It remains to be determined how spongioblasts and their derivatives relate topographically and morphologically to protoplasmic and fibrous astrocytes, as well as to type 1 and 2 astrocytes, categories that have been defined in vitro (see below).

Another issue relevant to the subject of glial neoplasia is gliogenesis in the adult. The subventricular zone persists in man and, at least with primates, retains a low level of cell proliferation (23). In rodents, the evolution of immature into mature glia has been observed in adult animals (24). There is, however, little information on this important subject in humans.

Most cells in the ventricular zone evolve into GFAP-negative ependymal cells, presumably by transition from elongated GFAP-positive cells entering the subventricular zone. It remains a subject of debate whether the latter cells, termed tanycytes, are derived directly from radial glia (13,37). It has been suggested that tanycytes are the origin of tanycytic ependymomas, as well as of astroblastomas.

The origin of oligodendroglia is uncertain, although evidence using retroviral vectors suggests that in the cerebral hemispheres they arise postnatally from a pool of cells in the subventricular zone (21,22). The concept that oligodendrocytes in the spinal cord are derived from radial glia is supported by the occurrence of cells transitional between radial glia and myelin-producing cells (4); an origin from cells migrating from the ventral cord has been suggested as well (43).

Complicating the genealogical investigation of the glial family tree is the observation of two glial lineages in vitro, one giving rise to an astrocyte class (type 1), the other to a progenitor (0-2A) that can develop into either an oligodendrocyte or another astrocyte class (type 2) (35). The two astrocyte types have been distinguished in culture by antigen expression and morphology. However, it is not yet clear how to correlate in vitro lineage schemes and astrocyte types with gliogenesis and astrocyte classes in vivo (2,27,32).

The development of the cerebellar hemispheres has attracted particular attention because of its relevance to the cytogenesis of medulloblastoma, a common tumor at that site. Much of the cerebellum, including the Purkinje cell layer, develops in a fashion similar to that of the cerebrum where neurons migrate outward from the subventricular zone. A notable exception, however, are the neurons of the internal granular cell layer which are not derived directly from the subventricular zone but are supplied from without, i.e., from the densely cellular external granular cell layer on the cerebellar surface (20). The original source is the rhombic lip. This external granular cell layer is subdivided into two layers: a deep, mitotically inactive lamina immunoreactive for the neuronal marker class III beta-tubulin and a superficial subpial layer which is mitotically active but immunonegative for the neural antigen marker (20). The small neurons descend the processes of the Bergmann glia to form the internal granular cell layer deep to the Purkinje cell layer. The external layer is therefore progressively depleted and is depopulated by the end of the first postnatal year (8). With regard to the histogenesis of medulloblastoma, the debate centers upon whether external granular cells are committed only to neuronal differentiation or retain the capacity also to produce glial cells. It also remains to be seen whether some medulloblastomas arise from neuroblasts following the traditional inside-out pattern of migration (20).

Normal Macroscopic Anatomy

The CNS lies protected within the skull and spine, invested by a tough, nearly acellular collagenous layer, the dura. Although adherent to the skull, the dura is largely unattached to the spine, except anteriorly where it is bonded to the posterior surfaces of vertebral bodies. The intracranial dura is reduplicated to form an arching midline fold, the falx cerebri, which partially separates the two cerebral hemispheres. A similar membrane forms a peaked septation, the tentorium cerebelli, which separates structures of the posterior from those of the middle fossa. In the anterior midline, a hiatus in the tentorium accommodates the midbrain and permits passage of cranial nerves and vessels. The tentorium serves as a landmark, conveniently placing most intracranial structures into either the supra- or infratentorial compartments. Infratentorial

structures include the cerebellum and most of the brain stem. The cerebrum, basal ganglia, thalamus, and hypothalamus are supratentorial. The configuration of the skull base permits further subdivision of supratentorial structures into those of the middle and anterior cranial fossae. The floors of these fossae support the temporal and frontal lobes, respectively.

Several localizing anatomic terms used frequently by neurosurgeons are worthy of note. These include the tuberculum sellae, dorsum sellae, and Meckel cave. The tuberculum sellae is, in essence, the top of the anterior wall of the sella turcica. Meningiomas are common in this region. The dorsum sellae is the sella's sloping posterior wall which bears the posterior clinoid processes. Within the middle cranial fossa is the Meckel cave, a medial recess housing the trigeminal nerve ganglion. This structure is also a common site for meningiomas.

From an anatomic and diagnostic standpoint (see Appendix G), intraspinal structures lie within one of three compartments: extradural (outside the dura but within the bony spinal canal), intradural-extramedullary (within the dura but outside the spinal cord), and intramedullary (within the spinal cord or its terminal extension, the filum terminale). The intradural-extramedullary compartment can be further subdivided into the subdural and subarachnoid spaces. Drop metastases and inflammatory states are usually confined to the latter. Regional epidural structures include vertebrae, intervertebral discs, segments of spinal nerve distant to the point at which they enter (posterior roots) or exit (anterior roots) the dural sac, and scant adipose tissue. It has been debated whether the epidural space normally contains lymphoid tissue, an understandable question given the occurrence of rare, seemingly primary epidural lymphomas. Structures assigned to the intradural-extramedullary compartment include the leptomeninges and the proximal portions of the spinal nerve roots. The spinal cord parenchyma, as well as lesions occurring within its substance, are termed intramedullary. As is the case for the brain as well, the blanket terms intra-axial and extra-axial are synonymous for lesions occurring within and without the CNS parenchyma.

To accommodate its expanse, the brain surface forms convolutions termed gyri in the cerebrum and folia in the cerebellum. Certain prominent clefts in the cerebrum serve as important

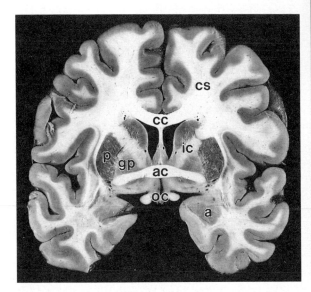
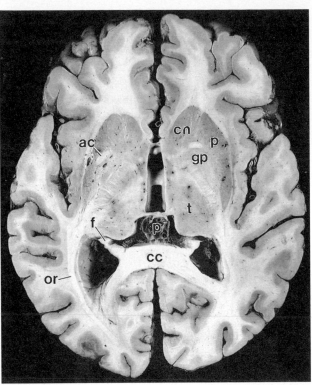

Figure 2-1
NORMAL BRAIN

The glistening white matter and the lusterless gray matter are sharply demarcated along the "gray-white junction" in coronal (left) and horizontal or axial (right) sections. On the left: cs-centrum semiovale; cc-corpus callosum; ic-internal capsule; ac-anterior commissure; oc-optic chiasm; p-putamen; gp-globus pallidus; a-amygdala. On the right: ac-anterior commissure; cn-caudate nucleus; p-putamen; gp-globus pallidus; t-thalamus; p-pineal; cc-corpus callosum; or-optic radiations; f-fornix.

anatomic landmarks. The generally horizontal Sylvian fissure delimits the superior border of the temporal lobe, while the central sulcus (Rolando fissure) angles somewhat posteriorly in the mid-portion of the cerebral hemisphere to separate the precentral or motor cortex of the frontal lobe from the postcentral or sensory cortex of the parietal lobe. The parietal and occipital lobes are partially demarcated by the short parieto-occipital fissure, a prominent structure on the medial surfaces of the cerebral hemispheres.

Generous surgical resections are possible, particularly in relatively "silent" areas. These include the frontal lobes anterior to the motor cortex, the anterior nonspeech-dominant temporal lobe, and the cerebellar hemispheres. Although homonymous hemianopsia results, large resections of the occipital lobe may be performed also. The parietal lobe, especially of the dominant hemisphere, the extraparietal speech areas

of the dominant hemispheres, the precentral region of the frontal lobe, the posterior limb of the internal capsule, and the sensory nuclei of the thalamus are charged with essential functions. As a result, these are only reluctantly disturbed for fear of significant postoperative neurologic deficits. Pathologists can expect small specimens from these regions.

In the normal adult brain, the deep white matter of the cerebral hemispheres (centrum semiovale) and compact pathways including the corpus callosum, fornices, anterior commissure, internal capsules, cerebral peduncles, and medullary pyramids, is glistening white and sharply demarcated from adjacent gray matter (fig. 2-1). Edema and infiltrating neoplasms rob these structures of their normal sheen, supplanting it with a dull yellow tinge or fine granularity (see figs. 3-5, left, 20-5). Since "deep nuclei," such as the globus pallidus and thalamus, are rich in myelin, they are mixed in

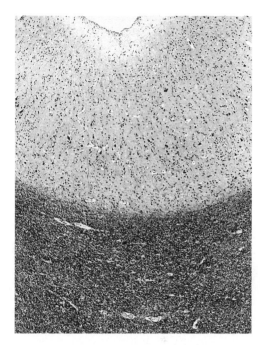

Figure 2-2
NORMAL BRAIN
The normal architecture of the cerebral cortex and underlying white matter is illustrated in adjacent sections stained by H&E (left) and H&E/Luxol fast blue methods (right). Myelin is darkly stained by the latter method.

macroscopic appearance. Nuclei of the brain stem are also indistinct given their small size and proximity to, or content of, myelinated fibers.

CNS contact with the outside world is mediated through cranial and spinal nerves. Of the former, the optic and olfactory "nerves" are not peripheral nerves but rather tracts of the CNS in which oligodendrocytes rather than Schwann cells are the myelinating element. The 10 remaining pairs of cranial nerves, or 11 if the vestigial cranial nerve zero on the undersurface of the frontal lobe is counted (11), are peripheral nerves with Schwann cell–derived myelin. As a result, these nerves, as well as their intraspinal counterparts, are potential sites of schwannomas. Of the intracranial nerves, only the eighth nerve is affected with any frequency. It is the vestibular, rather than acoustic, division which is the typical site of origin. The reason for this is not clear since the density of normal Schwann cells is the same in these two divisions (41).

The filum terminale, a thread-like terminal extension of the spinal cord, is composed largely of fibrous tissue, astroglia, and nests of ependymal cells. Small lobules of adipose tissue are found in about 10 percent of normal individuals (25). In a limited surgical exposure, the distinction of filum from nerve root may be difficult. A few peripheral nerve fascicles are often delicately adherent to its outer surface.

Normal Microscopic Anatomy

The normal microscopic anatomy of the CNS is a complicated subject, and a full description here is neither necessary nor possible. The following is limited to details referable to the origin and diagnosis of regional neoplasms. For further details, the reader is referred to a comprehensive treatise on the subject (15) and a brief review (10).

Gray Matter. Microscopically, gray matter is composed largely of neuronal cell bodies and their processes, particularly dendritic "trees" (fig. 2-2). Two general classes are recognized: large pyramidal cells and small round non-pyramidal cells. Dendrites of the pyramidal cells branch extensively and generally extend horizontally and toward the cortical surface. Axons are simpler in structure and usually emerge from the basilar portion of the cell. The finely

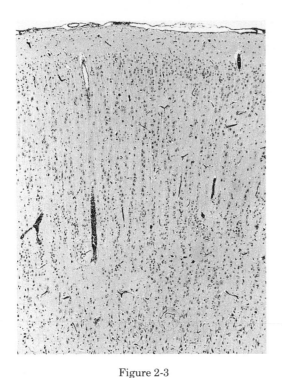

Figure 2-3
NORMAL CEREBRAL CORTEX
A prominent linear vertical orientation of neurons may be seen in certain cortical regions.

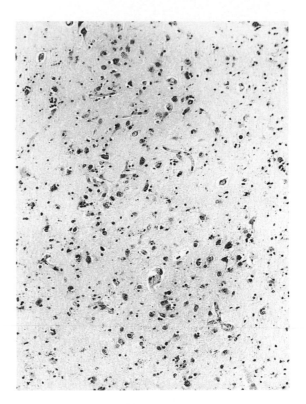

Figure 2-4
NORMAL AMYGDALA
Clustering of neurons, a normal anatomic feature in this region, should not be interpreted as evidence of hamartoma or of ganglion cell neoplasm.

fibrillar anuclear tissue seen between neuronal cell bodies is composed of these cell processes and is termed neuropil.

The organization of the cerebral cortex is of particular interest since it is frequently included in surgical specimens and must, in minute biopsies, be differentiated from ganglion cell tumors. Although not always obvious in fragmented surgical specimens, the cortex has both horizontal and vertical patterns of organization. Such lamination is seen well in the phylogenetically newer neocortex at such areas as the primary sensory and motor cortices. Horizontal layering results in the development of cortical laminae which vary in number with site. Best defined is the paucicellular molecular layer which lies immediately beneath the pial surface. Composed in part of astrocytic processes, its most superficial portion is intensely immunoreactive for GFAP. The vertical organization of the cortex is apparent as the columns of neurons described above (fig. 2-3). Large pyramidal neurons within these columns are distinctly polar and project conspicuous apical dendrites toward the pial surface. Although

such cells appear triangular in routine material, the angularity is to some extent artifactual since a more rotund configuration is observed in rapidly fixed specimens. The term ganglion cell is often applied to large neurons, many of which contain stacks of rough endoplasmic reticulum resulting in basophilic patches known as Nissl or tigroid substance. Polarity and lamination of large neurons are understandably absent in ganglion cell neoplasms whereas neuronal binucleation, a diagnostic feature of such tumors, is exceedingly rare in normal cortex.

At many supratentorial sites other than the cerebral cortex, neurons are less layered. This is especially true in the amygdala where clustering is normal and not to be interpreted as neoplastic or hamartomatous (fig. 2-4). The complicated architecture of the hippocampus may, particularly in tangential or oblique sections, cause similar confusion.

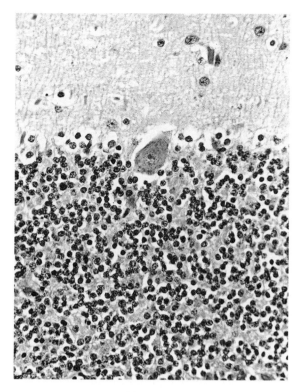

Figure 2-5
NORMAL CEREBELLAR CORTEX

The small neurons of the internal granular cell layer are juxtaposed to a bulbous Purkinje cell, seen at the top center of the illustration. Note the small fibrillar clearings within the densely cellular internal granular cell layer as well as the uniform roundness and hyperchromasia of normal granule cells.

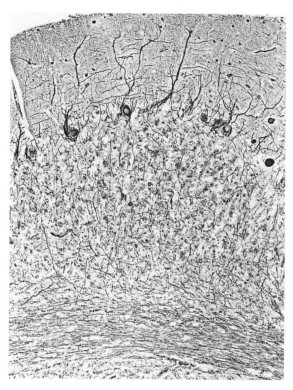

Figure 2-6
NORMAL CEREBELLUM

In this Glees stained section, the axons of Purkinje cells are seen at the bottom of the illustration, whereas dendrites of Purkinje cells fan out into the molecular layer at the top. The processes of the basket cells which envelop Purkinje cells are also seen. Note that Purkinje cells are uniformly distributed along the interface between the internal granular molecular layers.

The cerebellum illustrates the extremes of neuronal size by juxtaposing Purkinje cells with small hyperchromatic internal granule cells (fig. 2-5). Particularly in specimens studied at frozen section, care must be taken not to misinterpret the latter as a small cell neoplasm, especially medulloblastoma. The distribution of granule cells is such that their nuclei are interrupted by small synaptophysin-positive patches of neuropil which somewhat resemble the Homer Wright rosettes in medulloblastoma. Normal granule cells are smaller than those of small cell neoplasms, either primary or metastatic. Furthermore, they possess uniform round nuclei with distinct central nucleoli and lack mitotic activity.

Selective staining of neurons and their processes may be accomplished by either routine histochemical or immunohistochemical methods. Classic procedures include the Cresyl fast violet stain for cytoplasmic Nissl substance and the Bodian, Glees, Bielschowsky, or Holmes silver impregnation methods, all of which demonstrate axons. The Cresyl violet method highlights not only rough endoplasmic reticulum (Nissl substance) but chromatin and nucleoli as well. The previously noted silver impregnation methods for axons may be applied to paraffin-embedded tissues. They demonstrate axons as long dark threads of uniform thickness by depositing silver on their neurofilaments (fig. 2-6). It is the axons, rather than dendrites, that are predominantly stained. The noncommittal term neurite is used by some to designate a neuronal process, either axonal or dendritic, although the term is rigorously applied only to axons.

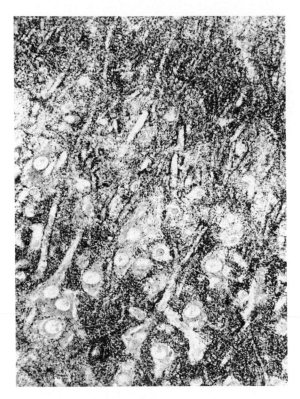

Figure 2-7
NORMAL HIPPOCAMPUS
Gray matter, as seen here in the Ammon horn of the hippocampus, exhibits a fine granular staining for synaptophysin.

Immunohistochemical stains are widely used for the identification of neurons. For instance, reactivity for specific neurotransmitters demonstrates the marriage of structure and function found throughout neuropathology. For practical application, however, the repertoire of reagents applied to surgical material is rather restricted and is used selectively to answer such practical questions as, "Is the cell a neuron or an astrocyte?" Staining for neuron-specific enolase (NSE) may be an initial step but provides less than conclusive evidence since nonspecific staining has been demonstrated in a variety of non-neural tissues, both normal and neoplastic. Nonspecificity aside, immunoreactivity for NSE is reliably present in gray matter, where staining is diffuse. Some neuronal cell bodies (perikarya) and their processes are intensely stained whereas adjacent neurons may be totally nonreactive. In contrast, immunopositivity for synaptophysin, a synaptic vesicle–associated protein, is considered neuron specific. It is reliably exhibited throughout gray matter where it appears as fine diffuse granularity. Unlike NSE, which often shows intense staining of cytoplasm and neuronal cell processes, synaptophysin usually produces only faint granular staining of the neuropil and, to a lesser extent, along perikarya (fig. 2-7). A granular surface staining is prominent in ganglion cell tumors, as is cytoplasmic staining for chromogranin (see figs. 4-3, right, 4-14). The latter is not seen in most normal neurons. Neurofilament protein reactivity using antibodies to phosphorylated epitopes is generally restricted to neurofilament-rich structures such as axons, rather than to perikarya or dendrites. The cell body is better stained with antibodies to non-phosphorylated neurofilament protein. Other reacting antibodies are microtubule-associated protein-2 (MAP-2) and tau. Antibodies to three neurofilament components, differing in molecular weight, are available. Antibody "cocktails" directed toward all three are in common use. Reactivity to neurofilament proteins (NFP) is taken as prima facie evidence of neuronal differentiation.

Other constituents of gray matter include axons, glial cells of astrocytic and oligodendroglial type, and blood vessels. As throughout most of the brain, with the notable exception of the choroid plexus stroma, fibrous tissue is scant and confined to the adventitia of blood vessels. Although the myelin content of gray matter is minimal when compared to that of white matter, widely separated myelinated fibers are seen within the cerebral cortex, basal ganglia, and brain stem. A prominent horizontal layer of myelinated fibers, the "outer stripe of Baillarger" or "stripe of Gennari," serves as a macroscopic marker of the primary visual or striate cortex of the medial occipital lobes. A final cell type in gray matter, the microglia, is discussed separately.

The nuclei of astrocytes within the gray matter are round and, although considerably smaller than those of large cortical neurons, approximate those of smaller neurons both in size and chromatin density. These astrocytes are referred to as protoplasmic, since their processes more frequently branch than those of the fibrillary astrocytes of white matter. Fewer intermediate (glial) filaments are found in them as well. Normal cortical astrocytes are positive for glutamine synthetase but are often only weakly reactive for GFAP. Reactive astrocytes, on the other hand, are strongly labeled with GFAP, highlighting their symmetric radial array of branching processes.

Eye-catching astrocytic products apparent in gray matter, but less so in white matter, are polyglucosan bodies or corpora amylacea. These slightly basophilic, PAS-positive, faintly laminated structures are contained within the terminations of astrocyte processes and are therefore most prominent in the subpial, subependymal, and perivascular regions. Corpora amylacea are argyrophilic (including methenamine-silver or Grocott stain) and PAS positive and should not be confused with fungi such as *Cryptococcus*.

A prominent finding in certain neoplasms and reactive states is an intracytoplasmic, hyaline, often corkscrew-shaped structure known as a Rosenthal fiber. In neoplasms, it is found principally in pilocytic astrocytomas (see fig. 3-78). In common reactive states it appears most frequently in gliosis around the third ventricle (see fig. 15-7), in the pineal body (see fig. 6-18), cerebellum (see fig. 7-6), tegmentum of the brain stem, and spinal cord, all the same general regions favored by pilocytic astrocytomas. This congruence in distribution raises the possibility that there is a subpopulation of astrocytes to which this form of gliosis or neoplasm can be attributed. Rosenthal fibers are not unique, however, to these lesions and may be seen in other areas, such as subpial astrocytes and in occasional diffuse or fibrillary astrocytic neoplasms (see fig. 3-14).

Elongated astrocytes, the Bergmann glia, are also found in the cerebellar cortex where they are confined to the layer that includes two types of neurons, the Purkinje and basket cells. The nuclei of Bergmann glia are larger and less dense than those of the underlying internal granule cells but smaller than those of Purkinje cells. Bergmann glia react to injury, especially loss of Purkinje cells by hypertrophy and hyperplasia.

In small numbers, oligodendrocytes are also normal inhabitants of gray matter. They are relatively restricted in distribution, several hovering about each large neuron, particularly in deep cortical layers (fig. 2-8). The presence of such "satellite oligodendroglia" should not be over-interpreted as perineuronal satellitosis due to infiltrating glioma. Smaller size, greater nuclear uniformity, more delicate chromatin, and delicate nucleoli distinguish normal satellite oligodendrocytes from their neoplastic counterparts.

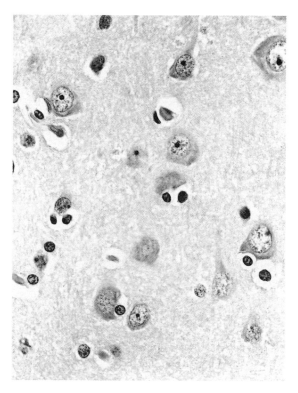

Figure 2-8
NORMAL CEREBRAL CORTEX
Many large neurons in the cerebral cortex are associated with small, dark, satellite oligodendroglia. These normal, well-differentiated cells should not be misinterpreted as those of an infiltrating glioma.

White Matter. Since it only transmits rather than initiates chemoelectric impulses, white matter is simpler than gray matter in its cellular composition and organization. It is composed largely of axonal processes and their accompanying myelin sheaths. Although occasional neurons are encountered in normal cerebral white matter, particularly that of the temporal lobe, they are few and largely concentrated beneath the cortical ribbon. Such neurons should not be interpreted as evidence of hamartoma or ganglion cell neoplasm.

Myelin, the lipid rich "insulation" applied to axons by the wrapping of oligodendrocytic processes, is highlighted with a variety of special stains. The Luxol fast blue method is best known and is generally combined with either the periodic acid–Schiff (PAS) or hematoxylin and eosin (H&E) method (see fig. 2-2, right). Immunohistochemically, antibodies for galactocerebroside, myelin basic protein, and Leu-7 can also be used (31). In diagnostic frozen sections stained with aqueous methods, such as toluidine blue, myelin sheaths exhibit irregular tubular profiles which superficially may resemble fungal hyphae.

Oligodendrocytes, whose somewhat hyperchromatic round nuclei are abundant in white matter, are, in fortuitous sections, found in rows or "fascicles" as they orient themselves to fiber pathways (fig. 2-9). Oligodendrocytes are prone to autolysis during which they imbibe fluid to produce a "fried egg" appearance similar to, although less prominent than that seen in oligodendrogliomas. Autolytic changes of astrocytes differ by being limited to the perivascular processes. The process of water imbibition produces clearing about small vessels.

Astrocytes are also abundant in the white matter where they are referred to as fibrillary or fibrous astrocytes. They are presumed to be the precursors of the common infiltrative fibrillary, fibrous, diffuse, or ordinary astrocytomas discussed in the next chapter. Although the nuclei of these astrocytes are somewhat larger and less hyperchromatic than those of oligodendrocytes, there is a degree of overlap in their nuclear characteristics (fig. 2-10). As a result, it is often difficult to assign individual cells to the astrocytic or oligodendroglial categories on the basis of H&E stained sections alone. On the other hand, in reactive lesions such as the response to metastatic tumor, infection, infarction, or demyelination, the cytoplasm of astrocytes becomes hypertrophic and their processes are readily evident (see fig. 3-18, right). In this setting, the two cell types are easily distinguished, particularly in sections stained with Luxol fast blue combined with H&E; the pink cytoplasm of reactive cells is seen well in contrast to the blue background of myelin sheaths. Astrocytes are also readily identified by their immunoreactivity for GFAP (fig. 2-11).

Ependyma. Among glia, ependymal cells are unique, since they form an epithelial layer lining the ventricular system as well as the discontinuous remnants of the central canal of the postpubertal spinal cord. Although in adults scattered cilia are found on ultrastructural examination, few if any persist at the light microscopic level. No basal lamina underlies the ependymal layer, which rests directly upon subependymal glial. At the anteroposterior ex-

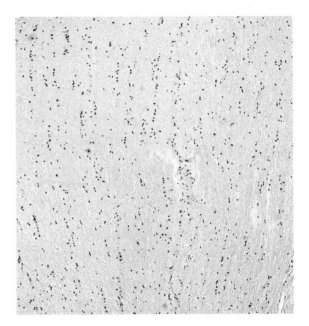

Figure 2-9
NORMAL CEREBRAL WHITE MATTER
Fortuitous sections catch oligodendroglia in short columns. This normal alignment should not be confused with infiltrating neoplastic cells.

tremes of the ventricular cavities as well as in the adult spinal cord, disorganized ependymal cell remnants are a normal anatomic feature and should not be interpreted as evidence of a glioma.

Immunohistochemically, normal ependyma is reactive for S-100 protein and, to a variable degree, for GFAP and epithelial membrane antigen (42). A special variant of the ependymal cell, the tanycyte, is an elongated tapered cell which, unlike ordinary columnar ependymal cells, extends via long basilar processes into the subependymal layer (37).

Choroid Plexus. Histogenetically related to ependyma, choroid plexus epithelium is a simple layer of cuboidal to columnar cells squarely seated upon a basement membrane. A well-defined papillary fibrovascular stroma underlies this layer (6,34,39). In distinction to ependyma, choroid plexus displays an apical rounded or "cobblestoned" profile (see fig. 3-166), and, at least by light microscopy, lacks cilia. Normal choroid plexus is immunoreactive for cytokeratins, particularly low molecular weight forms, vimentin, S-100 protein, and prealbumin (transthyretin) (16,20a,26). With age, circumnuclear masses of

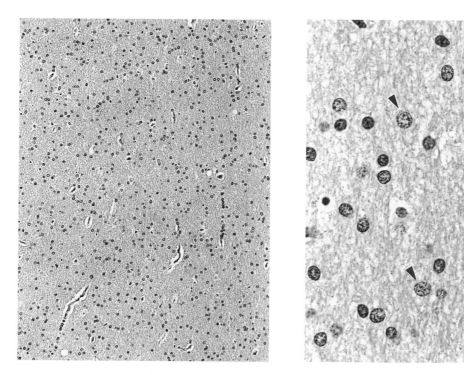

Figure 2-10
NORMAL CEREBRAL WHITE MATTER
Left: At low magnification, normal cerebral white matter exhibits a generally uniform distribution of cells in medium density.
Right: At high magnification, the larger, more vesicular nuclei of astrocytes (arrows) may often be distinguished from the smaller, darker ones of oligodendrocytes. In other instances, particularly in previously frozen tissue, the two cell types are indistinguishable.

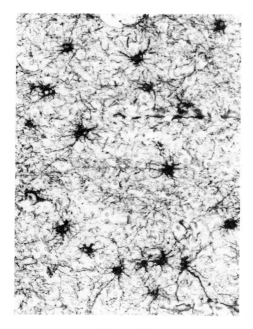

Figure 2-11
NORMAL CEREBRAL WHITE MATTER
An immunostain for GFAP demonstrates the normal fibrillary or fibrous astrocytes, with long processes inserting into the walls of blood vessels.

argyrophilic filaments, so-called Biondi rings, become prominent within choroid plexus cells (7).

Pineal Gland. During embryogenesis the pineal evolves from a biphasic organ consisting of two principal cell types. These include darkly pigmented, melanin-containing S-100–positive cells, and paler, NSE–reactive neurosecretory cells. In adults the gland is a more homogeneous structure composed of lobules of neurosecretory cells in which melanin may only occasionally be seen at the ultrastructural level (28). At any stage, a biopsy of the pineal gland may resemble a neoplasm, particularly when lobulation is not observed (see figs. 6-5, 6-6, 6-19). Regional astrocytes and ependymal cells are the sources of occasional gliomas in the pineal gland.

Meninges. The meninges include the pachymeninx or dura mater and the leptomeninx or pia-arachnoid (33). The former is a dense fibrocollagenous investment of low cellularity which is bilaminar in many areas. Sandwiched between the layers of the dura are branches of the middle meningeal artery, a terminal extension of the external carotid system. Branches of this vessel are commonly recruited to supply dura-based tumors such as meningioma and meningeal hemangiopericytoma, but are largely unaffected by intraparenchymal neoplasms, such as gliomas, which derive their vasculature principally from the internal carotid or vertebrobasilar systems. Determination of the vascular supply thus serves as a helpful neuroradiologic clue in the preoperative differential diagnosis of CNS neoplasms.

The dural venous sinuses are low pressure avalvular channels directing blood from cerebral veins to the internal jugular system. Blood from the cerebral cortex is channeled to the superior sagittal sinus, whereas that from deep cerebral structures passes to the straight sinus. These sinuses merge at the torcular, a point of confluence lying beneath a major bony landmark, the inion. Flow proceeds from the torcular, through the transverse and sigmoid sinuses, to exit the cranium and to return, via the internal jugular veins, to the heart. Venous blood from the temporal lobe cortex passes directly into the adjacent transverse and sigmoid sinuses. Two large veins on the brain convexity serve as both landmarks to the surgeon and, on occasion, as obstacles to en bloc resection: the veins of Labbé and Trolard. The former passes from the Sylvian fissure inferiorly to the transverse sinus while the latter courses superiorly along the general region of the central sulcus to the superior sagittal sinus and is generally well defined.

Protruding into venous sinuses as small botryoid masses are arachnoid villi which convey cerebrospinal fluid from the subarachnoid space to the venous system. These structures become prominent with age and are then termed Pacchionian granulations. When large, they induce small pits, foveolae granulares, on the inner table of the skull. Occasionally, these are large enough to mimic a pathologic condition (36a). Arachnoidal cells play an active role in fluid transport since they line the villi and abut the lumina of venous sinuses. These same cells also fan out diffusely over the surface of the arachnoid membrane as an inconspicuous covering. With age, arachnoidal cell aggregates become sufficiently prominent to be grossly apparent as white flecks. Whorls, psammoma bodies, and intranuclear pseudoinclusions identical to those

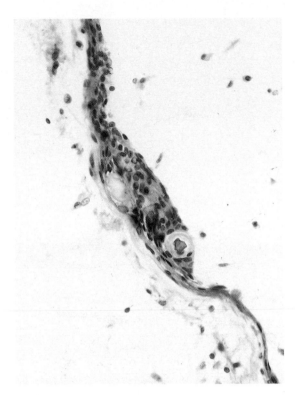

Figure 2-12
NORMAL MENINGOTHELIAL CELLS
With age, meningothelial cells become prominent as small clusters. Neoplastic transformation produces meningiomas. Note the presence of a psammoma body.

of the meningioma are common features, both in granulations and arachnoidal cell clusters (fig. 2-12). Meningothelial cells are uniformly immunoreactive for vimentin and epithelial membrane antigen and, to a lesser extent, for cytokeratin and S-100 protein (38,45). Their epithelial ultrastructural features include well-formed desmosomes and tonofilaments (46), seen also in meningiomas.

In contrast to the dura, the arachnoid membrane is delicate and transparent, particularly in early age. As life proceeds, it gradually succumbs to clinically insignificant fibrosis, particularly over the convexities of the cerebral hemispheres. This process should be distinguished from pathologic opacification due to neoplastic or inflammatory cell infiltrates. Normally, the membrane strips readily from the brain. The far more delicate pia mater lies adjacent to the glia

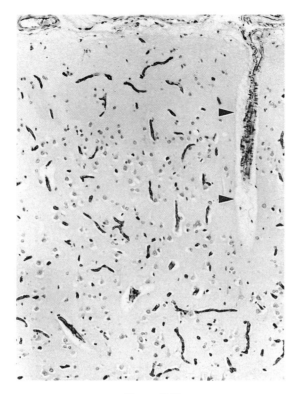

Figure 2-13
NORMAL CEREBRAL MICROVASCULATURE
The rich network of small vessels in the cerebral cortex is readily apparent after staining with HAM-56. Note the perivascular space around the vessel at the top right of the illustration (arrows).

limitans of the brain formed by the expansions of subpial astrocytes which fan out over the surface of the brain. The cells of this specialized astrocytic layer may be related to the histogenesis of a special form of superficial glioma, the pleomorphic xanthoastrocytoma, since basal laminae are common to both the normal cells and to the neoplasm. The pia is also reflected to form a cuff around vessels; although often considered subarachnoid in location, these vessels are actually separated from it by the pia (1,18).

The arachnoid membrane is composed, in large part, by arachnoid cells as well as by specialized fibroblasts which form trabeculae within the subarachnoid space. The outer surface or roof of the space consists of horizontally oriented arachnoidal cells; the tight junctions of these cells act as a barrier similar to that of the brain's vasculature. This arachnoid barrier layer is joined to the innermost layer of the dura, the dural border layer. Despite the commonly observed separation of the arachnoid membrane from the dura, both at surgery and at autopsy, the "subdural space" is an artifactual cleft produced by cleavage within the dural border layer (14).

In histologic sections, the subarachnoid space extends into the brain as a perivascular sleeve known as the Virchow-Robin space (fig. 2-13). Its depth corresponds approximately to the midportion of the cortical ribbon. Although microscopic studies suggest that this space does not normally communicate directly with the subarachnoid space, in practice it is patent to neoplastic cells (see figs. 3-58, 9-43, 20-11, 20-12), inflammatory elements, and microorganisms (18).

Blood Vessels. The brain is richly vascular, being supplied by both the internal carotid (anterior) and vertebrobasilar (posterior) circulations, which are joined by the posterior communicating arteries. After entering the intracranial cavity, the arteries traverse the subarachnoid space to penetrate the substance of the nervous system. In contrast to other body sites, the media of intraparenchymal vessels is so thin as to be scarcely discernible. Arteries with a well-defined muscular coat are, almost by definition, limited to the subarachnoid space, a feature that helps identify this compartment when overrun by neoplasm or inflammation (see fig. 4-10). In superficial cortical biopsies, the normally rich vasculature of the subarachnoid space may be artifactually compressed to simulate a vascular malformation (see fig. 10-4). In contrast to malformed vessels, these juxtaposed but otherwise orderly vessels possess a normal complement of smooth muscle.

The structure of intraparenchymal vessels can be highlighted by a number of methods. These include the trichrome stain which demonstrates adventitial connective tissue; the reticulin and PAS stains, and type IV collagen immunostain, all of which highlight basement membranes; and factor VIII–related antigen immunostains, *Ulex europaeus* preparations, and HAM-56 which highlight endothelial cells (fig. 2-13) (44). Pericytes are recognized by their myoid characteristics, which are apparent both ultrastructurally and on immunostaining for muscle-specific actin. Special features of the cerebral vasculature include paucity of smooth muscle, absence of an external elastic lamina in arteries, the presence of tight junctions between endothelial cells, and the apposition of astrocytic foot processes to vessel walls. Endothelial tight junctions are the basis of the blood-brain barrier which requires metabolites, drugs, and toxins to pass through, rather than between, endothelial cells. At the light microscopic level, the space occupied by the astrocytic processes abutting vessels appears as an artifactual clear zone, an effect produced by their autolytic imbibition of water.

Microglia. These mesenchymal cells of monocyte/macrophage lineage are so inconspicuous and morphologically nonspecific in terms of their histologic appearance that for decades their very existence was debated. Reactivity of these cells on immunohistochemical (lysozyme) or lectin (Ricinus communis agglutinin-1) stain leaves no doubt of their presence, although the histogenesis of microglial cells remains a matter of debate (5,17). In standard H&E stained sections microglia are seen to be ubiquitous but inconspicuous. Their small thin nuclei are about as long as those of endothelial cells but are considerably thinner. Lectin staining visualizes their cytoplasm as bipolar extensions which branch, somewhat at right angles, to permeate the adjacent brain (fig. 2-14).

In pathologic states associated with tissue destruction, microglia "round up" to assume the conventional shape of actively phagocytic cells. In large lesions, they are joined and greatly outnumbered by hematogenous macrophages. When engorged with debris, both cell types become vacuolated to form gitter cells. Lipid-rich gitter cells are particularly abundant in demyelinating disease and infarcts (see figs. 19-4–19-6, 19-13). The superficial similarity between gitter cells and oligodendrocytes is discussed later in the text. The macrophage nature of the former is readily demonstrated by immunohistochemical stains with antisera to HAM-56 or KP-1 (see figs. 19-9, 19-16). The rare neoplastic transformation of microglial cells is discussed in the section on microgliomatosis.

Lymphocytes. Very few lymphocytes are seen in the normal CNS. Even a few, generally about vessels, are evidence of disease.

Central Nervous System (CNS)–Peripheral Nervous System (PNS) Junction. With the exception of the eighth or vestibulo-acoustic nerve, the zone of transition between the CNS

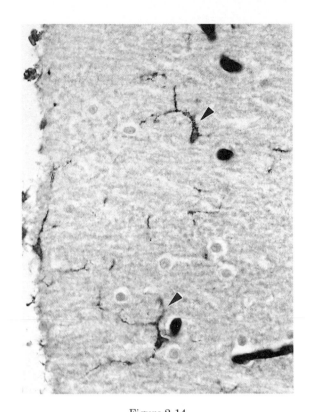

Figure 2-14
NORMAL MICROGLIA
The cytoplasm of microglia, which is inconspicuous in H&E stained sections, can be demonstrated by lectin staining for Ricinus communis agglutinin-1.

(with its oligodendrocytes) and the PNS (with its Schwann cells) is positioned within a millimeter or two of the brain's external, or pial, surface. In the eighth nerve, the transition zone is situated 1 cm more laterally, placing the junction in the internal auditory meatus. Acoustic schwannomas begin, therefore, in the auditory canal and, only with subsequent enlargement, reach the cerebellopontine angle. Largely because of the resolution of magnetic resonance imaging, many schwannomas are now detected at the intracanalicular stage. In spinal nerve roots, the CNS-PNS transition zone is situated close to the pial surface (fig. 2-15). A short unmyelinated segment, the Obersteiner-Redlich zone, is interposed between the terminal domains of PNS and CNS at this point.

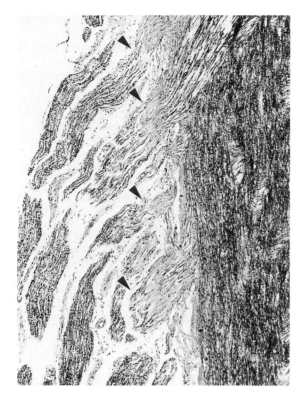

Figure 2-15
NORMAL CENTRAL NERVOUS SYSTEM–
PERIPHERAL NERVOUS SYSTEM JUNCTION

With the exception of the eighth cranial nerve, the junction between the central and peripheral nervous systems occurs within several millimeters of the pial surface. As seen in the spinal cord, the darkly-staining myelin of nerve roots (left) terminates abruptly at a transitional zone (arrows), which is itself sharply defined from the spinal cord (right). (Hematoxylin and eosin/Luxol fast blue stains).

REFERENCES

1. Alcolado R, Weller RO, Parrish EP, Garrod D. The cranial arachnoid and pia mater in man: anatomical and ultrastructural observations. Neuropathol Appl Neurobiol 1988;14:1–17.
2. Cameron RS, Rakic P. Glial cell lineage in the cerebral cortex: a review and synthesis. Glia 1991;4:124–37.
3. Choi BH. Glial fibrillary acidic protein in radial glia of early human fetal cerebrum: a light and electron microscopic immunoperoxidase study. J Neuropathol Exp Neurol 1986;45:408–18.
4. _____. Myelin-forming oligodendrocytes of developing mouse spinal cord: immunocytochemical and ultrastructural studies. J Neuropathol Exp Neurol 1986;45:513–24.
5. Dickson DW, Mattiace LA, Kure K, Hutchins K, Lyman WD, Brosnan CF. Microglia in human disease, with an emphasis on acquired immune deficiency syndrome. Lab Invest 1991;64:135–56.
6. Dohrmann GJ, Bucy PC. Human choroid plexus: a light and electron microscopic study. J Neurosurg 1970;33:506–16.
7. Eriksson L, Westermark P. Characterization of intracellular amyloid fibrils in the human choroid plexus epithelial cells. Acta Neuropathol 1990;80:597–603.
8. Friede RL. Dating the development of human cerebellum. Acta Neuropathol (Berl) 1973;23:48–58.
9. _____. Gross and microscopic development of the central nervous system. Developmental neuropathology. 2nd ed. Berlin: Springer-Verlag, 1989:2–20.
10. Fuller GN, Burger PC. Central nervous system. In: Sternberg S, ed. Histology for pathologists. New York: Raven Press, 1992:145–67.
11. _____, Burger PC. Nervus terminalis (cranial nerve zero) in the adult human. Clin Neuropathol 1990;9:279–83.
12. Galileo DS, Gray GE, Owens GC, Majors J, Sanes JR. Neurons and glia arise from a common progenitor in chicken optic tectum: demonstration with two retroviruses and cell type-specific antibodies. Proc Natl Acad Sci USA 1990;87:458–62.
13. Gould SJ, Howard S, Papadaki L. The development of ependyma in the human fetal brain: an immunohistological and electron microscopic study. Brain Res Dev Brain Res 1990;55:255–67.
14. Haines DE. On the question of a subdural space. Anat Rec 1991;230:3–21.
15. Haymaker WE, Adams RD, eds. Histology and histopathology of the nervous system. Springfield, IL: Charles C. Thomas, 1982.
16. Herbert J, Wilcox JN, Pham KT, et al. Transthyretin: a choroid plexus-specific transport protein in human brain. The 1986 S. Weir Mitchell award. Neurology 1986;36:900–11.
17. Hulette CM, Downey BT, Burger PC. Macrophage markers in diagnostic neuropathology. Am J Surg Pathol 1992;16:493–9.
18. Hutchings M, Weller RO. Anatomical relationships of the pia mater to cerebral blood vessels in man. J Neurosurg 1986;65:316–25.
19. Kadhim HJ, Gadisseux JF, Evrard P. Topographical and cytological evolution of the glial phase during prenatal development of the human brain: histochemical and electron microscopic study. J Neuropathol Exp Neurol 1988;47:166–88.
20. Katsetos CD, Frankfurter A, Christakos S, Mancall EL, Vlachos IN, Urich H. Differential localization of class III β-tubulin isotype and calbindin-D28k defines distinct neuronal types in the developing human cerebellar cortex. J Neuropathol Exp Neurol 1993;52:655–66.
20a.Lach B, Scheithauer BW, Gregor A, Wick MR. Colloid cyst of the third ventricle. A comparative immunohistochemical study of neuraxis cysts and choroid plexus epithelium. J Neurosurg 1993;78:101–11.
21. Levison SW, Goldman JE. Astrocyte origins. In: Murphy S, ed. Astrocytes: pharmacology and function. San Diego: Academic Press, 1993.
22. _____, Goldman JE. Both oligodendrocytes and astrocytes develop from progenitors in the subventricular zone of postnatal rat forebrain. Nature, 1993. In press.
23. Lewis PD. Mitotic activity in the primate subependymal layer and the genesis of gliomas. Nature 1968; 217:974–5.

24. McCarthy GF, Leblond CP. Radioautographic evidence for slow astrocytic turnover and modest oligodendrocyte production in the corpus callosum of adult mice infused with ^{3}H-thymidine. J Comp Neurol 1988;271:589–603.

25. McLendon RE, Oakes WJ, Heinz ER, Yeates AE, Burger PC. Adipose tissue in the filum terminale: a computed tomographic finding that may indicate tethering of the spinal cord? Neurosurgery 1988;22:873–6.

26. Miettinen M, Clark R, Virtanen I. Intermediate filament proteins in choroid plexus and ependyma and their tumors. Am J Pathol 1986;123:231–40.

27. Miller RH, David S, Patel R, Abney ER, Raff MC. A quantitative immunohistochemical study of macroglial cell development in the rat optic nerve: in vivo evidence for two distinct astrocyte lineages. Dev Biol 1985;111:35–41.

28. Min KW, Seo IS, Song J. Postnatal evolution of the human pineal gland. An immunohistochemical study. Lab Invest 1987;57:724–8.

29. Misson JP, Takahashi T, Caviness VS Jr. Ontogeny of radial and other astroglial cells in murine cerebral cortex. Glia 1991;4:138–48.

30. Moore KL, ed. The developing human. Clinically oriented embryology. 4th ed. Philadelphia: WB Saunders, 1988.

31. Nakagawa Y, Perentes E, Rubinstein LJ. Immunohistochemical characterization of oligodendrogliomas: an analysis of multiple markers. Acta Neuropathol (Berl) 1986;72:15–22.

32. Noble M. Points of controversy in the 0-2A lineage: clocks and type-2 astrocytes. Glia 1991;4:157–64.

33. O'Rahilly R, Müller F. The meninges in human development. J Neuropathol Exp Neurol 1986;45:588–608.

34. _____, Müller F. Ventricular system and choroid plexuses of the human brain during the embryonic period proper. Am J Anat 1990;189:285–302.

35. Raff MC, Miller RH, Noble M. A glial progenitor cell that develops in vitro into an astrocyte or an oligodendrocyte depending on culture medium. Nature 1983;303:390–6.

36. Rakic P. Guidance of neurons migrating to the fetal monkey neocortex. Brain Res 1971;33:471–6.

36a. Rosenberg AE, O'Connell JX, Ojemann RG, Plata MJ, Palmer WE. Giant cystic arachnoid granulations: a rare cause of lytic skull lesions. Hum Pathol 1993;24: 438–41.

37. Sarnat HB. Regional differentiation of the human fetal ependyma: immunocytochemical markers. J Neuropathol Exp Neurol 1992;51:58–75.

38. Schnitt SJ, Vogel H. Meningiomas. Diagnostic value of immunoperoxidase staining for epithelial membrane antigen. Am J Surg Pathol 1986;10:640–9.

39. Shuangshoti S, Netsky MG. Histogenesis of choroid plexus in man. Am J Anat 1966;118:283–316.

40. Sidman RL, Rakic P. Neuronal migration, with special reference to developing human brain: a review. Brain Res 1973;62:1–35.

41. Tallon E, Harner S, Scheithauer BW, et al. Does the distribution of Schwann cell correlate with the observed distribution of acoustic schwannomas. Am J Otol 1993;14:131–4.

42. Uematsu Y, Rojas-Corona RR, Llena JF, Hirano A. Distribution of epithelial membrane antigen in normal and neoplastic human ependyma. Acta Neuropathol (Berl) 1989;78:325–8.

43. Warf BC, Fok-Seang J, Miller RH. Evidence for the ventral origin of oligodendrocyte precursors in the rat spinal cord. J Neurosci 1991;11:2477–88.

44. Weber T, Seitz RJ, Liebert UG, Gallasch E, Wechsler W. Affinity cytochemistry of vascular endothelia in brain tumors by biotinylated Ulex europaeus type I lectin (UEA I). Acta Neuropathol (Berl) 1985;67:128–35.

45. Winek RR, Scheithauer BW, Wick MR. Meningioma, meningeal hemangiopericytoma (angioblastic meningioma), peripheral hemangiopericytoma, and acoustic schwannoma. A comparative immunohistochemical study. Am J Surg Pathol 1989;13:251–61.

46. Yamashima T, Kida S, Yamamoto S. Ultrastructural comparison of arachnoid villi and meningiomas in man. Mod Pathol 1988;1:224–34.

❖❖❖

3

TUMORS OF NEUROGLIA AND CHOROID PLEXUS EPITHELIUM

ASTROCYTIC NEOPLASMS

FIBRILLARY OR "DIFFUSE" ASTROCYTIC TUMORS

Definition. Infiltrating neoplasms composed of fibrillary or fibrous astrocytes.

General Features. Comprising a significant proportion of all primary brain tumors, fibrillary or "diffuse" astrocytomas extend over a continuous morphologic spectrum of differentiation and tumor grade. Although these invasive and biologically malignant tumors occur in patients of all ages and arise at all levels of the neuraxis, they do not do so randomly. In adults, they usually appear in the cerebral hemispheres, whereas the same neoplasms in the pediatric population typically arise in the brain stem (2,3,43,73). Less common examples involve the spinal cord of both children and adults (22–24,33). The cerebellum is rarely affected at any age (20,29,47,70,111,130); most astrocytic tumors at this location are of pilocytic type. The same is true of the optic nerve where only a rare astrocytoma is a fibrillary or diffuse lesion (51). The distinction between fibrillary and pilocytic astrocytic neoplasms is extremely important given the divergent biologic behavior of these two classes of astrocytic neoplasms. The modifiers "diffuse" or "ordinary" are sometimes applied to the fibrillary lesions to help make this distinction clear.

Among fibrillary astrocytic neoplasms of the cerebral hemispheres, a correlation is observed between histologic grade and four clinical variables: patient age, duration of symptoms, neurologic performance status, and length of postoperative survival (11,18,89,124). With only occasional exceptions, lesions in older patients are more anaplastic, biologically aggressive, recently symptomatic, and destructive of neurologic function. In contrast, fibrillary or diffuse astrocytic tumors in younger patients tend to be better differentiated, more chronically symptomatic, less disruptive of neurologic function, and slower in their rate of growth (18,61,91,124,125).

A cardinal property of fibrillary astrocytomas is a propensity to undergo anaplastic change to a more malignant lesion, i.e., to increase in histologic grade (86,97,101). This process is common and relates somewhat to patient age since it occurs more often and appears more rapidly in older individuals. It is especially frequent in gemistocytic astrocytomas (104). This progression can be often seen when initial specimens are compared with those taken later in the course of the disease (86). The process is also frequently observed when a single specimen contains differing grades of neoplasm. Thus, tumors that are largely astrocytoma often include foci of anaplastic astrocytoma and even glioblastoma (figs. 3-1, 3-2) and many glioblastomas exhibit areas of

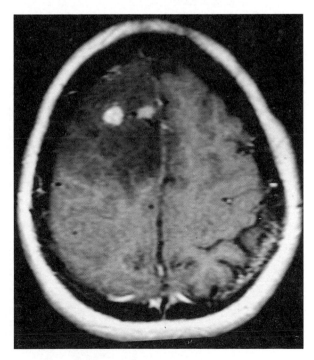

Figure 3-1
FIBRILLARY OR "DIFFUSE" ASTROCYTIC
NEOPLASM WITH DIFFERING DEGREES
OF DIFFERENTIATION
A large area of dark magnetic resonance signal representing low-grade astrocytoma is present in the frontal lobe on the left. Higher-grade foci are apparent as the two white contrast-enhancing foci within this darker zone.

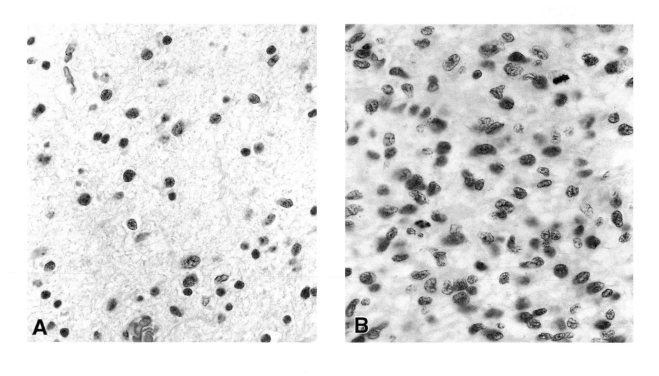

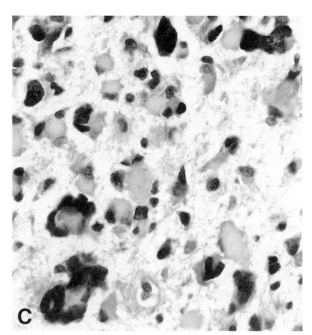

Figure 3-2
FIBRILLARY OR "DIFFUSE" ASTROCYTIC NEOPLASM WITH DIFFERING DEGREES OF DIFFERENTIATION
Varying histologic patterns were encountered in the surgical specimen from the case illustrated in figure 3-1: a paucicellular astrocytoma devoid of mitoses and with only minimal nuclear pleomorphism (A); a considerably more cellular and mitotically active anaplastic astrocytoma (B); and a focus with a degree of cytologic pleomorphism common to many glioblastomas (C).

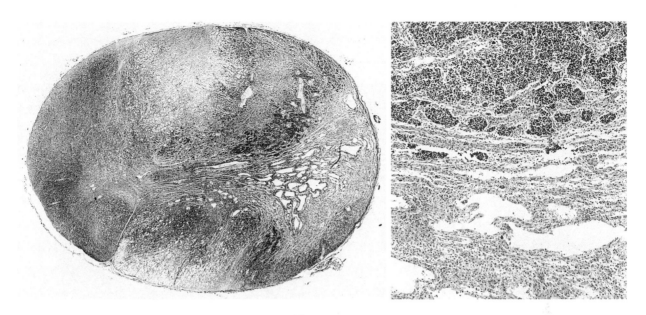

Figure 3-3
GLIOBLASTOMA MULTIFORME ARISING IN AN ASTROCYTOMA
Left: This spinal cord exhibits both a lightly staining microcystic astrocytoma as well as a darkly staining glioblastoma.
Right: At higher magnification, gemistocytic astrocytoma with microcystic change is apparent at the bottom of the illustration and cellular nodules of glioblastoma multiforme are seen at the top. The 6-year history of symptoms attested to the initially low-grade nature of this astrocytic tumor.

preexisting lower-grade tumor, either astrocytoma or anaplastic astrocytoma (figs. 3-3, 3-4). When incomplete, this progression from lower to higher grade produces borderline lesions that are difficult to grade.

Grading. The grading of astrocytomas represents an attempt to establish artificial and abrupt points of division in what is actually a continuum of neoplastic evolution, a process that takes place through a complicated series of steps, many unaccompanied by detectable morphologic changes. If this process, by which the tumors evolve towards glioblastomas, proceeds by accumulation of molecular events, molecular milestones may be detectable and may become part of routine pathologic analysis. In a sense, these events represent incremental increases in tumor grade; it may be possible to recognize tumor progression at an earlier focal cytologic stage before it can be detected using classic histologic criteria. Despite exciting innovations in tumor classification and grading, the following discussion of fibrillary astrocytic neoplasms focuses on classic morphologic criteria. Comments regarding newer methods are added only when they contribute to diagnosis and prognosis.

A number of histology-based systems have been devised that divide the spectrum of diffuse astrocytic tumors into prognostically meaningful grades. The goals and limitations of grading as it applies to diffuse astrocytic neoplasms can be found in an interesting article from 1964 by Sayre with its accompanying panel discussion (107). More recent articles emphasize the regional heterogeneity of tumor grade and its implications for prognosis and treatment (13,23a). Some of these grading systems are a priori schemes, whereas others are based upon the identification of histologic variables of prognostic significance. Favorable prognostic variables for the fibrillary astrocytic tumors include the presence of microcysts and the finding of better differentiated components (in an anaplastic astrocytoma or glioblastoma). Cytologic atypia, mitotic activity, vascular ("endothelial") hyperplasia, and necrosis are, on the other hand, prognostically unfavorable variables (11,18,27,91,115).

The early system of Bailey and Cushing was based on the superficial similarity of neoplastic cells to three perceived stages of glial cytogenesis. The resulting categories, in ascending degree

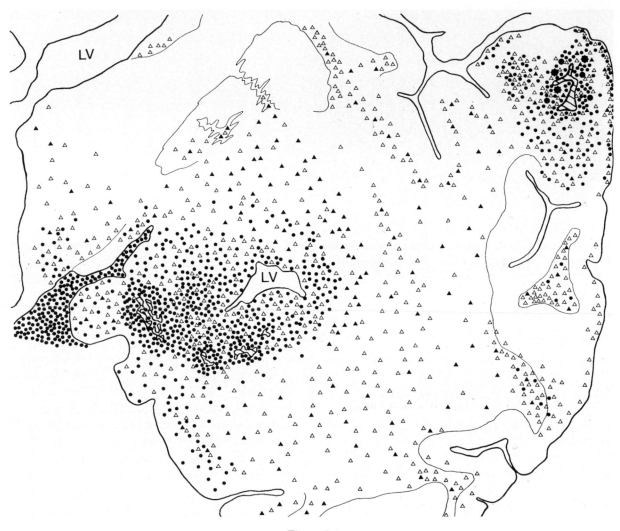

Figure 3-4
GLIOBLASTOMA ARISING IN AN ASTROCYTOMA
The diagram illustrates the astrocytoma component as low density regions of solid and open triangles; two foci of glioblastoma are shown as the densely populated regions. One glioblastoma surrounds the temporal horn of the lateral ventricle (LV) and the other expands the superior temporal gyrus at the top right of the illustration. The better differentiated component had been apparent clinically and radiographically for 6 years. (From Burger PC, Kleihues P. Cytologic composition of the untreated glioblastoma with implications for the evaluation of needle biopsies. Cancer 1989;63:2014–23.)

of malignancy were: astrocytoma, astroblastoma, and spongioblastoma multiforme.

Although a three-tiered system is still popular, the Bailey and Cushing approach was subsequently abandoned in favor of the four-tiered Kernohan system which appeared in 1949 (60, 61,133). Kernohan and his associates viewed astrocytomas as exhibiting different degrees of "dedifferentiation." Astrocytomas were designated as grades 1–4 in accordance with the popular four-tiered Broder classification which had

been applied successfully to tumors of other tissues. Kernohan and his associates, as well as many subsequent investigators, noted close correlations between patient age, tumor grade, and the length of postoperative survival. Although these successful correlations cemented the popularity of the system, current detractors note that Kernohan grade 1 tumors included both fibrillary and pilocystic astrocytomas. These two lesions are biologically distinct entities with significantly different prognoses. Furthermore, the classification equated glioblastoma with both grade 3 and 4 tumors while failing to provide clear criteria for their distinction.

The Ringertz system, which appeared in 1950, designated subdivisions by words rather than numbers and addressed a shortcoming in the Kernohan classification by consolidating all glioblastomas into one grade (100). It assigned fibrillary or diffuse astrocytic tumors to one of three grades: astrocytoma, an "intermediate lesion," and glioblastoma multiforme. The astrocytoma was well differentiated, with rare mitoses and no vascular proliferation. The intermediate lesion, although more cellular and mitotically active, showed little if any vascular proliferation or necrosis. The glioblastoma was pleomorphic, mitotically active, and exhibited neovascularization and necrosis. Like the Kernohan system and numerous subsequent systems, significant differences in survival were noted between patients in each grade.

The World Health Organization (WHO) employs a three-tiered system resembling the Ringertz scheme (64). Using Roman rather than Arabic numerals, it assigns the well-differentiated diffuse astrocytoma to grade II, the intermediate lesion or anaplastic (malignant) astrocytoma to grade III, and the glioblastoma to grade IV. Grade I is reserved for pilocytic astrocytomas and a small number of other low-grade or quasihamartomatous lesions.

The more recently introduced St. Anne-Mayo grading system was specifically designed for application to astrocytomas of the diffuse or fibrillary type. It employs a four-tiered format based on the presence or absence of four variables: nuclear atypia, mitoses, vascular proliferation, and necrosis (27). Rare tumors devoid of these features are designated grade 1, those demonstrating one variable are assigned grade 2, those with two variables are grade 3, and tumors with 3 or 4 features become grade 4. This simple system has been retrospectively applied to large series of similarly treated patients with long follow-up, is easily applied, and provides reproducible, prognostically useful results (27,62). Since the four parameters noted appear sequentially, the scheme actually lends itself to further simplification. In practice, grade 2 tumors show atypia alone, grade 3 tumors add mitoses, and grade 4 lesions acquire either or both vascular proliferation or necrosis. Since grade

1 tumors are rare, the system is essentially three-tiered, employing grades 2, 3, and 4.

While conceding that rare astrocytomas of the diffuse type are so well differentiated or low in grade as to deserve a separate fourth category (27), this volume recognizes only three lesions: astrocytoma, anaplastic astrocytoma, and glioblastoma (15,18,90,91). Use of the term "anaplastic" as an adjective to astrocytoma to denote the intermediate lesion can be challenged since, strictly speaking, the term anaplasia indicates maximal malignancy. Use of the obvious alternative term, malignant astrocytoma, poses a more significant problem in that it suggests the well-differentiated astrocytoma is benign, which it most certainly is not. The term atypical astrocytoma has been applied but fails to accurately reflect the malignancy of this tumor.

The approach used here is analogous to the Ringertz, St. Anne-Mayo, and WHO systems. The astrocytoma is equivalent to the grade 2 astrocytoma of the St. Anne-Mayo classification and the grade II astrocytoma of the WHO. The anaplastic astrocytoma is equivalent to the astrocytoma grade 3 and grade III of these same two systems, and the glioblastoma to grades 4 and IV. It is somewhat difficult to compare this classification with the Kernohan system since Kernohan's grade 1 tumors included pilocytic astrocytomas. Nevertheless, in this Fascicle astrocytoma is equivalent to the nonpilocytic tumors among Kernohan grade 1 lesions, as well as a portion of what Kernohan included under grade 2 neoplasms; anaplastic astrocytoma is equivalent to the remaining grade 2 neoplasms of the Kernohan system; and glioblastoma corresponds to astrocytomas of Kernohan grades 3 and 4.

The simultaneous use of these various systems is obviously confusing and it is important that clinicians and radiotherapists be familiar with the classification used at their institution. An unspecified "grade one astrocytoma" could refer to a Kernohan grade 1, a designation including both pilocytic astrocytoma and low-grade fibrillary astrocytoma, the very rare well-differentiated infiltrative lesions of the St. Anne-Mayo classification, or to ordinary low-grade astrocytomas of one of several other systems. The unqualified diagnosis of "grade three astrocytoma" is also ambiguous since it may refer to a glioblastoma in the Kernohan system

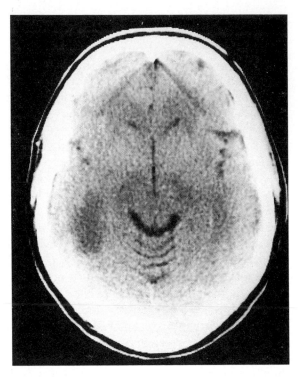
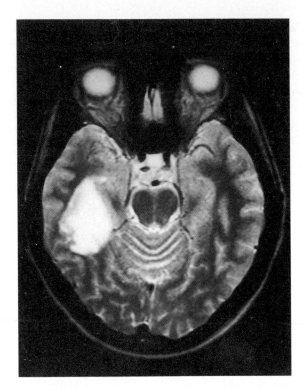

Figure 3-5

NEURORADIOLOGIC IMAGES OF A WELL-DIFFERENTIATED ASTROCYTOMA

Left: By computerized tomography, this "diffuse" or fibrillary astrocytoma is represented by a somewhat ill-defined area of low density within white matter.

Right: A T2-weighted magnetic resonance image from the same patient demonstrates the typical, rather discrete white area of high signal intensity.

or a variously defined anaplastic astrocytoma in other systems. For these reasons, we recommend that a diagnosis of astrocytoma include either an adjective such as "anaplastic" or a numerical grade and an indication of which system is being employed, e.g., astrocytoma, grade 3 (St. Anne-Mayo) or astrocytoma, grade III (WHO). Some practitioners report the grade using a numerator/denominator designation. The anaplastic astrocytoma described in this volume would be designated "astrocytoma grade 2/3" or "grade 2 (out of 3)."

Etiology. The etiology of the diffuse or fibrillary astrocytomas is unknown. Genetic predisposing factors, as in Turcot syndrome (21,46,71, 78) or ionizing radiation (63,74,96,106,123,129, 137,145), account for only occasional cases. Rare examples also occur in Ollier disease and Mafucci syndrome (81,99). Most radiation-induced gliomas are histologically malignant at the time of diagnosis; most are either anaplastic astrocytoma or glioblastoma. Fibrillary astrocytic neoplasms are rare among blacks (80).

Astrocytoma

Definition. A well-differentiated, diffusely infiltrative neoplasm of fibrillary astrocytes.

Clinical and Radiographic Features. Fibrillary astrocytomas favor the cerebral hemispheres of young to middle-aged adults (figs. 3-5, 3-6) and the brain stem of children (figs. 3-7, 3-8). Occasional examples occur in the cerebellum (47,111) or spinal cord (fig. 3-9) (24,33). At any site these astrocytomas must be distinguished from pilocytic astrocytomas. Out of precedent alone, astrocytomas of the optic nerve and brain stem are often simply designated gliomas: optic nerve glioma and brain stem glioma. In the optic nerve, virtually all such tumors are pilocytic astrocytomas, whereas in the brain stem most are of the fibrillary type. Cerebellar astrocytomas are usually pilocytic as well. Both pilocytic and fibrillary tumors occur in the spinal cord.

Just like any expanding intracranial mass, astrocytomas may produce nonspecific symptoms

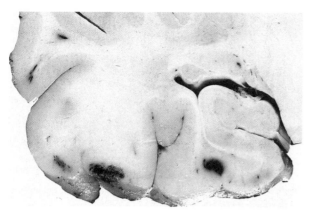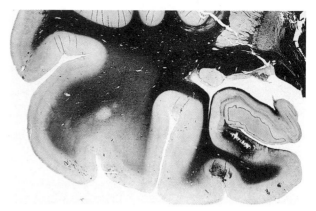

Figure 3-6
WELL-DIFFERENTIATED ASTROCYTOMA
Left: The brain of a 24-year-old who was fatally injured in an automobile accident contains an incidental well-differentiated fibrillary astrocytoma in the temporal lobe. The lesion forms an ill-defined expansion of the white matter associated with blurring of the gray-white junction and enlargement of an overlying gyrus. Note the contusions. The neoplasm's effect on the gray-white junction should be compared to the normal anatomy illustrated in figure 2-1.

Right: A histologic section stained for myelin illustrates the area of reduced staining typical of such lesions. (Courtesy of Dr. E.C. Gessaga, Aarau, Switzerland.)

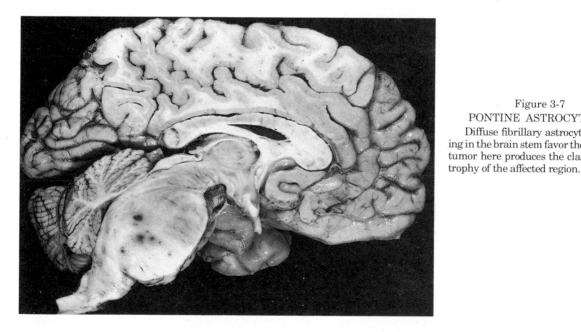

Figure 3-7
PONTINE ASTROCYTOMA
Diffuse fibrillary astrocytomas arising in the brain stem favor the pons. The tumor here produces the classic hypertrophy of the affected region.

of mass effect, seizures, and neurologic deficits reflecting the site of the tumor. Seizures are more common than functional deficits due to parenchymal destruction; the latter occur more frequently in association with tumors of higher grade. Astrocytomas in the brain stem produce neurologic signs reflecting dysfunction of cranial nerve nuclei and compression of sensorimotor tracts traversing the pons or medulla (135). In combination with radiographic evidence of brain stem enlargement or "hypertrophy," these symptoms are often considered sufficiently specific to justify radiotherapy without biopsy and histologic confirmation.

By computerized tomography (CT), astrocytomas of the cerebral hemisphere appear as ill-defined areas of low density with their epicenters in the white matter (fig. 3-5, left). In contrast to most high-grade astrocytic tumors, no enhancement is noted following the intravenous

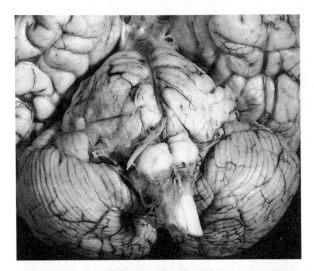

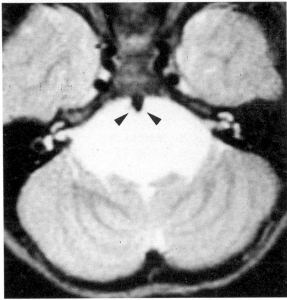

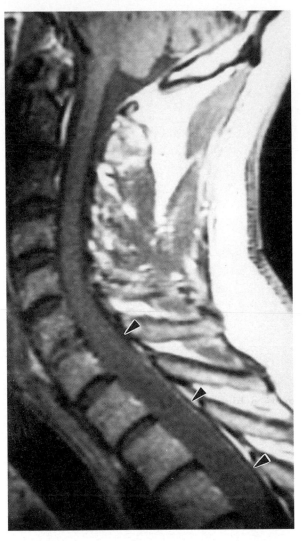

Figure 3-8
WELL-DIFFERENTIATED FIBRILLARY
ASTROCYTOMA OF THE PONS

Partial encirclement of the basilar artery is common in fibrillary astrocytomas of the pons (top). This distinctive feature is recognized readily in magnetic resonance images (bottom, arrows), as is the diffuse high signal intensity of this intrinsic pontine neoplasm. (Courtesy of Dr. James W. Langston, Memphis, TN.)

Figure 3-9
WELL-DIFFERENTIATED FIBRILLARY OR
"DIFFUSE" ASTROCYTOMA OF THE SPINAL CORD

The diffuse noncontrast-enhancing tumor (arrows) enlarges the spinal cord over multiple segments.

administration of an iodinated contrast agent. By magnetic resonance imaging (MRI), astrocytomas are rather ill-defined areas of low signal intensity on T1-weighted images; on T2-weighted images they appear better circumscribed with a high signal intensity because of their increased water content (fig. 3-5, right).

In the brain stem, astrocytomas are also low attenuating, nonenhancing lesions by CT and bright on T2-weighted MRIs (fig. 3-8, bottom). The presence of enhancement should suggest a higher-grade fibrillary astrocytic tumor or, especially if the lesion is bulky and dorsally exophytic, a pilocytic astrocytoma (see fig. 3-68).

Astrocytomas in the spinal cord can span one or many spinal segments (fig. 3-9), sometimes in association with a syrinx (see Appendix G). As in the intracranial compartment, well-differentiated astrocytomas of the cord are typically not contrast

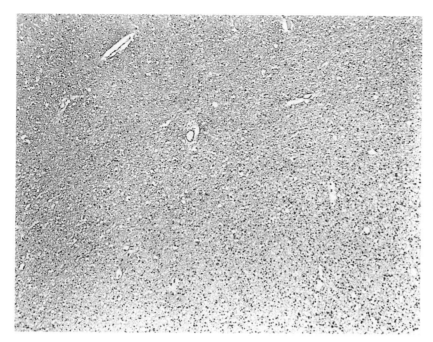

Figure 3-10
WELL-DIFFERENTIATED
FIBRILLARY ASTROCYTOMA
As illustrated in this section taken from the neoplasm seen in figure 3-9, the well-differentiated fibrillary astrocytoma produces an ill-defined region of hypercellularity which, through a gradient of decreasing cellularity, merges imperceptibly with the surrounding brain parenchyma.

enhancing. As at other sites, enhancement suggests a high-grade fibrillary astrocytic tumor, pilocytic astrocytoma, ependymoma, or other lesions such as hemangioblastoma. Pilocytic astrocytomas of the spinal cord are common; in children, they outnumber diffuse or fibrillary types.

Macroscopic Findings. Early in their evolution, deep-seated astrocytomas may be too subtle to be grossly apparent; later, they overtly expand the white matter and even the overlying cerebral gyri (fig. 3-6, left). A small, timidly obtained biopsy from expanded, yet not necessarily infiltrated, cortex overlying an astrocytoma may not yield diagnostic tissue. Upon incision, astrocytomas vary in texture. Some are firm, while others are softer than surrounding white matter, assuming an almost gelatinous quality. Intratumoral cysts filled with clear fluid are occasionally seen and help distinguish astrocytoma from glioblastoma, with its necrotic center and turbid hemorrhagic contents. At autopsy or in macroscopic sections of lobectomy specimens, astrocytomas are ill-defined expansions of white matter which blur the ordinarily well-demarcated gray-white junction (fig. 3-6, left).

Astrocytomas of the brain stem generally have their epicenter within the pons, which undergoes hypertrophy as it is forced to accommodate the proliferating cells (figs. 3-7, 3-8, top). This expanding structure encroaches posteriorly and superiorly on the fourth ventricle, often to the point of functional obstruction, while anteroinferior enlargement first displaces and then encircles the basilar artery. The latter results in a virtually diagnostic radiographic image (fig. 3-8, bottom).

Astrocytomas of the spinal cord produce an ill-defined fusiform enlargement. A fluid-filled cyst or syrinx may lie either within the tumor proper or extend from its rostral or caudal poles into noninfiltrated cord. Cyst formation is more frequent in pilocytic than in fibrillary astrocytomas.

Microscopic Findings. At low magnification, most astrocytomas are obvious regions of hypercellularity largely within white matter. Better differentiated lesions exhibit a modest increase in cellularity, approximately twice normal, and an infiltrative pattern of growth that overruns or incorporates preexisting axons, oligodendrocytes, and astrocytes over a large area (fig. 3-10). There may be little disturbance in the cytologic or architectural features of the affected tissue. The margin of such tumors is generally indistinct since tumor cells lie dispersed within fiber pathways. Spread of tumor cells is, however, often less apparent than in anaplastic astrocytoma or glioblastoma.

With time, astrocytomas extend beyond their original boundaries to enter overlying cortex or deep hemispheric structures. Proliferation in subpial, perivascular, perineuronal, and subependymal zones results in the formation of "secondary structures." Such characteristic patterns of tumor spread are usually more prominent in oligodendrogliomas, astrocytomas undergoing malignant change, or the so-called gliomatosis cerebri (113,114).

In all but the best differentiated neoplasms, astrocytoma cells are irregularly distributed as compared to the regimented composition of the normal white matter (fig. 3-11 in comparison to fig. 2-10). In addition to hypercellularity, which is often subtle, nearly all astrocytomas possess cells with enlarged, cigar-shaped, or irregular hyperchromatic nuclei.

The cytoplasm of astrocytoma cells varies considerably both in amount and configuration. In paucicellular lesions within which tumor cells lie isolated in virtually intact brain tissue, cytoplasm is scarcely visible ("naked nuclei"), and scant processes, if present, are lost in a fine fibrillar background. Such neoplasms are recognized as astrocytomas more on the basis of their nuclear atypia, irregular cell distribution, and increased cellularity than by the cytoplasmic configuration of their cells (fig. 3-11). In more classic cellular lesions, the cells possess a few asymmetric and often short processes which are the basis of the overt astrocytic quality of such tumors (fig. 3-12).

Only a minority of astrocytomas exhibit the prominent rotund configuration and abundance of eosinophilic cytoplasm necessary to justify the label gemistocytic (fig. 3-13). By definition, most cells in the gemistocytic variant of diffuse astrocytoma exhibit a plump, glassy cell body and a corona of short, stout to delicate processes. Aside from their population density, such cells when scattered and well differentiated can closely resemble reactive astrocytes. The principal distinguishing feature of reactive cells is their uniform distribution and symmetric stellate configuration; the long radiating processes of these cells are best seen in smear preparations or immunostains for glial fibrillary acidic protein (GFAP). The appearance in many gemistocytic astrocytomas of a complement of small, poorly differentiated cells with scant cytoplasm, and an

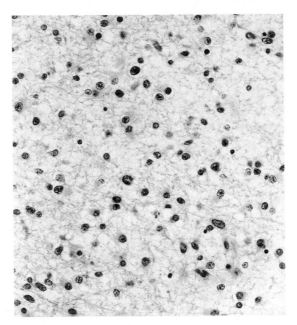

Figure 3-11
WELL-DIFFERENTIATED
FIBRILLARY ASTROCYTOMA
Higher magnification of the specimen shown in figure 3-10 shows a hypercellular lesion composed of cells with moderate pleomorphism and chromatin density. As is often the case, the cytoplasm is not conspicuous.

increased mitotic or proliferation index such as Ki-67 or bromodeoxyuridine (BrdU), indicates malignant transformation. Most gemistocytic tumors are therefore assigned to the next higher grade, i.e., anaplastic astrocytoma or, when vascular proliferation and necrosis are seen, to the ultimate grade, glioblastoma. We do not, however, believe that all gemistocytic astrocytomas should necessarily be classified as high-grade astrocytomas (anaplastic astrocytoma or glioblastoma), although we recognize the potential of these lesions to behave aggressively (67,126).

Microcystic spaces, hereafter referred to as microcysts in spite of their lack of an epithelial lining, are a distinctive and diagnostically helpful feature of gliomas (fig. 3-14). These round fluid-filled microcavities characterize well-differentiated gliomas of either astrocytic or oligodendroglial type, but are rarely, if ever, found in reactive gliosis. Varying in size and contour, and frequently filled with stainable mucin or proteinaceous fluid, they differ from the linear clefts produced by ice crystals formed during frozen section processing. Microcysts are, with few exceptions, seen in

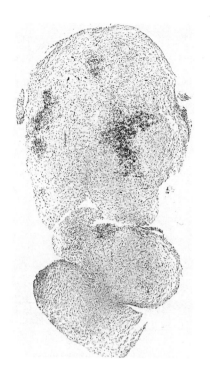

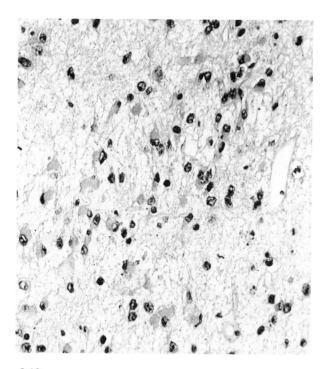

Figure 3-12
NEEDLE BIOPSY SPECIMEN OF FIBRILLARY ASTROCYTOMA
Left: The hypercellularity of this astrocytoma is apparent at low magnification.
Right: Irregular clustering of the cells with nuclear pleomorphism and scant eosinophilic cytoplasm is evident upon closer view.

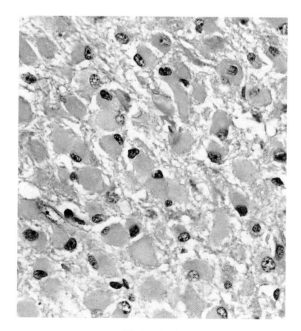

Figure 3-13
GEMISTOCYTIC ASTROCYTOMA
Eosinophilic cells with prominent glassy cytoplasm and eccentric, somewhat hyperchromatic nuclei are a typical feature of this type of diffusely infiltrative astrocytoma. Perivascular lymphocytes are common in gemistocytic lesions.

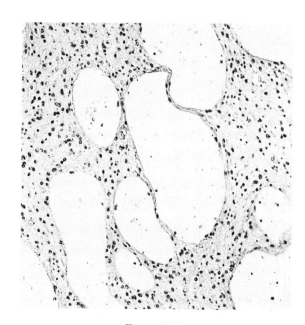

Figure 3-14
WELL-DIFFERENTIATED
FIBRILLARY ASTROCYTOMA
Microcystic spaces, often filled with proteinaceous fluid, may be seen in fibrillary astrocytomas, but are more frequent in oligodendrogliomas.

younger patients and, unless they are accompanied by clear evidence of malignant transformation, generally indicate a well-differentiated or low-grade glioma. Microcyst formation may be seen within either cortex or white matter, but is more prominent in the former.

Small numbers of perivascular lymphocytes are commonly observed in astrocytomas, particularly in those of gemistocytic type (fig. 3-13) (134). Germinal center formation is rarely noted.

The nuclei of astrocytomas vary with both type and degree of differentiation. Those in small, very well-differentiated tumors are uniformly round to oval, with little hyperchromasia or nuclear prominence. Aside from gemistocytic tumors in which nuclei are often round, those in more typical astrocytomas are elongated, irregular, and hyperchromatic. Prominent nucleoli are uncommon in fibrillary astrocytomas but small ones are common in gemistocytic tumors.

Almost by definition, mitoses are absent in astrocytoma. Even one, particularly if found in a small specimen, should call the diagnosis into question. In effect, the St. Anne-Mayo grading scheme actually uses their presence to distinguish grade 2 (astrocytoma) from grade 3 (anaplastic astrocytoma) lesions. Since well-differentiated astrocytomas rarely exhibit foci of coagulative necrosis, their presence alone, in the absence of other features of atypia or anaplasia, is not diagnostic of glioblastoma. Nonetheless, the presence of necrosis in a well-differentiated neoplasm, particularly one devoid of mitoses, should prompt reconsideration of the diagnosis, exclusion of other forms of glioma, and review of the patient's history in an effort to explain the finding. Prior radiotherapy, for example, will produce multiple small foci of parenchymal necrosis.

In histologic sections of astrocytomas, neoplastic cells are found most easily in areas identified as edematous by CT or MRI. Although it is generally difficult to determine the full extent of an infiltrating astrocytoma in histologic sections, careful study of such preparations and accompanying smear or squash preparations can identify single neoplastic cells in otherwise intact parenchyma (26). Such cells are distinguished from reactive astrocytes by their larger more irregular nuclei, hyperchromasia, cellular pleomorphism, and, as mentioned above, by the

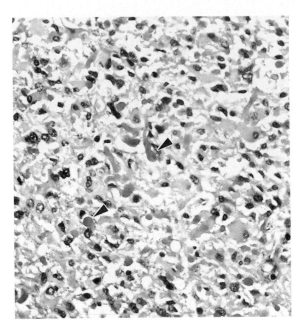

Figure 3-15
FIBRILLARY ASTROCYTOMA
WITH ROSENTHAL FIBERS
Rare fibrillary astrocytomas contain Rosenthal fibers (arrows), a feature far more characteristic of pilocytic astrocytoma.

characteristics of their processes: shortness, paucity, and random nonstellate configuration.

At any point in tumor progression, malignant transformation may add clones of new cells more prone to cortical infiltration and extension along white matter fiber pathways. At this point, even though cellularity may be low and mitoses difficult to find, the lesion usually satisfies the histologic criteria for anaplastic astrocytoma. Labeling indices are typically high in such diagnostically challenging tumors.

Cartilage is a rare feature of astrocytoma (59). An occasional diffuse or fibrillary astrocytoma, usually a gemistocytic variant, may be rich in Rosenthal fibers (fig. 3-15). These eosinophilic hyaline structures are much more commonly associated with pilocytic astrocytomas and are, accordingly, discussed in detail in that section.

Frozen Section. Although the typical features of astrocytoma are obvious in both permanent and frozen sections, variations in staining characteristics and section thickness complicate interpretation in the latter (figs. 3-16–3-18) (17, 108). The presence of ice crystals compounds the problem since the clefts mimic microcysts and

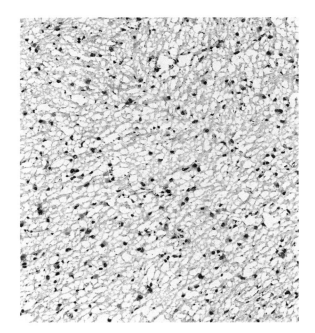

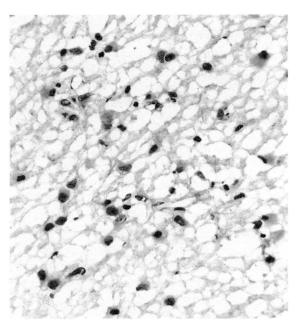

Figure 3-16
WELL-DIFFERENTIATED FIBRILLARY
ASTROCYTOMA: FROZEN SECTION
The cytologic features of this fibrillary astrocytoma are considerably altered in a cryostat section, but the tumor retains its hypercellularity and its irregular distribution of nuclei.

Figure 3-17
WELL-DIFFERENTIATED FIBRILLARY
ASTROCYTOMA: FROZEN SECTION
The neoplastic astrocytes are irregularly grouped and hyperchromatic, although some hyperchromasia and pleomorphism are artifacts of the freezing process.

compress intervening tissue to produce artifactual increases in cell density. The problem is especially acute in small specimens of the sort obtained by stereotactic needle biopsy. In such cases, adequate samples of nonfrozen tissue should be obtained for optimal processing. Every effort should be made to avoid freezing an entire specimen. Freezing distorts the nuclei of normal astrocytes and oligodendrocytes and, in both frozen and permanent sections, the contorted hyperchromatic nuclear profiles resemble those of astrocytoma. Furthermore, even if an astrocytoma seems apparent, it is nonetheless wise to make only a more general diagnosis of "low-grade infiltrating glioma" since it is often difficult to distinguish astrocytoma from oligodendroglioma based only on frozen sections.

In summary, a firm intraoperative diagnosis of infiltrative glioma requires an unequivocal increase in cellularity, irregularly distributed glial cells, and, in some instances, microcysts. If only slight hypercellularity and mild nuclear pleomorphism are seen, additional tissue should be requested and the diagnosis deferred to permanent sections.

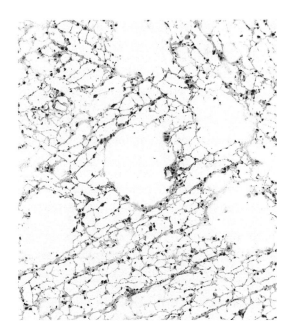

Figure 3-18
WELL-DIFFERENTIATED FIBRILLARY
ASTROCYTOMA: FROZEN SECTION
Ice crystals are difficult to avoid when freezing edematous gliomas. Here, the linearly oriented artifactual clefts can be distinguished readily from the round, diagnostically helpful, microcysts.

Cytology. Cytologic preparations of either smear or squash type are invaluable aids in diagnosis. Astrocytomas vary considerably in appearance depending not only upon their histologic subtype but upon their cellularity. When isolated cells are present in otherwise intact parenchyma, the nuclei, even on smear, usually appear "naked," without pink fibrillated cytoplasm. In contrast, when cellular tumors are smeared the often aggregated cells possess elongated cytoplasmic processes with variable fibrillarity. The nuclei are coarser and more irregular than those of normal brain cells (pls. IA, IB). The feltwork of glial processes that characterizes cellular tumors is more readily seen than in histologic sections. Often, these cellular extensions are delicate and cannot be related to a particular cell. Cytologic preparations of gliotic tissue, on the other hand, exhibit classic astrocytes with long, symmetrically radiating processes extending from the perikaryon (pl. IC). The nuclei of astrocytomas are generally more angulated and hyperchromatic than those of either oligodendroglioma or reactive gliosis. In chronic gliosis or irradiated tissue, however, nuclear abnormalities may be seen.

Needle Biopsy Findings. Since astrocytomas in needle biopsy specimens can be exceedingly difficult to interpret, a definitive diagnosis may have to await the study of permanent sections. In our experience, 1-cm-long trochar biopsies are preferable over the smaller, partly crushed specimens obtained from cup style forceps or aspirated in thin needles (see fig. 3-12).

Immunohistochemical Findings. The cytoplasm of fibrillary astrocytomas is positive for GFAP. In gemistocytic tumors, reactivity is usually prominent in the filament-rich periphery, the central organelle-containing region being largely nonreactive. Most astrocytomas are S-100 protein and vimentin immunoreactive (25, 48,66,118,144). Although the latter antigen is shared by so many cell types as to almost lack diagnostic utility, it is of use in demonstrating the antigenic viability of a specimen. For reasons not entirely clear, cytokeratin reactivity is also common (25). Scattered cells are immunoreactive for alpha-B-crystallin (54).

Ultrastructural Findings. The cells of astrocytoma vary greatly in size, configuration, content of organelles, and fibrillarity. Most show evidence of differentiation, particularly as cytoplasmic filaments and omnidirectional processes. Filaments vary in distribution. When parallel, they may fill processes or be disposed in skeins or whorls. Gemistocytic astrocytes are distinctive in having aligned subplasmalemmal filaments, as well as jumbled filaments among organelles within the center of the cell body (66,109,110). Randomly distributed, often poorly formed, intercellular junctions may be encountered.

Differential Diagnosis. Since the diagnosis of well-differentiated astrocytoma is often difficult and of obvious clinical importance, all available information should be used in this effort. This requires awareness of the neuroradiologic images. If the radiographic appearance of a lesion differs significantly from the "typical" astrocytoma described under Clinical and Radiographic Features, the diagnosis should be questioned (see Appendix C). Caution is also in order in the absence of mass effect. One should be extremely hesitant in the face of a contracting lesion, no matter what the histologic or cytologic appearance. The presence of contrast enhancement or a cyst-mural nodule architecture are also atypical of fibrillary astrocytoma and should prompt reconsideration of the diagnosis. In fact, the presence of a contrast-enhancing ring almost rules out a fibrillary astrocytoma since the pattern is more characteristic of glioblastoma, pilocytic astrocytoma, abscess, metastasis, infarct, or demyelinating disease. Even focal contrast enhancement in a diffusely infiltrative astrocytoma is strong presumptive evidence of malignant transformation.

Radiographic findings are important in the assessment of spinal cord lesions. The typical diffuse astrocytoma is an ill-defined mass unaccompanied by contrast enhancement (see Appendix C). Enhancement in an intramedullary astrocytic tumor of the diffuse type almost invariably represents a high-grade tumor (anaplastic astrocytoma or glioblastoma). Alternatively, enhancement is present in other spinal cord tumors, such as pilocytic astrocytoma, ependymoma, or hemangioblastoma.

With radiographic data in hand, histologic examination can focus on cellularity as a key to indicate the presence of an abnormality. Thereafter, histologic examination centers upon a search for nuclear atypia, microcysts, or cortical

PLATE I

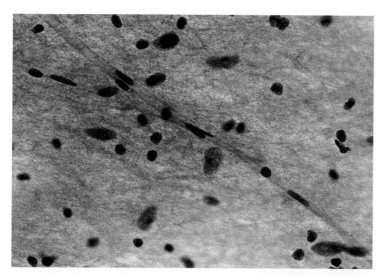

A. NORMAL GRAY MATTER
This smear preparation of normal cerebral cortex contains the small nuclei of glia and the larger, somewhat elongated nuclei of ganglion cells. Capillaries transverse the field.

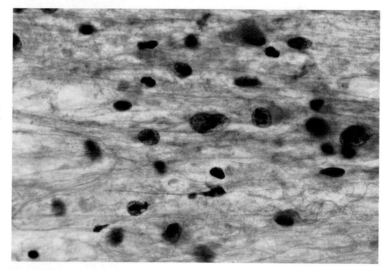

B. ASTROCYTOMA
Astrocytes with moderate hyperchromasia and nuclear pleomorphism sit in a finely fibrillar background characteristic of gliomas.

C. GLIOSIS
In contrast to the astrocytoma, the abundant omnidirectional processes of reactive cells reach out to define spherical domains. Multiple contacts with adjacent vessels are typical.

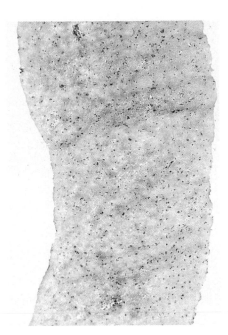 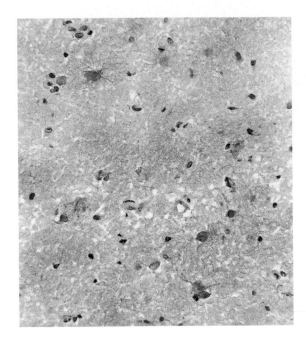

Figure 3-19
REACTIVE GLIOSIS
As in this needle biopsy specimen, astrogliosis lends an appearance of hypercellularity (left), but is more a reflection of cellular hypertrophy than of hyperplasia (right).

involvement with satellitosis and subpial tumor cell accumulation. The presence of any one of these features, even in the setting of minimal hypercellularity, clearly indicates an abnormality. Since reactive gliosis does not, as a rule, produce a substantial increase in cellularity, its histologic distinction from well-differentiated astrocytoma generally poses no difficulty (fig. 3-19). In all but the most florid examples of gliosis, reactive cells are noted more for nuclear uniformity and cellular hypertrophy than for hyperplasia. Uniform cell distribution, prominence of cytoplasm, and stellate symmetry of elongated processes are also characteristic. The cells are thus individually conspicuous but are not substantially increased in number. Furthermore, the cytoplasm of reactive astrocytes is exceptionally prominent in contrast to the usually limited cytoplasm of all but gemistocytic neoplastic astrocytes. Most astrocytomas, even if not patently "astrocytic" in appearance, are thus too cellular to suggest gliosis. Gliosis, although obviously astrocytic, is not particularly cellular. The infiltrating edge of a gemistocytic astrocytoma does, however, pose a diagnostic problem. As is discussed above under Microscopic Findings, paucicellular portions of this neoplasm can be

difficult to distinguish from active gliosis (figs. 3-20, 3-21). Smears and immunohistochemical staining for GFAP are both useful in this setting. The multiple long-tapering processes of reactive astrocytes contrast with the less symmetric, shorter, thinner, and more "pruned" branches of the less uniform neoplastic cells.

Caution is recommended when the sole abnormality is uniform hypercellularity in the absence of atypia or prominent cytoplasm. In this setting, consideration must be given to the possibility that the biopsy is simply a thickly cut section of normal brain. White as well as gray matter may be misleading since clustering of oligodendrocytes is accentuated about neurons and around vessels in thick sections.

The possibility of a non-neoplastic condition must always be considered in the differential diagnosis of fibrillary astrocytoma. Of special importance is demyelinating disease (fig. 3-22), histologically similar to astrocytoma and oligodendroglioma. An additional macrophage-rich lesion that can be misinterpreted as an astrocytoma is cerebral infarct. At low magnification, one is often alerted to the possibility of demyelinating disease by the perivascular cuffs of lymphocytes, a prominent

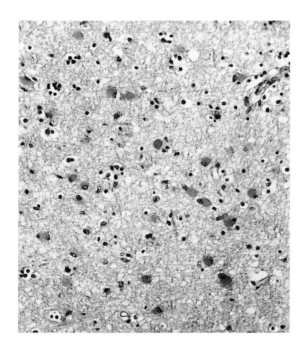

Figure 3-20
REACTIVE GLIOSIS
Hypertrophic reactive astrocytes may be difficult to distinguish from gemistocytic astrocytoma.

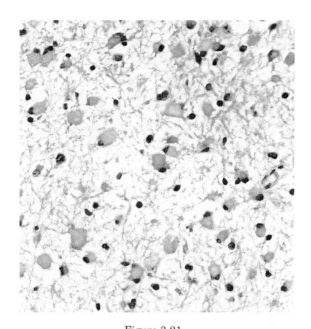

Figure 3-21
GEMISTOCYTIC ASTROCYTOMA
Paucicellular regions of gemistocytic astrocytoma may closely resemble reactive gliosis.

feature of the acute and subacute phases of demyelination. Key to the diagnosis of demyelinating disease and cerebral infarcts are the numerous foamy macrophages. These cytologically bland cells abound in the parenchyma, and as they return with phagocytized myelin debris, accumulate in perivascular spaces where they wait two or three cells deep to reenter the vasculature. Such cells are characterized by their roundness, discrete cell borders, uniform round nuclei, vacuolated cytoplasmic content of myelin debris, and immunoreactivity with macrophage markers. Macrophages are infrequent in brain tumors, even in malignant varieties.

When reactive conditions are excluded and a diagnosis of neoplasia is established, the two principal diagnostic considerations include oligodendroglioma and fibrillary astrocytic tumors of higher grade. Additional considerations include other varieties of astrocytoma, as well as a highly fibrillary ependymoma.

Oligodendroglioma deserves principal consideration since, like astrocytoma, it is an infiltrating, usually supratentorial glioma with a predilection for patients in the third and fourth decades of life. It generally poses little diagnostic

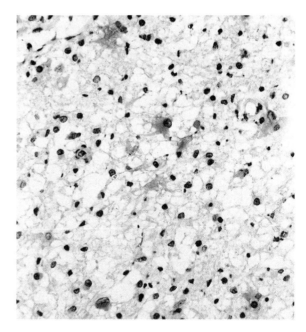

Figure 3-22
DEMYELINATING DISEASE
MIMICKING ASTROCYTOMA
The combination of hypertrophic reactive astrocytes and the hypercellularity imparted by macrophages produces a lesion superficially resembling an astrocytoma.

difficulty when hypercellular, rich in perinuclear halos, and marked by geometrically arranged, often intersecting, small vessels. Less cellular examples, or ones in which perinuclear halos are inconspicuous or absent, may be difficult to distinguish from a better differentiated astrocytoma (see fig. 3-118). In general, even astrocytomas in their best differentiated or lowest grade are noted for greater nuclear pleomorphism, more prominent cytoplasm, and process formation. Astrocytomas usually lack the calcification and cortical involvement with extensive perineuronal satellitosis so characteristic of oligodendrogliomas.

As is discussed in the sections on oligodendrogliomas and mixed gliomas, some oligodendrogliomas include cells with eccentric, eosinophilic, GFAP-positive cell bodies which lend a decidedly astrocytic appearance (see fig. 3-120). We neither consider these cells to be astrocytes, nor the lesions that contain them to be mixed gliomas, since the nuclei of such cells retain the roundness expected of oligodendrocytes. The eosinophilic cytoplasm of such "microgemistocytes" varies considerably. It may be glassy, coarsely fibrillar, or dotted with brightly eosinophilic granules which correspond ultrastructurally to minute Rosenthal fibers.

Some well-differentiated gliomas resemble astrocytoma-oligodendroglioma hybrids by straddling the morphologic boundaries of these neoplasms (see fig. 3-129). Such tumors have consistent cell size and nuclear roundness but contain angulated dark nuclei typical of those of astrocytoma. Perinuclear halo formation is present, but is restrained in degree and falls just short of making a definitive morphologic statement. Although the classification of such lesions is problematic, we usually assign them, admittedly somewhat arbitrarily, to the oligodendroglioma category.

It is extremely important to distinguish fibrillary astrocytomas from pilocytic astrocytomas (fig. 3-23). The former, even when well differentiated, are infiltrative, biologically malignant tumors for which surgery offers little promise of cure. The opposite is true of many pilocytic astrocytomas. These should be suspected on clinical and radiographic grounds, given their general, but not invariable, occurrence in young patients and the frequent cyst-mural nodule architecture. A salient microscopic feature is the pattern variation, often biphasic, varying from densely com-

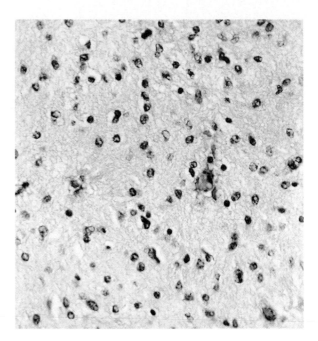

Figure 3-23
PILOCYTIC ASTROCYTOMA
RESEMBLING DIFFUSE ASTROCYTOMA
Small fragments from the edge of a pilocytic astrocytoma may closely resemble an infiltrative fibrillary astrocytoma. Radiographic features are helpful in alerting the pathologist to the likely diagnosis of a pilocytic neoplasm.

pacted elongated or piloid cells associated with Rosenthal fibers to a loose knit texture in which microcyst formation is accompanied by protein droplets or granular bodies. The significance of Rosenthal fibers, protein droplets, and granular bodies cannot be overemphasized. These are rare in fibrillary or diffuse astrocytomas. In contrast to fibrillary or diffuse astrocytomas, pilocytic lesions are more solid and considerably less infiltrative, although at high magnification there can be considerable overlap in the appearance of the two neoplasms (fig. 3-23).

Occasional ependymomas consist in large part of elongated fibrillar cells and phenotypically resemble astrocytoma (see figs. 3-136, 3-137). The presence of vague perivascular pseudorosettes or of obvious ependymoma in other portions of the lesion is sufficient justification for a diagnosis of ependymoma. We use the term mixed glioma only sparingly in the ependymoma category.

The distinction of astrocytoma from anaplastic astrocytoma may be a problem, depending upon the diagnostic criteria applied. In some classifications there are no absolute criteria that distinguish these two grades. Increased cellularity, increased nuclear hyperchromasia and pleomorphism, increased mitotic activity, and greater percentages of proliferating cells characterize anaplastic astrocytoma. In the St. Anne-Mayo system, mitoses are of great significance in the diagnosis since, even if rare, their presence elevates a lesion with nuclear atypia to a grade 3 (out of 4) status.

It seems likely that proliferation markers will, in time, augment histologic grading in distinguishing between astrocytoma and anaplastic astrocytoma. Some consensus may then be reached as to what level of cell proliferation divides, in a clinically meaningful manner, well-differentiated from anaplastic astrocytomas. The reported Ki-67 labeling indices of astrocytoma have generally been less than 2 percent, often 1 percent or less, but there is considerable variation from case to case (16,28,82b,98, 121,136,146). The bromodeoxyuridine labeling index of astrocytomas is generally less than 1 percent (68), a level that has been associated with a low mortality over a 180-week period (50). In contrast, an index above 1 percent is associated with an aggressive course, more typical of anaplastic astrocytoma. There is limited data for Ki-67, but in one study of fibrillary astrocytic neoplasms as a whole, a high level of staining (greater than 7.5 percent) was a poor prognostic sign (82b). Within the well-differentiated astrocytomas, there was suggestive evidence that patients were at higher risk for shorter survival if the index was equal to or greater than 3 percent. It remains to be seen whether further experience with more patients lowers this admittedly arbitrary cut-off point.

Some astrocytomas contain many cells with large hyperchromatic, seemingly hyperploid nuclei which suggest anaplasia, but are paucicellular and devoid of mitotic activity. They may also occur in younger patients as low density, non-contrast-enhancing lesions. Such tumors are generally assigned to the category of the well-differentiated astrocytoma, but generate concern because of their cytologic features and should prompt review of the biopsy site radiographically. On the other hand, some astrocytic tumors are paucicellular yet contain pleomorphic, elongated, hyperchromatic nuclei which prompt suspicion of a widely infiltrative malignant astrocytoma, perhaps even glioblastoma. In this setting, a high bromodeoxyuridine or Ki-67 labeling index is taken by some as evidence supporting a diagnosis of anaplastic astrocytoma. In other situations, there is such a disparity between cellularity and cytologic features, that it is appropriate to communicate the quandary to clinicians who must then make a therapeutic decision based on the clinical, radiologic, and pathologic findings. Such worrisome lesions often have a rapid evolution or exhibit foci of radiographic contrast enhancement, features which when coupled with histologic data strongly suggest, but do not permit, a diagnosis of high-grade malignancy.

Treatment and Prognosis. Although well-differentiated astrocytomas appear indolent when compared to the overtly malignant glioblastoma and the only slightly less aggressive anaplastic astrocytoma, most patients with astrocytoma of the cerebral hemispheres (27) and, far less commonly the cerebellum (47,111), are dead within 10 years (97). The median survival in one series was 8.2 years (139) and 7.25 years in another (79). At present, the precise frequency of progression of astrocytomas to tumors of higher grade is unknown, but in patients whose astrocytomas are biopsied or resected a second time, the majority of specimens show increased anaplasia (128,139). Progressive anaplasia is usually apparent as foci of contrast enhancement on CT and MRI scans or as hypermetabolic foci on positron emission tomography (35). The presence of gemistocytes is a poor prognostic sign (126), and all gemistocytic astrocytomas are considered anaplastic by some observers (67). This is not our practice, however.

As might be expected, given the close relationship between age and prognosis in patients with diffuse or fibrillary astrocytic neoplasms, younger individuals with better differentiated astrocytomas do considerably better than patients presenting later in life (79). Progression to high-grade malignancy is also more likely in older patients in whom it occurs more precipitately. Complicating therapeutic decisions is the fact that astrocytomas in the second decade of life may remain stable for years, showing neither clinical nor radiographic evidence of tumor progression. In two studies, tumor-related deaths were found only in patients with progression of the tumor to a higher grade; none of the patients died of progressive low-grade disease (79,139).

There are several situations with either little or frankly confusing available prognostic data. For instance, the course, resectability, and prognosis of small cerebral hemispheric astrocytomas now detectable by MRI remain to be established.

It is difficult to generalize about the prognosis of brain stem astrocytomas since most published studies appear to combine diffuse and pilocytic tumors. Patients with the latter lesions, not surprisingly, do significantly better (2,127). In general, diffuse intrinsic, radiographically infiltrative, and presumably fibrillary astrocytomas have an extremely poor prognosis: most patients die within 1 year (36,132). Malignant degeneration of such tumors is common and may be accompanied by seeding of the subarachnoid space.

There are few long-term studies of spinal cord astrocytomas in which an important distinction is made between fibrillary and pilocytic lesions. Some suggest a 5-year survival of less than 50 percent for patients with fibrillary types, whereas other studies suggest a more favorable outlook (82a,103a).

The role, dose, distribution, and timing of radiotherapy for diffuse astrocytoma of the cerebral hemispheres are much debated (126), particularly when the tumor has, at least by radiologic criteria, been "totally excised." Treatment may be held in reserve in such cases and administered upon recurrence, often at a point when malignant transformation is apparent as foci of contrast enhancement. A beneficial effect on survival of doses greater than 5300 rads was noted in one study (126). An additional study also found an apparent benefit of radiation therapy, while noting a better prognosis for younger patients and for those whose tumors had little or no mass effect (126a). Radiation is administered with less hesitation when residual disease is radiographically apparent, particularly if the patient is symptomatic.

Anaplastic Astrocytoma

Definition. An astrocytic tumor of fibrillary type which is intermediate in differentiation between the better differentiated astrocytoma and glioblastoma.

Clinical and Radiographic Features. Since anaplastic astrocytomas occur in the same locations as astrocytoma and glioblastoma, the majority affect the cerebral hemispheres. In accord with the statistical relationship between grade and patient age in diffuse astrocytic neoplasms, anaplastic astrocytomas generally occur in patients a decade older than those with better differentiated astrocytomas and a decade younger than those with glioblastomas. Whereas the peak incidence of cerebral examples is in the fifth decade, the pontine lesions typically occur in children.

Given its varying histologic definition, it is no surprise that a precise radiographic characterization of anaplastic astrocytoma has been difficult to achieve. Some lesions partially enhance following the intravenous administration of contrast agents. The ring pattern of enhancement surrounding a central area of necrosis noted with glioblastoma, however, is not seen. As is previously noted and further discussed below, some malignant astrocytic neoplasms with ring enhancement may be diagnosed as anaplastic astrocytoma, or even astrocytoma, if tissue sampling is limited to the infiltrating edge of the glioblastoma or to a preexisting low-grade component.

Macroscopic Findings. Intraoperatively, anaplastic astrocytomas are usually sufficiently cellular to produce a discernible mass which is generally tough or, if sufficiently cellular, soft. Cortical involvement results in firmness, pallor, and gyral expansion (fig. 3-24).

Microscopic Findings. The anaplastic astrocytoma, although clearly an astrocytic neoplasm, is one that typically exceeds well-differentiated astrocytoma in terms of cellularity, nuclear pleomorphism, and hyperchromasia (fig. 3-25). Lacking is the marked cellularity and necrosis of glioblastoma. Although vasculature may be prominent and tangles of well-formed capillaries lined by a delicate single layer of epithelium may be seen, multilayered vascular proliferation is not observed. The diagnostic significance of vascular proliferation varies with the classification employed. Understandably, there may be considerable overlap at either end of the spectrum of lesions designated anaplastic astrocytoma. Mitotic figures are encountered, although sometimes in small number.

The significance of necrosis in malignant astrocytic neoplasms depends to a certain extent on the classification and grading system employed.

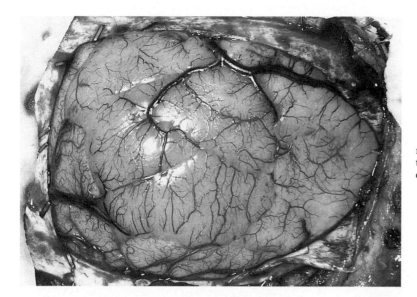

Figure 3-24
ANAPLASTIC ASTROCYTOMA
As in this specimen from a 40-year-old man with a recent onset of seizures, anaplastic astrocytoma may infiltrate the cerebral cortex to expand and deform gyri.

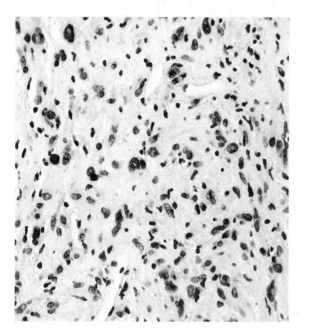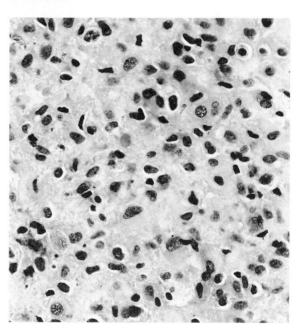

Figure 3-25
ANAPLASTIC ASTROCYTOMA
Seen at low (left) and high (right) magnification, this degree of cellularity and pleomorphism warrants the diagnosis of anaplastic astrocytoma.

In the modified Ringertz system, upon which this section is largely configured, necrosis in an anaplastic diffuse astrocytoma is indicative of a glioblastoma. In the St. Anne-Mayo system, a tumor showing necrosis and only one other variable, usually cytologic atypia, technically represents a grade 3 lesion, one roughly equivalent to the anaplastic astrocytoma in this discussion. In

practice, however, this is an unusual situation since most necrosis-containing malignant diffuse astrocytic neoplasms easily qualify as grade 4 (glioblastoma).

Microcysts may be seen in mitotically active anaplastic astrocytomas but their presence should make the pathologist cautious about the diagnosis since these structures are a more common feature

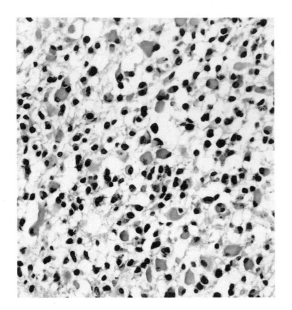

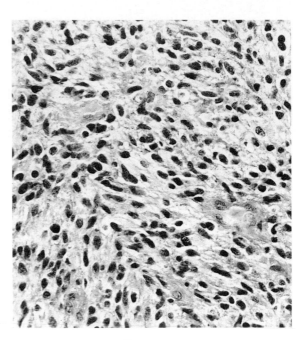

Figure 3-26
ANAPLASTIC ASTROCYTOMA
Gemistocytic tumors frequently exhibit small cells with scant cytoplasm and dark nuclei. This ominous finding suggests early anaplastic transformation.

Figure 3-27
ANAPLASTIC ASTROCYTOMA
Some anaplastic astrocytomas are composed in large part of a dense population of small cells with scant cytoplasm. The diagnosis is appropriate when adequate tissue sampling excludes the presence of vascular proliferation and necrosis, but a comment about the degree of anaplasia is warranted.

of better differentiated astrocytoma, pilocytic astrocytoma, or oligodendroglioma.

Some anaplastic astrocytomas have a pronounced gemistocytic component accompanied by dispersed or clustered small hyperchromatic cells (fig. 3-26). As was discussed, in contrast to some observers (67), we do not consider gemistocytic cytology alone sufficient for a diagnosis of anaplastic astrocytoma. On the other hand, gemistocytic lesions often are mitotically active and have a small cell component so that they are then appropriately placed in the anaplastic astrocytoma category. Gemistocytic astrocytomas are especially prone to malignant degeneration and in large specimens foci of glioblastoma, often multifocal, with vascular proliferation and necrosis are frequent (13,104).

The diagnosis of anaplastic astrocytoma, or grade 3 astrocytoma according to the St. Anne-Mayo system, is usually not difficult since it requires finding only two variables. Most qualify on the basis of nuclear atypia and mitotic figures alone. In practice, particularly with small specimens, the diagnosis is sometimes reached in the absence of mitoses and in the face of high cellularity and overt nuclear atypia.

The key factor underlying a meaningful diagnosis of anaplastic astrocytoma is the extent to which the specimen is representative. A well-selected specimen obtained by CT- or MRI-guided stereotactic biopsy, preferably serial biopsies along a trajectory, is often more informative than one timidly obtained by open biopsy or generously resected but missing the most malignant area. Many cellular tumors with mitotic activity presumably represent "near misses" of a glioblastoma (fig. 3-27). In such instances, one would assume that additional tissue cores would demonstrate either or both vascular proliferation or necrosis. There are, particularly in younger patients, occasional cellular small cell neoplasms which, even in large specimens, do not demonstrate either vascular proliferation or necrosis and qualify for the anaplastic astrocytoma designation.

A frequent diagnostic problem is presented by a highly infiltrating and cytologically malignant, but paucicellular, neoplasm. Finding mitoses and a high proliferation index generally elevates these tumors into the anaplastic category.

Frozen Section. Anaplastic astrocytomas are hypercellular and exhibit both hyperchromatic nuclei and mitotic activity.

Cytology. The appearance of anaplastic astrocytoma in smears is highly variable. In tumors of low or moderate cellularity only nuclear atypia and rare mitoses may be evident. In cellular lesions, on the other hand, cells become loosely cohesive and their processes entwine to form a fibrillary background which is the sine qua non of glioma. Nuclei are typically hyperchromatic and variably pleomorphic (pl. IIA). When such atypia is marked, consideration should be given to the possibility of a glioblastoma.

Immunohistochemical Findings. The immunohistochemical features of anaplastic astrocytoma are those of glioblastoma multiforme and astrocytoma and include positivity for GFAP and S-100 protein (see Appendix H). Reactivity for vimentin, sometimes impressive in degree, is of little diagnostic significance, but gives assurance that the specimen's antigenic viability has not been compromised by fixation and tissue processing. Many cells are reactive for alpha-B-crystallin (54).

Differential Diagnosis. In most cases, anaplastic astrocytoma is sufficiently infiltrative and cellular to indicate an abnormality; normal brain or reactive gliosis are not considered diagnostic alternatives. However, the possibility of reactive gliosis always must be considered for the sake of completeness, but it is quickly dismissed since anaplastic astrocytomas are substantially more cellular, pleomorphic, and mitotically active. Considerable nuclear pleomorphism may be observed in gliosis, particularly in the subacute or chronic reactions seen in demyelinating diseases, progressive multifocal leukoencephalopathy, the environs of craniopharyngioma, or tissue previously subjected to irradiation.

Demyelinating lesions, such as occur in multiple sclerosis, are occasionally approached surgically. Due mainly to their cellularity and the presence of occasional mitoses, plaques can resemble an infiltrating glioma. The diagnosis of demyelinating disease is primarily dependent upon recognition of its principal cells as phagocytes. Phagocytes have discrete cell borders, nuclear uniformity, foamy cytoplasm filled with myelin debris, and a tendency to angiotropism. The granular periodic acid–Schiff (PAS) positivity of macrophages as well as immunoreactivity for histiocyte markers such as HAM-56 or KP-1 also is diagnostic.

In the clinical setting of immunosuppression, with AIDS as the most common example, progressive multifocal leukoencephalopathy (PML) must be included in the differential diagnosis. This demyelinating process of viral etiology is characterized by pleomorphic astrocytes that can appear neoplastic because of their markedly hyperchromatic nuclei. The nature of the lesion is most readily recognized by its high content of foamy macrophages or gitter cells and the purple ground glass viral inclusions within the nuclei of enlarged oligodendrocytes. These are most evident at the margin of the lesion.

Principal neoplasms in the differential diagnosis of anaplastic astrocytoma include other gliomas, particularly oligodendroglial tumors, and the most closely related astrocytic neoplasms of lower and higher grade: astrocytoma and glioblastoma. Anaplastic astrocytomas share a number of histologic features with oligodendrogliomas, not only with anaplastic oligodendrogliomas but with even better differentiated examples that were subjected to freezing (see fig. 3-119). The characteristically round nuclei of neoplastic oligodendrocytes are deformed in the process, becoming angulated and hyperchromatic. In sections of tissue not previously frozen, distinctive oligodendroglial qualities are preserved, namely, nuclear uniformity and roundness. This contrasts with nuclear pleomorphism, not necessarily marked, in most anaplastic astrocytomas. Another feature of oligodendrogliomas is heavy cortical involvement with perineuronal satellitosis and subpial accumulation of tumor cells.

Although, ostensibly, the presence or absence of GFAP positivity would be definitive evidence in distinguishing an anaplastic astrocytoma and an oligodendroglial tumor, this is not the case. GFAP positivity is observed in a number of cellular oligodendrogliomas and should not be overinterpreted as evidence of an astrocytic neoplasm. Such reactivity usually highlights a small hyaline or fibrillar plump body of paranuclear cytoplasm. While it can be argued that these GFAP-positive cells are astrocytes, we consider them oligodendrocytes when they possess the nuclear characteristics of oligodendroglioma and

PLATE II

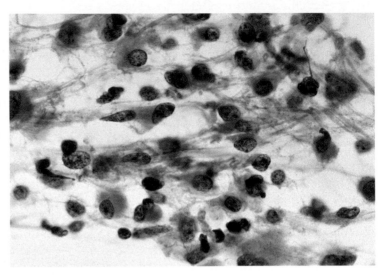

A. ANAPLASTIC ASTROCYTOMA

The cells are clearly astrocytic because of the eosinophilic cytoplasm with processes, but are more crowded and hyperchromatic than those of the well-differentiated astrocytoma illustrated in plate IB.

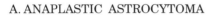

B. GLIOBLASTOMA MULTIFORME

Characteristic of most glioblastomas are small cells with elongated nuclei and bipolar processes. As here, the chromatin is generally not markedly dense nor are nucleoli usually prominent.

C. GLIOMATOSIS CEREBRI

Uniform, somewhat elongated nuclei of intermediate density are typical. Note the incorporated reactive astrocyte at the right with its prominent radiating processes.

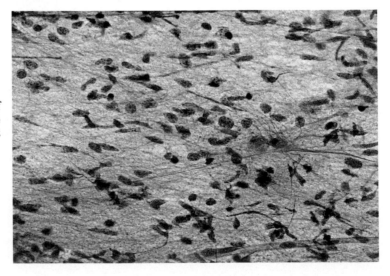

represent, as they often do, only a portion of what is otherwise a typical oligodendroglioma.

In light of the progressive transformation that characterizes diffuse astrocytic tumors, it is not surprising that anaplastic astrocytoma merges imperceptibly with astrocytoma and glioblastoma and that there is, short of arbitrary definitions, no obvious histologic or cytologic lines of demarcation between these lesions. If confirmed, the observation that overexpression of the epidermal growth factor receptor occurs only in glioblastoma, could provide a means to distinguish anaplastic astrocytoma from glioblastoma. Unfortunately, amplification is noted in less than half of glioblastomas (6,53), but, when present, could be of use in identifying high-grade tumors, particularly in a small or nonrepresentative specimen.

Classic anaplastic astrocytomas are moderately and diffusely hypercellular and lack both vascular proliferation and necrosis. From this point, there is a graded spectrum of lesions with increasing cellularity and other features of glioblastoma. Although the point of separation between anaplastic astrocytoma and glioblastoma is not precise, we consider the presence of necrosis as one point of distinction. Whether a similar assignment can be made on the basis of vascular proliferation alone is debatable, but markedly cellular lesions with this vascular change are classified by many observers as glioblastomas. Indeed, patients whose "anaplastic astrocytomas" exhibit vascular proliferation, or greater than 1 mitosis per 10 high-power fields, do less well than those whose tumors do not contain these features (37). It is important, too, that the highly reproducible St. Anne-Mayo grading system for diffuse astrocytic tumors makes a distinction between mere hypervascularity and telangiectatic vessels on the one hand, and multilayer vascular proliferation on the other. The latter had the same prognostic significance as necrosis in a multivariant analysis of nearly 300 uniformly treated tumors (27).

Sometimes, in small specimens such as those obtained by stereotactically-directed needle biopsy, a neoplasm that is extremely cellular but lacks both necrosis and vascular proliferation is seen. Although we are reluctant to diagnose glioblastoma in the absence of these two features, there comes a point at which hypercellularity

and, often, pleomorphism and mitoses become so overt that a diagnosis of glioblastoma is intuitively obvious, even in the absence of requisite histologic features. Thus, although the point is not quantifiable, there are clearly cases in which a diagnosis of anaplastic astrocytoma does not do justice to a lesion's malignancy and, bowing to common sense, we consider such tumors glioblastomas. As an alternative, a comment can be added to a diagnosis of anaplastic astrocytoma indicating that "hypercellularity is so marked as to suggest the tumor may be a glioblastoma." Since the treatment of the glioblastoma and anaplastic astrocytoma is similar, if not identical, this distinction is of little therapeutic importance. In this setting, clinicians can synthesize salient clinical, radiographic, and histologic data and advise patients regarding prognosis and therapeutic options.

Treatment and Prognosis. Anaplastic astrocytoma is a highly malignant tumor with a median survival, following surgery and radiation therapy, of approximately 2 to 3 years (18,27,90,91). Survival is favorably affected by presentation early in life, maximal resection, and by the extent of anaplasia. The utility of labeling indices, such as Ki-67, in assessing prognosis in patients with anaplastic astrocytoma is not clear. Not surprisingly, the reported ranges of proliferation indices are quite variable; considerable overlap is seen with those of glioblastomas (27,46,176,211,253). In regard to cytofluorometry, in one study patients with aneuploid tumors did better than those with euploid lesions (192). The role for chemotherapy remains unsettled, but its efficacy appears to be better established for anaplastic astrocytoma than for glioblastoma.

Glioblastoma Multiforme

Definition. A highly malignant glioma most closely related to fibrillary or diffuse astrocytic neoplasms.

General Comments. We consider glioblastomas to be astrogliomas since most are patently astrocytic or associated with lower-grade astrocytic neoplasms. Without question, some are so poorly differentiated that they provide no histologic evidence of an astrocytic precursor lesion. Under rare circumstances, others evolve from oligodendroglioma by acquisition of a preponderant astrocytic element, a late-phase process. While some malignant ependymomas assume features of a glioblastoma, most remain rather monomorphous. Thus, vaguely ependymal tumors are better classified as malignant ependymoma than glioblastoma.

Glioblastomas that contain large distinct areas of differentiated astrocytic tumor have been referred to as "secondary glioblastomas" (see figs. 3-3, 3-4) (13,112–114). More commonly, well-differentiated and anaplastic cells are admixed making it difficult to appraise this evolution but there seems little reason to doubt that in such cases the small and poorly differentiated cells arise in transition from obvious astrocytes (13). Other glioblastomas are densely cellular and homogeneously anaplastic, exhibiting none of the less cellular and better differentiated components seen in "secondary" tumors. It remains a matter of debate whether these "primary glioblastomas" arise de novo as malignant or have overrun and obscured a small precursor lesion. Studies using molecular biological markers are, at this point, few and preliminary but do support the notion of primary and secondary glioblastomas (140).

Clinical and Radiographic Features. Glioblastoma is by far the most common glioma. It affects principally the cerebral hemispheres in adults and the brain stem in children (30). It therefore shares the same topographic distribution as better differentiated diffuse or fibrillary astrocytomas. The cerebellum is far less often involved, and patients of all ages may be affected (20,29,47,70,111). Pilocytic astrocytomas outnumber diffuse astrocytic tumors at this location. In the optic nerve and cerebellum, glioblastomas are even more overshadowed by pilocytic neoplasms (1). The spinal cord is an uncommon site (22).

In the cerebral hemispheres, glioblastomas appear at any age but are most frequent after the fifth decade and comprise most diffuse astrocytic neoplasms in patients aged 70 and above. Most glioblastomas are solitary, but occasional examples are geographically separate in the same patient and warrant the designation "multicentric" (5). True multicentricity is difficult to establish, however, even at autopsy.

By CT, glioblastoma usually appears as a central area of hypodensity surrounded by a ring of contrast enhancement and a penumbra of cerebral edema. By MRI, the lesion typically has an enhancing ring seen in T1-weighted images with gadolinium enhancement and a generally broad surrounding zone of edema apparent in T2-weighted images (fig. 3-28). The central hypodense core represents necrosis, the contrast-enhancing rim is composed of highly cellular neoplasm with abnormal vessels permeable to contrast agents, and the peripheral zone of nonenhancing low attenuation is vasogenic edema containing varying numbers of isolated tumor cells (12,26,57). Although glioblastomas appear cystic given their low density centers, untreated tumors are rarely fluid filled. Indeed, a diagnosis of glioblastoma should be reconsidered if a cyst of significant size is observed. Primary brain tumors with central, fluid-filled cavities are usually well-differentiated, prognostically favorable lesions, such as pilocytic astrocytoma, ganglion cell tumor, or pleomorphic xanthoastrocytoma (see Appendix D). By MRI, glioblastomas are surrounded by a variable, but frequently extensive, "bright" or white signal in T2-weighted images. This edematous zone, for the most part, contains isolated infiltrating tumor cells within intact parenchyma.

The presenting symptoms of glioblastoma are similar to those of better differentiated diffuse astrocytomas, although accompanying neurologic deficits are generally more abrupt in onset and rapid in evolution. Unlike lower-grade lesions in which infiltration of intact parenchyma is a conspicuous feature, glioblastomas produce greater mass effect and tissue destruction, the result being focal neurologic deficits. Acute hemorrhage underlies the onset of symptoms in occasional cases (65).

Macroscopic Findings. When the dura is reflected by the surgeon to expose the brain, some glioblastomas are apparent by the expansion of cortical gyri. Tumors that actually infiltrate the cortex produce grossly apparent irregularity, firmness, and abnormalities of the surface vasculature (fig. 3-29). Some become attached to, and superficially vascularized from, the dura. As the operation proceeds and the brain is entered, a gray fleshy rim corresponding to the region of contrast enhancement may be encountered. With further dissection, a necrotic

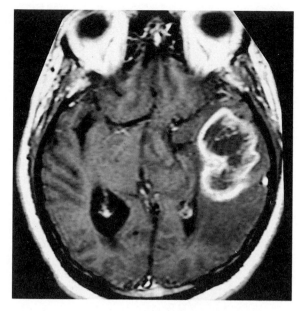 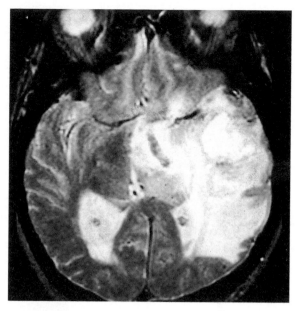

Figure 3-28
GLIOBLASTOMA MULTIFORME
Left: As seen here by magnetic resonance imaging, the glioblastoma multiforme usually exhibits a "ring" or "ring-like" zone of contrast enhancement around a dark central area of necrosis.
Right: Surrounding the densely cellular, contrast-enhancing portion of the lesion is a broad zone of cerebral edema best seen in a T2-weighted image.

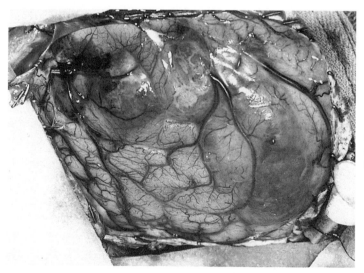

Figure 3-29
GLIOBLASTOMA MULTIFORME
As seen at surgery, the cortical involvement of this glioblastoma produces irregular thickening and discoloration of the gyri. Many glioblastomas are not apparent on gross external inspection.

core becomes evident and provides strong presumptive evidence of the diagnosis. Similarly, in transected lobectomy specimens as well as in postmortem whole brain sections, glioblastomas appear as largely necrotic masses with a peripheral zone of fleshy gray tissue (fig. 3-30). The thickness of this viable rim varies from case to case, thick in some and almost absent in others.

Surrounding white matter may be firm and granular, indicating gross neoplastic involvement, or simply wet and dull with loss of demarcation at the gray-white junction as a consequence of edema. The ordinarily glistening, ivory-colored white matter acquires a faint yellow hue.

Glioblastomas appear either diffusely infiltrative, particularly in cases in which a central fleshy

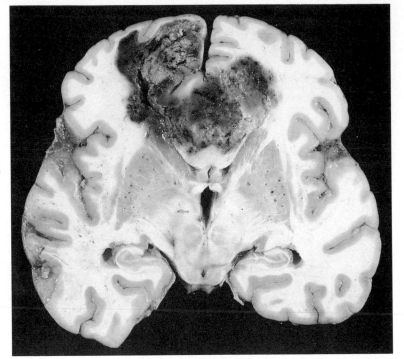

Figure 3-30
GLIOBLASTOMA MULTIFORME
This typical untreated glioblastoma, here
with the classic "butterfly" configuration, is
a necrotic hemorrhagic mass. (Courtesy of
Dr. Rodney D. McComb, Omaha, NE.)

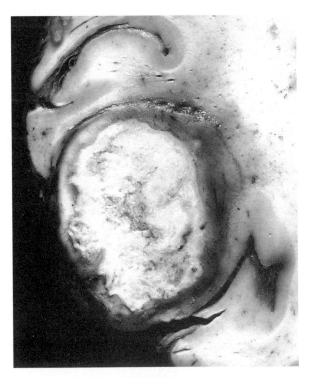

Figure 3-31
GIANT CELL GLIOBLASTOMA MULTIFORME
Some glioblastomas, such as this giant cell variant, are
discrete firm masses which clinically and radiographically
simulate metastatic carcinoma.

or necrotic area is lacking, or sufficiently circumscribed as to mimic metastatic carcinoma. Confusion with the latter is especially likely in the
rare giant cell variant of glioblastoma, a tumor
often so well demarcated as to prompt the disbe-
lieving surgeon to dismiss a frozen section diagnosis of glioma (fig. 3-31). Glioblastoma, nonetheless, remains the principal consideration, given
the tumor's deep-seated location. The epicenter
of most metastatic carcinomas is in the cortex
near the gray-white junction.

Glioblastomas of the brain stem share the
hemorrhage and necrosis of the supratentorial
counterparts. Extension along fiber pathways,
such as the middle cerebellar peduncles, is common (fig. 3-32).

Microscopic Findings. Glioblastomas are
cellular masses with varied tissue patterns as
described below. Depending somewhat upon the
disposition of white matter tracts within and
around the tumor, it appears either infiltrative
or discrete. Tumors affecting nearby gray matter
may be diffusely infiltrative, exhibiting many of
the features of gliomatosis cerebri (see fig. 3-43).

In light of the almost endless intra- and intertumoral heterogeneity of glioblastoma (fig. 3-33),
it is unrealistic to characterize all variations of

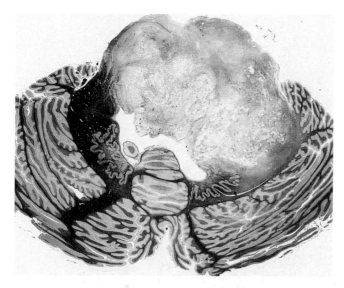

Figure 3-32
GLIOBLASTOMA MULTIFORME
OF THE BRAIN STEM
A glioblastoma has overrun the brain stem and formed an expansile, largely necrotic mass. Note extension of the lesion into the middle cerebellar peduncle (at the right) and the edema-related pallor of the cerebellar white matter.

this polymorphic glioma. Nevertheless, certain tissue patterns are sufficiently common or diagnostically important to warrant description. Some of the rarer variants deserve space out of proportion to their incidence since they can mimic other neoplasms and thus present problems in differential diagnosis.

The most common form of glioblastoma develops in transition from a better differentiated diffuse astrocytoma. Cytologically, the constituent cells of such tumors vary greatly in size, configuration, fibril content, and extent of process formation, but share a common astrocytic quality attributable largely to their pink cytoplasm. An element of polymorphism is the rule (fig. 3-33A, B). In fibrillary tumors, cytoplasm varies in quantity and is attenuated within processes whereas gemistocytic lesions exhibit plump cell bodies with scant process formation. As previously noted, gemistocytic tumors often acquire small, hyperchromatic, undifferentiated-appearing cells, a cardinal feature of transformation to glioblastoma.

At the other end of the spectrum lie highly infiltrative glioblastomas that are less "multiforme," but composed of monotonous, small, largely GFAP-negative cells which congregate in high density (fig. 3-33C, D). Nearly undifferentiated, such small cell lesions are the classic primary glioblastomas: tumors unassociated with a better differentiated or lower-grade lesion. Necrosis with pseudopalisading is often prominent and mitotic activity is high. A somewhat better

differentiated small cell glioblastoma is composed of GFAP-positive cells with short, delicate, often bipolar processes (fig. 3-33E).

Among the numerous other tissue patterns, one composed primarily of tumor giant cells is highly distinctive (fig. 3-33F). Since many glioblastomas contain such cells, no clear distinction can be drawn between truly giant cell variants and tumors containing more limited numbers of such elements. Nonetheless, in some lesions the cells are so monstrous and numerically overwhelming that it is hard to avoid placing the tumor in a distinct histologic category. Intercellular reticulin or even collagen deposition may be sufficiently abundant to produce induration. This, when combined with a degree of discreteness, can produce macroscopic similarity to a metastatic carcinoma or sarcoma (discussed above). Indeed, such lesions were once termed "monstrocellular sarcoma," a designation abandoned since their glial nature was demonstrated by immunoreactivity for GFAP (77,119).

In addition to multiforme glioblastomas consisting of a pleomorphic melange of cells, some tumors exhibit either a fascicular pattern resembling sarcoma (fig. 3-33G) or stellate cells in a myxoid stroma (fig. 3-33H). It is not always clear whether such lesions are simply glioblastoma variants or represent distinct clinicopathologic entities. Other variants are lipid rich (102) or have well-defined granular cytoplasm resembling macrophages (see Granular Cell Astrocytic Neoplasms).

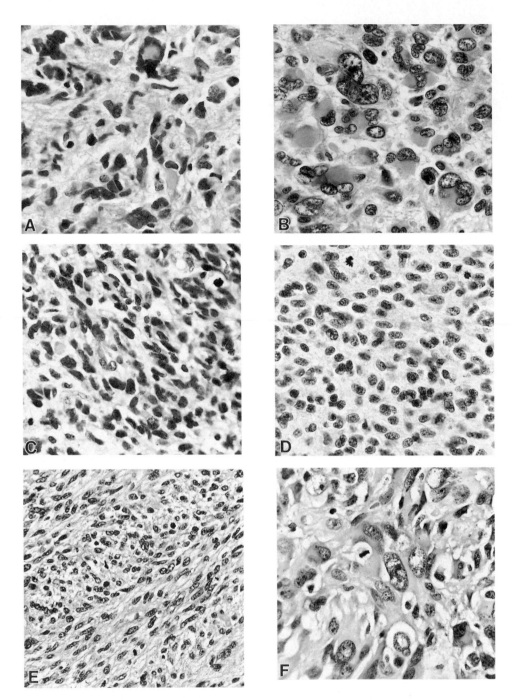

Figure 3-33
GLIOBLASTOMA MULTIFORME: VARIATIONS IN HISTOLOGIC APPEARANCE

The panels illustrate the great histologic and cytologic variation in this most common primary brain tumor. A shows a frequent pattern with nuclear angulation, hyperchromatism, and pleomorphism. These features, in association with the fibrillar background, help distinguish such a glioblastoma from other diagnostic considerations such as metastatic carcinoma and lymphoma. In B, the neoplastic cells are plumper and somewhat more epithelioid in their appearance, yet the lesion is recognized as a glioma by the glassy cytoplasm, cytoplasmic processes, and fibrillar background. A common small cell variant (C), is formed of mitotically active cells with hyperchromatic elongated, although not greatly anisomorphic, nuclei. The small, bland, monomorphic nuclei in other glioblastomas (D) can, in regions of lesser cellularity, misrepresent the lesion as a lower-grade neoplasm. Glioblastomas with a fascicular pattern (E) can resemble sarcoma. There is little evidence of invaded brain in occasional cases composed of closely packed, large pleomorphic cells (F). Such lesions must be distinguished, by mitoses, necrosis, and vascular proliferation, from the pleomorphic xanthoastrocytoma.

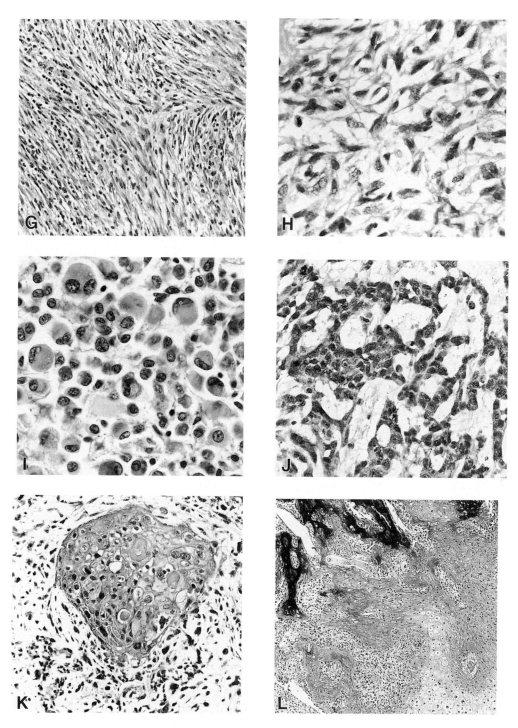

Figure 3-33 (continued)

GLIOBLASTOMA MULTIFORME: VARIATIONS IN HISTOLOGIC APPEARANCE

Compacted masses of bipolar cells are occasionally seen (G). Stellate cells lend a somewhat myxoid appearance to some lesions (H). As seen in I, cells in other glioblastomas can resemble metastases (especially malignant melanoma) when cell borders are discrete and the nuclei are round and contain prominent nucleoli. In the absence of a clearly infiltrative component or more typical histologic features, the diagnosis in such settings often depends on immunohistochemistry (GFAP). Glandular and ribbon-like epithelial structures (J) can also be confused with metastatic carcinoma. Islands of squamous differentiation (K) are seen rarely in glioblastomas and gliosarcomas. Unusual "metaplastic" elements in some malignant gliomas are bone and cartilage (L). The diagnosis of gliosarcoma is appropriate when the mesenchymal components are neoplastic.

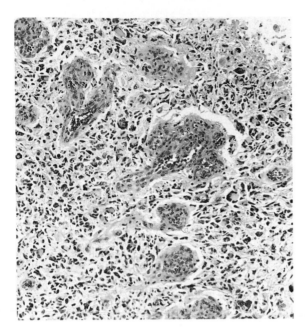 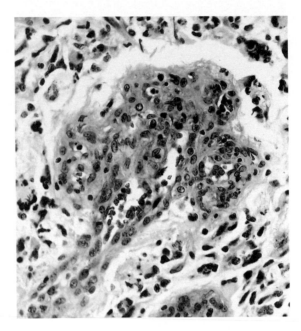

Figure 3-34
GLIOBLASTOMA MULTIFORME

Left: Vascular proliferation, a common feature of glioblastoma, produces tufts which often grow directionally. Here, as is often the case, they are oriented toward a focus of necrosis (top right).

Right: At high magnification, the neovascular tuft is a mass which, as can be confirmed by immunohistochemistry, is formed of both endothelial cells and smooth muscle cells (pericytes).

Some glioblastomas have a carcinoma-like appearance produced by plump epithelioid cells with discrete cell borders (fig. 3-33I). Other glioblastomas with epithelial metaplasia are even more diagnostically challenging (58,83,84). Such unexpected tissue components may arise in conventional glioblastomas but are more prone to occur in gliosarcoma. The epithelial structures vary in appearance from ribbons of poorly differentiated epithelial cells somewhat resembling medulloepithelioma (fig. 3-33J) to glandular clusters or islands of squamous cells replete with keratin pearls (fig. 3-33K). Not surprisingly, such cells are often immunoreactive for cytokeratins, a finding underscoring caution when keratin immunostains are used to distinguish glioblastoma from metastatic carcinoma. Other non-neoplastic metaplastic tissues include bone and cartilage (fig. 3-33L).

For any of the variants of glioblastoma there are two features of great prognostic significance and requisite to the diagnosis: hyperplasia of vascular cells and necrosis. The relative weight given to these two variables in the grading of diffuse astrocytic neoplasms has been discussed. Although it is often inferred that the vascular reactions of glioblastoma are endothelial in nature (endothelial proliferation), immunohistochemical studies indicate that many of the cells are reactive for smooth muscle antigens and that only the cells lining vascular spaces are positive for factor VIII–related antigen (45,82,116,141). Pericytes or smooth muscle cells therefore presumably contribute to the hyperplasia which in this Fascicle is referred to as vascular ("endothelial") proliferation. Cells containing muscle antigens are also a component of gliosarcomas (44). The vascular cells, whose true hyperplasia has been established by bromodeoxyuridine labeling (88), produce multilayered small vessels which in advanced states form coiled masses closely resembling glomerular tufts of the kidney (fig. 3-34). Such proliferation is often conspicuous about foci of necrosis and may exhibit directional growth or tropism, as illustrated by arcades of glomeruloid tufts apparently aligned in response to unseen tissue factors. Such arrays may be seen at the periphery of cellular zones and

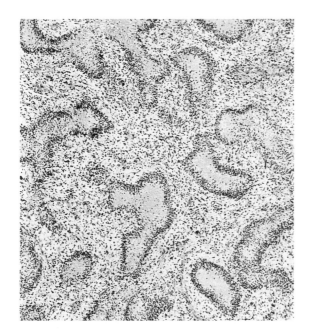

Figure 3-35
GLIOBLASTOMA MULTIFORME

In many instances, necrosis is surrounded by a distinctive collar of cells, which are often smaller than those in surrounding neoplastic tissue. The phenomenon is referred to as pseudopalisading.

necrotic foci, along anatomic boundaries, or even in remote portions of the leptomeninges, as within the spinal leptomeninges in cases of cerebral glioblastoma. Enlargement or hypertrophy of vascular cells is common in malignant gliomas but does not qualify as vascular proliferation. It should nevertheless prompt a search for vessels with the prognostically important hyperplasia. Telangiectatic vessels without multilayered hyperplasia are also common in malignant gliomas, and are seen as well in indolent neoplasms such as pilocytic astrocytoma. They do not have the prognostic significance of the true vascular proliferation just described.

Additional vascular changes without the prognostic significance of multilayered vascular proliferation include collagenous thickening, telangiectasis, and gaping, closely-packed abnormal channels.

The second cardinal feature of glioblastoma is necrosis, which takes the form of either large confluent areas destructive of parenchyma and vasculature, or small, often multiple and serpiginous foci. Large confluent regions are evident on CT or MRI scan as the tumor's hypodense central core. A distinctive feature present about necrosis, but most conspicuous about the smaller foci, is a peripheral, somewhat radially oriented accumulation of cells called pseudopalisading (fig. 3-35). This is a highly distinctive feature, seen almost exclusively in high-grade gliomas. Only rarely is it encountered in other tumors such as medulloblastoma or supratentorial embryonal tumors. When present in an oligodendroglioma, however, it should not be the basis of a reflex change in diagnosis to glioblastoma.

Since the brain vigorously attempts to clear necrotic debris after vascular or traumatic insults, it is somewhat surprising that the necrosis of glioblastoma usually does not attract many macrophages, although these cells can be identified readily by specific markers (85,103). Inflammatory cells, primarily T lymphocytes, are particularly common in tumors with gemistocytic features (7,8,11,94,103,131).

Frozen Section. A diagnosis of glioblastoma is most easily made on specimens straddling the enhancing cellular area and, if present, the adjacent hypodense necrotic core. One can confidently say that the contrast-enhancing area, whether of a glioblastoma or other enhancing lesions, has obviously not been sampled if the specimen is so modestly cellular to suggest reactive gliosis or a better differentiated infiltrating glioma.

Specimens from the contrast-enhancing rim consist of markedly cellular neoplasm, usually with a fibrillarity attributable to tumor cell processes (17,108). Reactive astrocytes, conspicuous by their symmetric stellate configuration, are noted in hypocellular areas but may be less obvious in cellular portions of the tumor. Prognostically important features such as mitoses, vascular proliferation, and necrosis must be carefully sought (fig. 3-36) (17,26,108). The proliferating vessels are readily identified with the hematoxylin and eosin (H&E) method which shows capillary tangles as well as larger caliber vessels expanded by their content of multilayered endothelial cells. Necrosis may be difficult to identify in frozen sections where it is readily confused with normal, albeit artifactually altered, white matter. Aqueous staining methods more readily demonstrate the amorphous granular debris that characterizes necrosis. The alignment of nuclei so typical of pseudopalisading is a helpful low-power feature since it demarcates

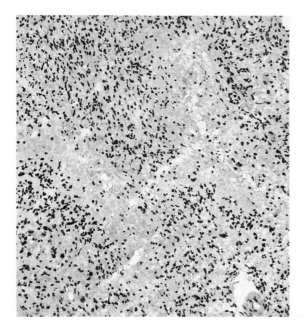

Figure 3-36
GLIOBLASTOMA MULTIFORME: FROZEN SECTION
The diagnostically welcome feature, necrosis, is not always immediately apparent.

zones of necrosis. In the setting of an infiltrating glial neoplasm, palisading necrosis is virtually diagnostic of glioblastoma, except for occasional malignant oligodendrogliomas.

Cytology. Intraoperative cytologic preparations are of great assistance in distinguishing glioblastoma from two principal differentials: metastatic carcinoma and malignant lymphoma. They are also useful in excluding cellular, reactive, or vascular lesions.

Most glioblastomas are formed of cells with conspicuous processes. Squash or smear preparations are well suited to demonstrate these cellular extensions since the processes form a finely fibrillar background that can readily be resolved (pl. IIB, p. 48). Such fine cellular extensions are not seen in any neoplasm other than those of glial or neuronal origin, including metastatic carcinoma and lymphoma. In lesions with astrocytic differentiation, the glassy cytoplasm of neoplastic cells is also observed.

Cytologic preparations demonstrate a wide range of nuclear abnormalities and underscore the frequent presence of small cells with somewhat elongated nuclei. Chromatin in these cells is only moderately dense and nucleoli are not

usually prominent. These somewhat long, often bipolar cells are distinctive of glioblastoma and further exclude considerations of carcinoma, lymphoma, and malignant oligodendroglioma.

Needle Biopsy Findings. Evaluation of a glioblastoma specimen obtained by stereotactically-directed needle biopsy must be done with an awareness of neuroradiologic findings and in close communication with the surgeon. Although stereotactic biopsy systems have a high theoretical degree of precision, in practice the needle or trochar may stray from its intended target on the contrast-enhancing rim and come to rest in an adjacent less cellular area of edema. Specimens from such "misses" often show only a paucicellular infiltrate or simply edematous brain with reactive gliosis. Understandably, such a report comes as a surprise to the surgeon. Numerous anatomic studies have shown a significant proportion of glioblastomas to be relatively circumscribed over some portions of their periphery. This permits a needle, passing the target point by only a millimeter or two, to fall outside the lesion (13,26). The issue reemphasizes the importance of communication between the pathologist and surgeon, and underscores the importance of radiographic findings so that discrepancies are resolved before the biopsy procedure is concluded. A nonrepresentative biopsy prompts additional sampling, sometimes after calculation of a new target point. Difficulties in sampling may cause glioblastomas to be undergraded. The result is a rise in the ratio of anaplastic astrocytoma to glioblastoma among patients whose tumors are diagnosed by needle biopsy (fig. 3-37) (41).

Grading and Subclassification. The grading and subclassification of glioblastomas remain controversial subjects. Kernohan divided glioblastomas into lesions of grades 3 and 4, with the distinction resting upon the extent of cellular differentiation, necrosis, and vascular proliferation. While there are studies that support Kernohan's contention that one can identify a somewhat better differentiated glioblastoma, such division represents unnecessary "fine tuning" and is difficult to reproduce (91). Indeed, survival differences are marginal and the distinction in no way affects therapy. We do not subdivide glioblastomas, preferring to adhere to a simple all-encompassing definition.

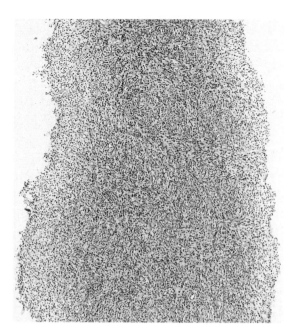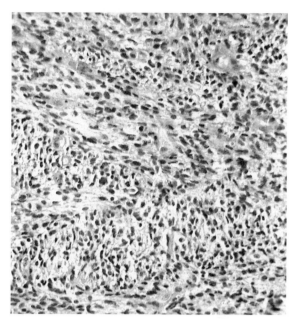

Figure 3-37
GLIOBLASTOMA MULTIFORME
Although this densely cellular and largely undifferentiated lesion technically merits a diagnosis of anaplastic astrocytoma, it is, for practical purposes, a glioblastoma.

Giant cell glioblastoma with radiographic and microscopic circumscription should be recognized in light of its somewhat more favorable prognosis. Furthermore, it must be distinguished from pleomorphic xanthoastrocytoma.

An important issue, of more theoretical than practical interest, relates to the histogenesis of glioblastoma. It is agreed that glioblastoma is glial, but controversy remains as to whether it is derived exclusively from astrocytes or has its origin also from oligodendrocytes or ependymal cells. As discussed above, the relationship of many glioblastomas to astrocytes seems apparent. The relationship of glioblastoma to the oligodendrocyte is a more difficult issue, one that cannot be resolved in all instances. This is particularly the case in frankly malignant gliomas with abundant glomeruloid vascular changes and necrosis but only vague oligodendroglial overtones. When fully malignant, some oligodendroglial tumors exhibit features common to glioblastoma, namely, high cellularity, brisk mitotic rate, vascular proliferation, and necrosis with pseudopalisading (see figs. 3-125, 3-126). If the neoplastic cells exhibit obvious oligodendroglial features, we classify the tumor as malignant oligodendro-

glioma. However, for some neoplasms that began as, or contain, clearly defined oligodendrogliomas, but elsewhere are largely undifferentiated or assume overt astrocytic characteristics, the term *glioblastoma multiforme* may be applied. These differences are largely semantic as both highly malignant oligodendrogliomas and glioblastomas arising in an oligodendroglioma behave in a similar aggressive fashion. The relationship between oligodendroglioma and glioblastoma is discussed later in this chapter in the section on oligodendroglial neoplasms.

Occasional lesions with the definite clinicopathologic characteristics of an ependymoma illustrate marked cellularity, vascular proliferation, and necrosis with pseudopalisading. We consider such tumors to be malignant ependymomas.

Immunohistochemical Findings. The immunophenotype of glioblastoma includes reactivity for GFAP (fig. 3-38), vimentin (25,117), and cytokeratin (see Appendix H). Less common variants are reactive for epithelial membrane antigen (121). While vimentin reactivity is entirely nonspecific and of little diagnostic significance, it does indicate the immunoviability of the specimen. On the other hand, immunoreactivity for GFAP within

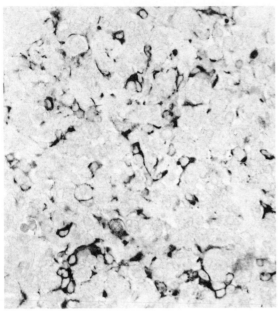

Figure 3-38
GLIOBLASTOMA MULTIFORME
In most glioblastomas some neoplastic cells are positive
for GFAP.

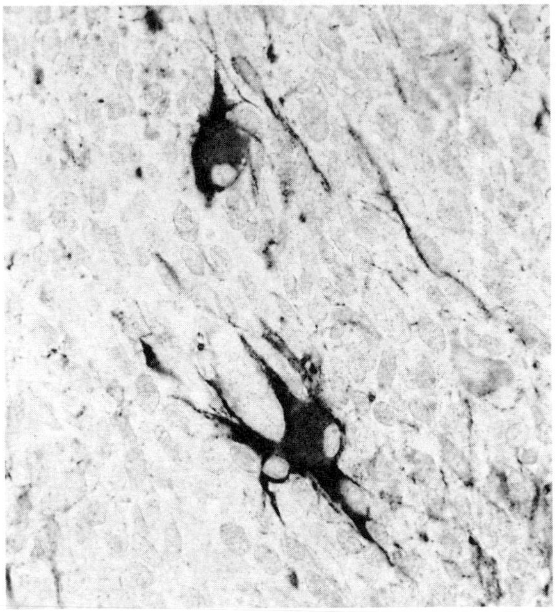

Figure 3-39
GLIOBLASTOMA MULTIFORME
Trapped reactive astrocytes are large, stellate, often peri-
vascular, and intensely reactive for GFAP.

neoplastic cells clearly establishes the tumor as a glioma, although not necessarily one of astrocytic type. Many glioblastomas are also positive for S-100 protein and alpha-β-crystallin (54).

As might be expected, the degree and geographic extent of GFAP reactivity in glioblastoma is highly variable (117). Generally, astrocyte-like cells are strongly positive, while small undifferentiated elements, as well as giant cells, are often negative or only weakly staining. Between these extremes, however, generalization is not possible. Some very "astrocytic" lesions may be largely negative for GFAP, whereas some small cell tumors, particularly those whose cells extend into fine bipolar processes, may be strongly and diffusely positive. S-100 reactivity is often stronger and more widespread than that of GFAP. Reactivity for this admittedly less than specific antigen provides indirect support for a diagnosis of glioblastoma.

Distinguishing between neoplastic and reactive astrocytes within glioblastomas is not always easy. Reactive cells are strongly GFAP positive and are firmly anchored in space by long, symmetrically disposed, tapering processes which grasp nearby vessels (fig. 3-39). Neoplastic cells are often less reactive for GFAP, generally do not

exhibit the star-like symmetry of their processes, and do not terminate extensively and exclusively upon blood vessels. It is unfortunate that in largely undifferentiated glioblastomas where immunoreactivity is most diagnostically crucial, it may be exceedingly difficult to relate GFAP-positive processes or even cytoplasm to neoplastic nuclei. One must be conservative in this effort, accepting as diagnostic only unequivocally GFAP-reactive cells with nuclear features of malignancy.

Although immunoreactivity for epithelial markers such as cytokeratins seems alien to astrocytes, such staining is frequently seen in both neoplastic and reactive cells (48a). Obviously, this seriously compromises the diagnostic value of the antibody for distinguishing glioblastoma from metastatic carcinoma. Staining for cytokeratins should be done therefore in concert with staining for GFAP and epithelial membrane antigen or other epithelial markers. Positivity for cytokeratins is most misleading in those rare metaplastic glioblastomas and gliosarcomas exhibiting true squamous or glandular differentiation. Such tumors are also immunopositive for epithelial membrane antigen.

Ultrastructural Findings. The ultrastructural findings in glioblastomas are in accord with the light microscopic degree of differentiation (110). Intermediate filaments are abundant in obviously astrocytic cells, but are often sparse or absent in ones that appear undifferentiated. In contrast to most metastatic carcinomas with their well-formed desmosomes, intercellular contacts in glioblastoma and other astrocytomas are poorly formed. In poorly differentiated lesions, junctions consist of little more than ill-defined opposed submembrane densities ("intermediate" junctions). Tonofilament bundles, either cytoplasmic or desmosome-associated, are also lacking in astrocytoma and glioblastoma.

Differential Diagnosis. Establishing the diagnosis of glioblastoma begins by determining that the neoplasm under study is primary rather than metastatic. It then proceeds by identifying it as a malignant astrocytic neoplasm, and concludes by distinguishing the glioblastoma from other gliomas, particularly anaplastic astrocytoma, the related tumor one grade removed.

The primary, rather than metastatic, nature of a glioblastoma is generally inferred from its infiltrative nature and glial appearance in H&E stained sections. In the absence of these features, immunoreactivity for GFAP is confirmatory. Infiltration is manifest by the overrunning of brain parenchyma, both gray and white matter. This is most evident at the periphery of the neoplasm where underlying brain tissue is most evident. Residual parenchyma may be difficult to identify in biopsies from the contrast-enhancing rim where underlying tissue is largely destroyed. Loss of normal architecture is evidenced first by disappearance of myelin and then by dropout of axons.

In contrast, metastatic neoplasms evolve from the tumor microembolus stage into large cohesive masses that displace rather than diffusely infiltrate brain tissue. By tracking along blood vessels they can infiltrate tissues and appear similar to a glioma (fig. 20-9), but the extent of this infiltration is generally limited. Isolated neoplastic cells are occasionally seen around some metastases but only in the immediate environs. Astrocytes are much less commonly incorporated into metastases than gliomas. When they are, they occur in small number about vessels, particularly at the periphery of the lesion.

Even if an infiltrating nature is difficult to establish, the cytologic composition of glioblastoma aids in the exclusion of metastatic carcinoma. Features particular to glioblastoma include small poorly differentiated cells; cells distinctly astrocytic or even oligodendroglial in appearance, showing little or no tendency to nuclear molding; and, in some cases, remarkable cellular and nuclear pleomorphism. The small cells of the glioblastoma, which are often smaller than those of small cell carcinoma, lie within a fine fibrillar background representing a meshwork of neoplastic cell processes or remnants of normal neuropil. When evident, the astrocytic nature of some cells is recognized by the fibrillated or glassy eosinophilic cytoplasm. The latter is the hallmark of gemistocytic astrocytoma, a tumor in which transitions are frequently noted from plump unequivocal astrocytes to small undifferentiated cells.

There are, nevertheless, monomorphous, highly cellular and compact glioblastomas that appear to exclude recognizable preexisting elements and raise the question of a metastasis. Carcinoma becomes even more suspect when glioblastomas contain compact epithelioid cells with discrete borders or when there is epithelial differentiation (see fig. 3-33J, K). It is of utmost importance to inspect biopsy fragments carefully, seeking peripheral infiltrative portions of the lesion. When these are not present, the distinction between glioblastoma and metastatic carcinoma awaits immunohistochemical analysis. In theory, immunohistochemistry should distinguish metastatic carcinoma from largely undifferentiated glioblastoma since the latter, at least focally, exhibits GFAP reactivity. This is usually the case, although incorporated normal astrocytes should not be interpreted as neoplastic. Such reactive elements, usually perivascular in location, are characterized by a degree of differentiation out of proportion to the anaplastic appearance of surrounding cells. Since it may be difficult to determine whether GFAP-positive processes emanate from neoplastic or reactive astrocytes, identification of the former is more reliable when their nuclei are identical to those of obviously neoplastic cells. The cytoplasm of poorly differentiated, particularly small cell, astrocytes is often scant and barely discernible. In other instances, it consists of an eccentric skirt of eosinophilic cytoplasm. Although it may be difficult to establish a diagnosis of malignant glioma on the basis of immunohistochemistry, the presence of GFAP-reactive cells deep within the interior of the lesion provides presumptive evidence of its primary glial nature.

Immunohistochemical markers of epithelial differentiation, although useful in the differential diagnosis of metastatic carcinoma, should be interpreted with caution and in concert with staining for GFAP. As discussed above, epithelial differentiation rarely occurs in otherwise typical glioblastoma or gliosarcoma. Despite the fact that epithelial neoplasms typically exhibit cytokeratins and epithelial membrane antigen, reactivity may be observed with other cell types, particularly for cytokeratins that have a tendency to stain cells containing intermediate filaments. Thus, both reactive and neoplastic astrocytes may be immunoreactive, and positive staining does not establish a lesion as epithelial unless it is simultaneously negative for GFAP and perhaps positive for epithelial membrane antigen (48a). The problem of nonspecific keratin reactivity in glial cells is best illustrated in brain tissue adjacent to metastatic carcinoma where not only the neoplasm but also reactive astrocytes can be cytokeratin positive.

Cerebral lymphoma enters into the differential diagnosis of glioblastoma, particularly when an older patient presents with a contrast-enhancing intracerebral mass. Lymphoma becomes even more suspect with a multicentric or subependymal process. Lymphomas typically have a high attenuation (hyperdense) appearance on CT, even without the administration of a contrast medium, and show homogeneous contrast enhancement. Ring enhancement may be seen in lymphomas with necrosis, particularly those associated with immunosuppression, as in AIDS, but the classic radiographic image of sporadic lymphomas is a solid (homogeneous) rather than hollow (ring-enhancing) lesion. In frozen sections, lymphoma is characterized by patchy hypercellularity due largely to its angiocentricity, conspicuous reactive gliosis, frequent single cell necrosis, histiocytic reaction, and general lack of vascular proliferation. Lymphomas can, however, appear similar to malignant gliomas if general nuclear roundness is artifactually altered by the freezing process (see fig. 12-7).

Cytologic preparations can be useful in excluding lymphoma. In brief, the cells of lymphoma detach as individual elements with scant, discrete cytoplasm and generally round or reniform vesicular nuclei.

Extent and Spread. The extent of a glioblastoma is a subject of great practical interest, particularly in regard to radiation therapy planning. It is perhaps fortunate for pathologists that a detailed study of surgical margins is infrequently requested, since it is a difficult and laborious task to determine tumor extent by tissue sections alone. For therapeutic purposes, tumor topography is inferred from radiographic images, and dosimetry is calculated largely on the size and configuration of the cellular contrast-enhancing component. Maximal radiation is delivered to the contrast-enhancing area plus a rim of arbitrary size, usually 2 or 3 cm.

Although it is neither practical nor possible to completely stage most glioblastomas, the distribution of their neoplastic cells is not entirely random since they exhibit a well-known tendency to spread along compact fiber pathways such as the corpus callosum, optic radiation, anterior commissure, fornix, and subependymal regions (figs. 3-40, 3-41). Such dissemination underlies the poor prognosis associated with neoplasms positioned near these anatomic siphons. Extension along these structures produces tumors with three-dimensional profiles and a complexity belied by the generally smooth contours seen in contrast-enhanced CT or MRI. The cells extending along these pathways are typically small, largely undifferentiated polar cells (fig. 3-42) which can partially regain an astrocytic phenotype when they come to rest around vessels or in the subpial region. In the cortex, highly infiltrative lesions produce so-called "secondary structures" such as perineuronal satellitosis and aggregation in the subpial and perivascular spaces (fig. 3-43) (113,114).

Several studies have established that much of the edematous zone around the tumor mass, as defined by hyperintensity of T2-weighted MRIs, contains infiltrating tumor cells (55–57). Only an occasional glioblastoma is sufficiently localized and detected early enough in its evolution that aggressive local therapies are curative.

Effects of Therapy. In many instances radiotherapy checks the rapid enlargement of glioblastoma and enforces a postradiation phase of remission or quiescence. The interlude is marked by stability, if not regression, in neurologic

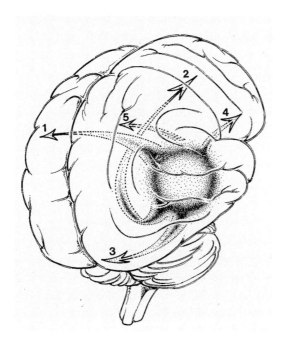

Figure 3-40
SPREAD OF GLIOBLASTOMA MULTIFORME
Common routes of tumor extension include: (1) the corpus callosum, (2) fornix, (3) optic radiation, (4) association pathways, and (5) anterior commissure. (Modified from fig. 4 from Burger PC. Classification, grading, and patterns of spread of malignant gliomas. In: Apuzzo ML, ed. Malignant cerebral gliomas. Park Ridge, Ill: American Association of Neurological Surgeons, 1990:3–17.)

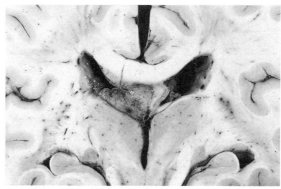

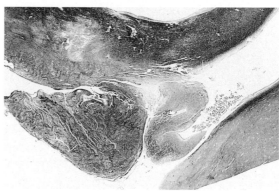

Figure 3-41
RECURRENT GLIOBLASTOMA MULTIFORME
As seen macroscopically (top) and in a histologic section (bottom), this glioblastoma has entered and enlarged the fornix from its origin in the corpus callosum.

deficits, as well as diminution in the size of the contrast-enhancing mass. In other patients, the tumor seems almost unaffected by radiotherapy and continues to enlarge unabated. Any period of response is unfortunately short-lived since within a year the tumor reasserts itself, as evidenced by clinical deterioration and the appearance of an expansile focus, or foci, of new contrast enhancement. Recurrence usually appears in the margins of the original tumor bed, but can appear in sites far removed from the original lesion. In the face of a life-threatening recurrent mass, reoperation may be contemplated. Debulking may be worthwhile, particularly if radionecrosis, rather than recurrent tumor, is suspected as the cause of clinical and radiographic deterioration. Positron emission tomography has proven useful in this important distinction, with recurrent tumor but not radionecrosis being metabolically active ("hot") in studies using fluorodeoxyglucose (fig. 3-44) (42).

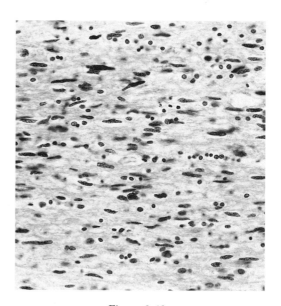

Figure 3-42
GLIOBLASTOMA MULTIFORME
Elongated tumor cells escape the primary site by tracking along a fiber pathway.

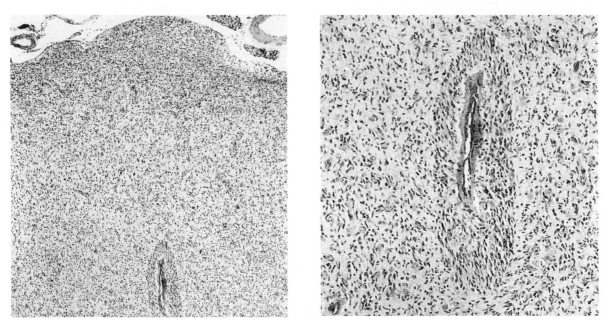

Figure 3-43
GLIOBLASTOMA MULTIFORME

Left: Some glioblastomas are especially infiltrative of the cerebral cortex where subpial, perivascular, and perineuronal accumulations are prominent.

Right: Higher magnification reveals the small cell nature of such tumors.

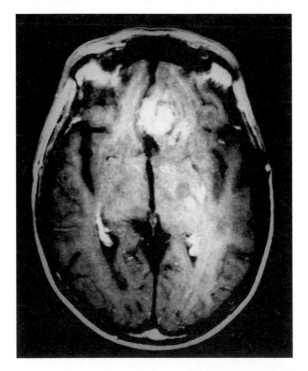
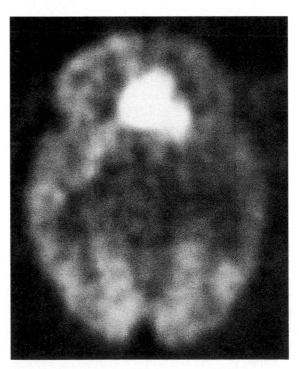

Figure 3-44
RECURRENT GLIOBLASTOMA MULTIFORME

Left: Recurrent glioblastomas produce expansile foci of contrast enhancement. These imaging features are nonspecific, however, and may be due to radionecrosis rather than recurrent tumor.

Right: Positron emission tomography resolves this issue in favor of recurrent tumor when an intensely active or "hot" focus of metabolic activity is noted. (Courtesy of Dr. John M. Hoffman, Durham, NC.)

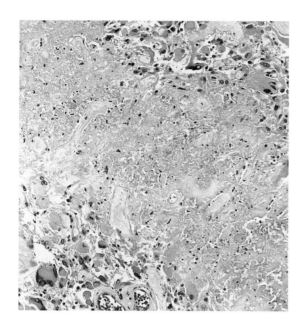

Figure 3-45
GLIOBLASTOMA MULTIFORME
Glioblastomas studied in their postirradiation phase of "quiescence" are paucicellular lesions with marked cellular atypia and foci of coagulation typical of radionecrosis.

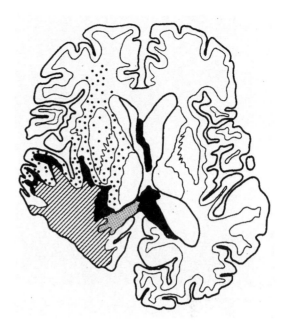

Figure 3-46
RECURRENT GLIOBLASTOMA WITH
RADIATION-ASSOCIATED CHANGES
The diagram illustrates common tissue reactions encountered in radiated patients at the time of tumor recurrence. The solid black areas represent a highly cellular malignant neoplasm which has both crossed the corpus callosum and extended along the ipsilateral fornix. The isolated solid circles represent zones of infiltrating neoplasm within largely intact white matter, a classic feature of diffuse gliomas. The finely stippled regions represent a paucicellular tumor with the cellular pleomorphism typical of the "quiescent" phase of glioblastoma. Areas of radionecrosis are diagonally hatched.

Biopsies taken during the "quiescent" post-treatment phase often appear significantly different from those of the pretreatment period. The tumor may be paucicellular and notable for conspicuous pleomorphic astrocytes. Some of these cells are radiation-affected tumor cells, others are reactive astrocytes with radiation atypia (fig. 3-45) (10,14,39,40,120). Small cells with markedly hyperchromatic nuclei and inconspicuous cytoplasm may be present, but only in such low numbers that biopsy interpretation is difficult. Such lesions are glioblastomas, but are best characterized as "persistent" or "quiescent" rather than "recurrent," since the latter term suggests an active proliferation and a justification for additional therapy. Since widely scattered cells in such regions may be positive for bromodeoxyuridine or Ki-67, some presumably represent neoplastic cells that survived radiotherapy with their capacity for growth intact.

The surroundings of previously irradiated gliomas are often punctuated by foci of coagulation necrosis which represent the brain's delayed expression of radiation injury. Additional changes attributable to radiation include fibrinoid necrosis and vascular thickening or hyalinization necrosis.

When they occur in the tumor bed, these changes represent desirable consequences of radiotherapy and, as such, are more appropriately designated radiation effect rather than the pejorative term radionecrosis (10,14). In most instances in which a previously irradiated tumor is biopsied and radiation effect is evident, viable tumor is also apparent. Only in a few instances does the contrast-enhancing mass consist solely of radionecrosis.

Since small foci of actively growing tumor, gliosis, irradiated quiescent neoplasm, radiation effect, and radiation necrosis can coexist in a specimen, the pathologist is frequently not in a position to define which single factor, or combination of factors, underlies the clinical and radiographic picture (figs. 3-46, 3-47). Radiation-induced changes notwithstanding, the finding of even a focal, small cell, mitotically active lesion,

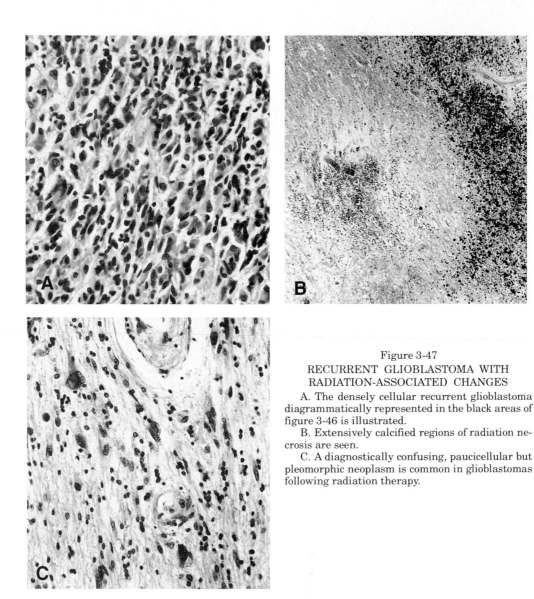

Figure 3-47
RECURRENT GLIOBLASTOMA WITH
RADIATION-ASSOCIATED CHANGES
A. The densely cellular recurrent glioblastoma diagrammatically represented in the black areas of figure 3-46 is illustrated.
B. Extensively calcified regions of radiation necrosis are seen.
C. A diagnostically confusing, paucicellular but pleomorphic neoplasm is common in glioblastomas following radiation therapy.

particularly one with necrosis with pseudo-palisading, is a poor prognostic sign. In the absence of such cells, for instance in cases in which the biopsy shows only pleomorphism and paucicellularity, we do not make a diagnosis of active tumor recurrence, although neoplastic cells are clearly present and only a rare patient is cured. It is perhaps appropriate that such patients be observed rather than treated with chemotherapy. Our diagnosis for the lesion shown in figure 3-45 would be glioblastoma multiforme, with a comment that the tumor is typical of a radiated glioblastoma in a phase of quiescence and not one of active recurrence.

Clinically significant radionecrosis usually follows external beam radiation by a 6- to 18-month interval and affects the general environs of the tumor bed (10). Obviously, the demonstration of a neoplastic focus does not establish that the recurrent tumor is a significant contributor to the contrast-enhancing area. Similarly, the histologic demonstration of radionecrosis is no guarantee that recurrent neoplasm is not present elsewhere in the lesion. Even if careful analysis of clinical, radiographic, and pathologic findings is undertaken, it can be difficult to determine which is the predominant lesion. As previously noted, both recurrence and radionecrosis are evident in most cases.

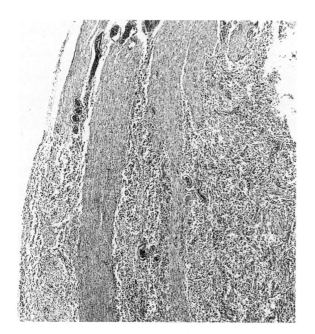 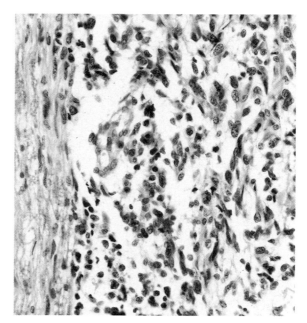

Figure 3-48
CEREBROSPINAL DISSEMINATION OF GLIOBLASTOMA MULTIFORME
As seen at low (left) and high (right) magnification, the small undifferentiated-appearing cells of this glioblastoma are drop metastases colonizing the nerve roots of the cauda equina.

As might be expected, the implantation of radioactive sources (brachytherapy) produces massive radionecrosis in a pattern in accord with the dose distribution. Unlike radionecrosis following conventional external beam therapy which appears after 6 to 18 months, the necrosis following brachytherapy often appears within the first 6 months and often requires surgical debulking. Specimens from such lesions consist largely of necrotic tissue with few if any interspersed islands of viable neoplasm or vasculature. The tumor may take the form of either a pleomorphic and paucicellular irradiated tumor or an actively proliferating small cell neoplasm. The presence of pseudopalisading around necrotic foci establishes beyond question the presence of recurrent tumor since radionecrosis lacks this feature.

The effects of chemotherapy upon the cytologic and histologic appearance of glioma cells is poorly understood.

Most glioblastomas recur in and around the original tumor bed (49,72) but contralateral recurrence is commonly seen with lesions close to the corpus callosum (fig. 3-46). Occasional cases recur far from the original site. This seems especially likely when prolonged local control is achieved by aggressive radiotherapy. At the time of death, therefore, foci of densely cellular tumor are seen usually about the original tumor site, frequently with involvement of adjacent fiber tracts such as the corpus callosum, fornix, or anterior commissure (see fig. 3-41) (9,113,114). These pathways in their normal state are illustrated in figure 2-1. Extensive subependymal spread is also common. Cerebrospinal dissemination occurs in about 10 percent of cases (fig. 3-48) (34,69,93,122) and may be more common in patients with long postoperative survival periods (138). Only a rare lesion metastasizes to a systemic site (4,31,32,38,52,75,76,87,92,95, 103b), and it is not surprising that vascular invasion is only uncommonly found (75,103b).

Treatment and Prognosis. Glioblastomas have frustrated almost every attempt at successful therapy. This is mainly because the tumor is well beyond the reach of local control when it is first detected clinically or radiographically. The emergence of resistant clones has interfered with chemotherapeutic approaches. Despite external beam radiotherapy, the median survival period of patients with cerebral glioblastoma is approximately 12 months. Longer survivals are

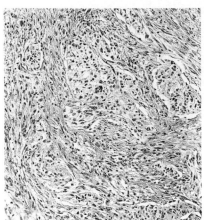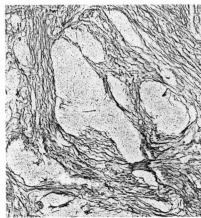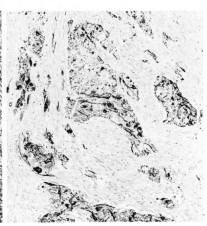

Figure 3-49
GLIOSARCOMA
The somewhat less dense, more fibrillar islands of glial tissue evident in the H&E stained section (left) are more obvious in adjacent sections after staining for reticulin and GFAP. The islands are characteristically free of reticulin (center) and stain darkly for GFAP (right).

most often noted in younger patients and, to a certain extent, among those in whom a better differentiated astrocytoma was a precursor lesion (secondary glioblastoma) (11,112,113,142). The especially poor outlook for elderly patients with a glioblastoma is well known (57a). Although difficult to confirm, the extent of resection also appears to affect survival (1a,89,142, 143). Patients with tumors of giant cell type appear to fare somewhat better (19). The prognosis for glioblastoma of the brain stem is understandably poor (132); dissemination in the subarachnoid space is common (93). Short survival periods are also expected for patients with glioblastomas of the spinal cord (82a).

Interstitial radiation extends the survival of patients with recurrent neoplasms by perhaps 1 year, as well as that of selected patients treated initially by this method. Survival periods of up to 2, 3, and even 5 years have been noted in some instances but permanent cure is rarely achieved.

The subclassification of glioblastomas for prognostic purposes by way of molecular biologic methods is a subject of active interest. There is contradictory evidence for example, whether amplification of the epidermal growth factor receptor gene portends a less favorable prognosis (6,53). The Ki-67 labeling indices vary greatly, and while generally in the 5 to 10 percent range, are greatly influenced by tissue sampling and counting methods (16,28,98,146). Indices based

upon bromodeoxyuridine labeling also vary greatly, ranging from 3.2 to 38.1 percent in one study (68). It remains to be seen whether proliferation indices have prognostic value in patients with glioblastomas.

Gliosarcoma

Definition. A neoplasm containing both malignant glial and mesenchymal tissues. Although the glial component is oligodendroglial in some cases, the lesion is discussed here under astrocytic neoplasms since most are glioblastoma/sarcomatous lesions.

Clinical Features. Approximately 2 percent of glioblastomas have this eye-catching, although prognostically insignificant, sarcomatous component and are appropriately designated gliosarcoma (148,155). Such tumors may occur anywhere in the brain but favor the same sites affected by glioblastomas.

Macroscopic Findings. A relatively discrete mass is the consequence of the reticulin- and collagen-rich mesenchymal component.

Microscopic Findings. Considerable histologic variation may be seen. In some cases, the sarcoma is a spindle cell proliferation with a herringbone architecture typical of well-differentiated fibrosarcoma (fig. 3-49). In other instances, it is disorganized and sufficiently pleomorphic as to resemble malignant fibrous

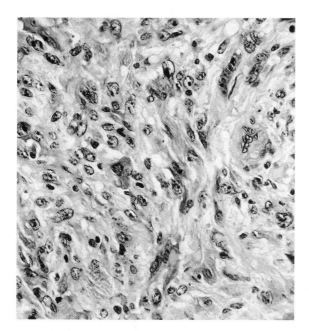

Figure 3-50
GLIOSARCOMA
The mesenchymal component of this gliosarcoma closely resembles malignant fibrous histiocytoma.

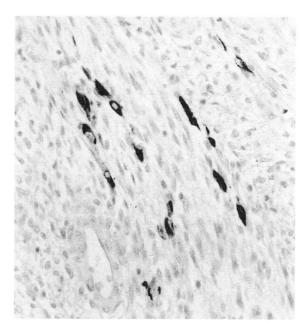

Figure 3-51
GLIOSARCOMA
The glial components of this gliosarcoma are widely dispersed and are identified only by their immunoreactivity for GFAP. Attention to cytologic features is still required for the diagnosis since trapped islands of reactive glia may be seen in rare sarcomas affecting the nervous system.

histiocytoma (fig. 3-50) (151,158). Many lesions fall between these extremes. The mesenchymal cells in most tumors are not only topographically related to blood vessels but appear to be proliferating vascular or adventitial elements. Meningeal mesenchymal cells also may be transformed. Immunohistochemical studies have suggested a smooth muscle component in the neoplastic mesenchymal tissue in some cases (150,152). Other reported lines of differentiation include striated muscle (147), bone, and cartilage (150a,159,160). As is discussed below, some "gliosarcomas" are an intricate mixture of mesenchymal and glial elements with isolated glial cells surrounded by meningeal tissue. This has given rise to the suggestion that gliosarcomas are only intensively desmoplastic malignant gliomas (152). While it is possible that some of these lesions are not gliosarcomas, many other mixed lesions have two clearly defined components, glial and mesenchymal, and deserve the designation gliosarcoma.

In most gliosarcomas, the glial component is astrocytic and in every way resembles glioblastoma. Typical lesions have a periphery of glioma surrounding a sarcomatous center, an arrangement that supports the view that the sarcoma arises secondarily within the proliferating vasculature of a high-grade glioma. The neoplastic glia can be inconspicuous in advanced lesions where they lie trapped in the sarcoma as clusters or even as single cells (fig. 3-51). With time, the sarcoma may so overgrow the parent glioma that it appears solid and sharply demarcated and the only obvious glial component is that which clings to the surface of the excised mass. Immunohistochemistry is required to detect the internal trapped glial cells in these instances. In some cases, glial cells are organized in such a way that they are misdiagnosed as carcinoma, particularly when they form epithelial arrangements like the tubules and canals that characterize adenoid gliosarcomas (153).

Although some gliosarcomas are obviously biphasic mesenchymal/glial neoplasms, the nature of the mesenchymal component in some desmoplastic malignant gliomas is, while exuberant, not clearly neoplastic. Such lesions demonstrate active microvascular proliferation with perivascular zones of plump adventitial or fibroblast-like cells. Away from the immediate perivascular zone, the proliferation appears to stabilize or regress as nuclear-cytoplasmic ratios, mitotic rate, and nuclear atypia all diminish at the same time as collagen deposition increases. Such specimens are not regarded as gliosarcoma. The same is true of gliomas, nearly all malignant, which secondarily involve the dura to incite intense desmoplasia mimicking sarcoma. In practical terms, the identical prognoses of glioblastoma and gliosarcoma relieve the pathologist of the sometimes difficult and arbitrary distinction between gliosarcoma and glioblastoma associated with exuberant, reactive mesenchymal proliferation.

It has been suggested that, in rare instances, the temporal relationship between glioma and sarcoma that is presumed to exist in gliosarcomas is reversed: that is, a preexisting sarcoma is the exciting stimulus and the glioma is the induced tumor, a lesion combination termed *sarcoglioma* (154). The case for such a sarcoma-glioma sequence can be made convincingly in some instances, although the possibility of coincidence must be considered. It can be supported when a glioma appears at the edge of a preexisting sarcoma of some chronicity, and is even more likely in cases in which the "inciting" tumor is well differentiated, e.g., meningioma, although the term sarcoglioma would no longer apply. Since in some cases the glial changes about a sarcoma more closely resemble atypical hyperplasia than clear-cut neoplasia, one must exercise caution in making a diagnosis of sarcoglioma, particularly on the basis of histologic changes alone.

Immunohistochemical Findings. Reactivity for GFAP readily identifies the glial component, whether disposed in large lobules or as isolated cells (figs. 3-49 right, 3-51) (149,155). Staining for alpha-1-antitrypsin and alpha-1-antichymotrypsin has been noted in the mesenchymal component of gliosarcomas (149,158) but alpha-1-antichymotrypsin reactivity may also be expressed in glioblastomas. Reactivity for myoid markers has been reported (150).

Ultrastructural Findings. In addition to poorly differentiated cells, cells resembling fibroblasts, histiocytes, and myofibroblasts have also been noted (151).

Treatment and Prognosis. Although there are reports indicating that the sarcomatous component of gliosarcoma may metastasize to extracranial sites, one large study failed to note a difference in survival between patients with gliosarcoma and glioblastoma (156). Occasional gliosarcomas erode through the skull into cephalic soft tissues (157).

Protoplasmic Astrocytoma

Definition. An astrocytoma composed of cells resembling the protoplasmic astrocytes of gray matter.

Clinical and Radiographic Features. Little is known about this uncommon and poorly defined entity, which to some observers is not a definite tumor entity but a pattern seen in such tumors as pilocytic astrocytoma. Most appear in children or young adults as superficially, sometimes cortically based cystic masses (161).

Macroscopic Findings. The lesion appears somewhat gelatinous and is, unlike "ordinary" fibrillary astrocytoma, relatively well circumscribed.

Microscopic Findings. Protoplasmic astrocytomas exhibit low to moderate cellularity and are noted for a cobweb architectural pattern created by small, poorly fibrillated cells with limp radiating processes enmeshed in a mucoid stromal matrix that contributes to the formation of often prominent microcysts (fig. 3-52). The nuclei are rather uniform in size, round to oval, and exhibit little if any mitotic activity. In common with pilocytic astrocytomas, these lesions may exhibit glomeruloid vessel proliferation, particularly within their cyst walls.

Immunohistochemical Findings. The lesions are weakly reactive for GFAP, with positivity confined to small paranuclear areas.

Differential Diagnosis. Unlike pilocytic astrocytomas, protoplasmic tumors lack the biphasic pattern, Rosenthal fibers, granular bodies, and hyalinized vessels. Oligodendrogliomas frequently exhibit similar loose textured components, microcysts, and scant GFAP immunoreactivity. More classic oligodendrogliomatous components should be sought to aid in making the distinction.

Treatment and Prognosis. The biologic behavior of this lesion is not well characterized. The possibility of malignant degeneration in some cases has been emphasized (161).

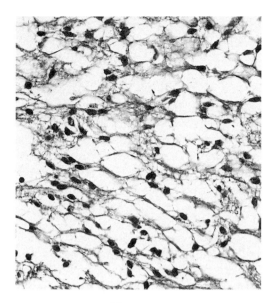

Figure 3-52
PROTOPLASMIC ASTROCYTOMA

This rare tumor features cellular uniformity and a microcyst-containing loose-textured network of relatively afibrillar astrocytes. Unlike the microcystic component of the often better demarcated pilocytic astrocytomas, protoplasmic astrocytomas lack abundant granular bodies.

Granular Cell Astrocytic Neoplasms

Definition. Intraparenchymal astrocytic neoplasms with a prominent component of granular cells.

General Comments. Infrequently, large numbers of granular cells are seen within otherwise typical diffuse or fibrillary astrocytic neoplasms. More commonly, such cells are found in pilocytic tumors. Astrocytic tumors containing granular cells are neither clinical nor pathologic entities, and should be classified according to conventional criteria. Granular cell–containing tumors are mentioned here only to avoid confusing them with non-neoplastic processes such as cerebral infarcts, granular cell tumor of the infundibulum (a presumably pituicyte-derived neoplasm), and granular cell tumors of peripheral nerves. Most of this discussion relates to diffuse astrocytomas, generally ones of high grade, with conspicuous granular cell changes.

Clinical and Radiographic Features. The clinical presentation, patient profile, and neuroradiologic aspects of these tumors are not unique since they are basically those of the underlying astrocytic neoplasm. Since granular cell

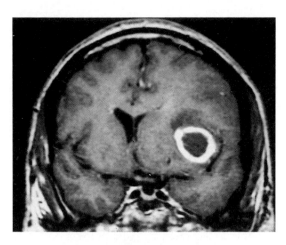

Figure 3-53
MALIGNANT GRANULAR CELL
ASTROCYTIC NEOPLASM

Malignant gliomas with a granular cell appearance are usually variants of glioblastoma and therefore present as a contrast-enhancing mass with a "ring" configuration.

change in "ordinary" astrocytomas often accompanies increased cellularity, degenerative changes, or necrosis, the tumors usually appear as contrast-enhancing masses (fig. 3-53). Most granular cell neoplasms arise in the cerebral hemispheres but some have been reported in the spinal cord and brain stem. Granular cell–containing pilocytic astrocytomas occur most often in young patients and are contrast-enhancing, demarcated lesions differing in no way from pilocytic tumors.

Macroscopic Findings. Diffuse astrocytomas with granular cell components are rare enough that no general statements about macroscopic findings can be made. Some do, however, exhibit the necrotic character of malignant gliomas.

Microscopic Findings. The lesions contain a prominent population of distinctive cells with discrete borders and finely granular cytoplasm (fig. 3-54). Their nuclei vary with the grade of the tumor, being generally larger and more coarsely constructed than those of normal astrocytes, yet lacking the marked hyperchromasia and pleomorphism seen in malignant glioma cells. The distinctive granularity of these cells is due to PAS-positive granules which often displace the nucleus. Histochemical stains for lipids are negative. Cytologic transitions from the granular cell pattern to conventional diffuse fibrillary astrocytoma are often noted.

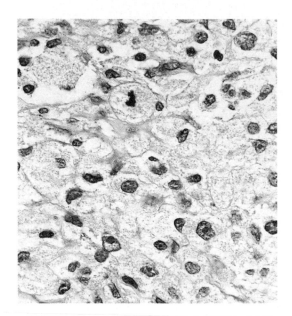

Figure 3-54
MALIGNANT GRANULAR CELL
ASTROCYTIC NEOPLASM
Granular cell astrocytic neoplasms consist of coarsely granulated, mitotically active cells. Distinguishing such a tumor from an infarct or demyelinating disease is based upon the neoplasm's nuclear pleomorphism, and the finding of at least some neoplastic cells with typical cytologic features of astrocytes.

Ultrastructural Findings. The cytoplasm of the granulated cells is filled with secondary lysosomes (162,164–167).

Immunohistochemical Findings. Granular cells are generally negative for GFAP, but faint staining has been observed in some (162–164,166). It is of note that immunoreactivity for macrophage markers, such as lysozyme, alpha-1-antitrypsin, and HAM-56, is negative.

Differential Diagnosis. Since granular cells may closely resemble macrophages, their appearance usually prompts consideration of cerebral infarction and demyelinating disease. In most instances, however, the nuclei are more hyperchromatic than those of macrophages and transitions to neoplastic astrocytes are readily identified. As noted above, immunohistochemical procedures aid in the distinction and serve to exclude a macrophage origin.

Treatment and Prognosis. Diffuse or fibrillary astrocytomas with granular cells behave like ordinary malignant gliomas of similar grade: despite radiation therapy, most patients with malignant examples die within 2 years of surgery

(163,164). Patients with pilocytic astrocytomas exhibiting granular cell elements have the favorable prognosis of the pilocytic tumor.

Gliomatosis Cerebri

Definition. A remarkably diffuse infiltrating glioma which may involve the supratentorial compartment, posterior fossa, or even intraspinal parenchyma, sometimes in continuity.

General Comments. It is debated whether gliomatosis cerebri is a pathologic entity or simply a group of histogenetically diverse tumors related only by a tendency to widespread infiltration. The term is generally reserved for lesions in which the infiltrative capability is seemingly out of proportion to both the degree of anaplasia and the inclination to form cellular masses. The definition is broad enough to encompass any diffuse glioma, although most appear to be fibrillary astrocytic neoplasms (168,170–172). Even sizable infiltrating neoplasms that also possess a solid, often necrotic core are not included in the gliomatosis category. As discussed under Differential Diagnosis, the entity overlaps histologically with another poorly defined lesion, so-called microgliomatosis.

Historically, the diagnosis of gliomatosis was made at autopsy when a widespread infiltrating lesion often involving more than one hemisphere was seen (173,174). At present, the diagnosis, if gliomatosis is accepted as an entity, is facilitated by sensitive neuroradiologic techniques. For instance, MRI demonstrates a diffuse increase in the T2 signal.

The lesion is discussed under astrocytic neoplasms since most examples are so derived, but occasional highly diffuse oligodendroglial neoplasms also qualify for the term "gliomatosis."

Clinical and Radiographic Features. Patients of all ages are affected. By definition, gliomatosis is radiographically widespread, with the lesion occupying the greater part of a hemisphere, if not both sides of the brain, and other structures in continuity. In exceptional cases, the brain stem and cord are also involved. As expected from the histologic features of a typical case, the lesion can be noncontrast enhancing and appear in T2-weighted images as an area of high signal intensity (fig. 3-55) (176).

Macroscopic Findings. The lesion is not only widely invasive and ill defined but may not be grossly evident even in a generous lobectomy

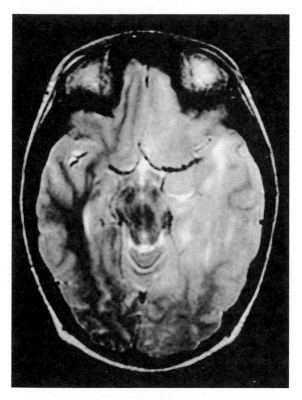

Figure 3-55
GLIOMATOSIS CEREBRI
As is evident in this T2-weighted image, gliomatosis cerebri diffusely involves large regions of the brain, as seen on the right side of the illustration.

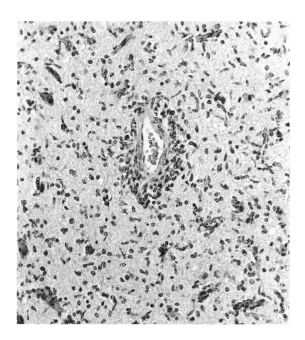

Figure 3-56
GLIOMATOSIS CEREBRI
The cells are diffusely infiltrative and exhibit angiotropism as well as perineuronal satellitosis.

specimen. In some cases, local mass effects are present and are a reflection of neoplastic hypertrophy of affected regions. As previously mentioned, the process is sufficiently diffuse in some cases to involve all levels of the central nervous system.

Microscopic Findings. Given the loose definition of gliomatosis, it is not possible to summarize the full spectrum of histologic findings; a wide variety of cytologic and histologic features and considerable variation in cellularity are found. Generally the infiltrate attains a moderate cellularity at best, the proliferation varying from virtually benign cells associated with little apparent cytoplasm to frankly malignant fibrillary astrocytic elements. The cells form secondary structures (fig. 3-56): the accumulation of neoplastic cells around vessels and neurons, and in the subpial and subependymal regions. In contrast to highly cellular malignant gliomas, gliomatosis produces little destruction of preexisting parenchyma.

Cytologically, the nuclei of gliomatosis cerebri cells vary greatly from round through oval to elongated. Chromatin is often moderately dense, but no absolute statement can be made since in some cases the nuclei are cytologically benign and, in others, small and coarsely hyperchromatic. Although cytoplasm is hardly discernible in many instances, particularly in sections stained with H&E, elongated processes are observed on special stains and in cytologic preparations. In other lesions or parts of lesions, the cells possess more cytoplasm or obvious processes and are overtly astrocytic. Mitoses are generally infrequent and vascular proliferation and necrosis are absent. The cytologic features in most cases, therefore, are not those associated with a high-grade lesion but those of a highly infiltrative, hypocellular low- to medium-grade process (fig. 3-57). Cellular foci of anaplastic transformation may be seen in some cases. Occasional lesions reported as gliomatosis cerebri appear oligodendroglial (169).

Frozen Section and Cytology. Cellular details, including nuclear elongation, are well preserved in frozen sections, but are more evident in cytologic preparations (pl. IIC, p. 48).

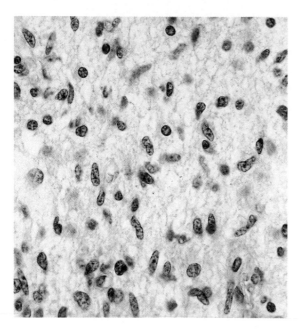

Figure 3-57
GLIOMATOSIS CEREBRI
The cells are often elongated and, while some are hyperchromatic, cytologic malignancy is usually lacking.

Because of the rarity of gliomatosis, the controversy surrounding its status as an entity, and the need for radiologic correlation, an intraoperative diagnosis is difficult. A diagnosis of "infiltrating glioma" or "primary neoplasm, most likely glioma" should suffice in most instances.

Immunohistochemical Findings. The elongated cell processes so inconspicuous in H&E stained sections are sometimes positive for GFAP. Stellate cells obviously more astrocytic in phenotype are GFAP positive. Reactivity for the latter is best seen in areas of secondary structure formation, sites in which the cells are more numerous and likely to acquire visible cytoplasm and processes.

Differential Diagnosis. The principal lesion in the differential diagnosis is the fibrillary, diffuse, or ordinary astrocytoma, although its distinction, as indicated above, is a somewhat philosophical issue. Oligodendroglioma is also a consideration since, like gliomatosis, it infiltrates not only white but also gray matter where it forms secondary structures. In tissues not subjected to freezing, however, oligodendrocytes are round rather than elongated, and their nuclei are usually surrounded by artifactual perinuclear

halos. Nevertheless, as indicated above, some reported cases of gliomatosis cerebri exhibit strikingly uniform nuclei, suggesting an oligodendroglial component (169). Malignant astrocytic neoplasms may also be highly infiltrative of gray matter and, when their cells squeeze through neuropil, may accumulate beneath the pia to produce a picture resembling gliomatosis (see fig. 3-43). The cells of most infiltrative astrocytic tumors are less narrow and elongated, and both more cytologically malignant and mitotically active. In addition, high-grade fibrillary astrocytic tumors often contain foci of cellular tumor seen either radiographically or macroscopically.

Microgliomatosis, an exceedingly rare and poorly understood lesion, is difficult to exclude on histologic grounds alone but is readily identified if the neoplastic cells are immunostained for macrophage markers. It is not known how many previously reported cases of gliomatosis cerebri were actually examples of microgliomatosis. One should be particularly suspicious in cases of "gliomatosis" in which marked cellular elongation is a feature, a characteristic also seen in the rod cells in reactive processes.

Treatment and Prognosis. Given the problems inherent in defining gliomatosis cerebri and distinguishing cases from look-alikes, it is difficult to generalize regarding its biologic behavior on the basis of published reports. As would be expected from its infiltrative character, gliomatosis is not cured by surgical resection (175). It is also not surprising that its clinical course varies considerably, with survival periods of months to many years, given the variety of lesions included under this diagnosis. Examples with cytologic malignancy and high mitotic indices can be expected to behave more aggressively than those with cytologically bland nuclei, unassociated with mitoses.

Meningeal Gliomatosis

Definition. A glioma residing primarily in the leptomeninges.

General Comments. The diagnosis of meningeal gliomatosis is rigorously applied only to leptomeningeal gliomas for which, despite careful search, no intraparenchymal source is found. In practice, however, it is used for neoplasms which, though largely leptomeningeal, are associated with a parenchymal component small

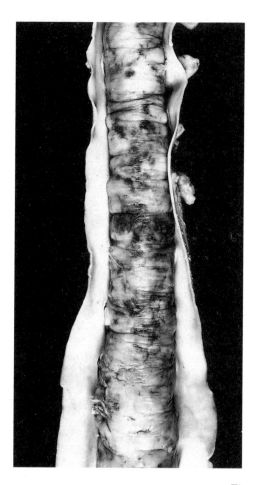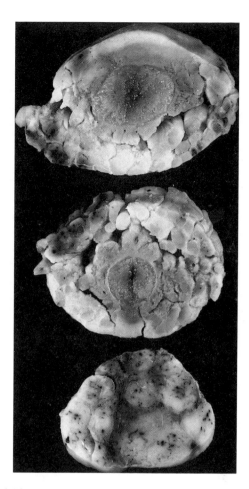

Figure 3-58
MENINGEAL GLIOMATOSIS
Left: In this spinal example, the tumor fills the subarachnoid space as a soft, gray, focally hemorrhagic infiltrate.
Right: On cut section, tumor surrounds the spinal cord, thickens the subarachnoid space, and encases nerve roots. No intraparenchymal primary site was discovered despite histologic sampling at multiple levels.

enough to be considered an ingrowth from the meningeal lesion. The term meningeal gliomatosis is not applicable to a large tumor obviously arising in the brain or spinal cord which has broken through the pia and spread locally within the subarachnoid space (184,189). Without a careful autopsy it is impossible to determine whether any gliomas are truly primary in the leptomeninges. Even then, skeptics would assume that the intraparenchymal primary site had escaped detection. Rare intracranial (187) and intraspinal (179,181,185) examples, however, have been described in which careful study failed to identify a parenchymal source.

Primary diffuse meningeal gliomas may be derived from small heterotopic nodules or protrusions

of glia in the subarachnoid space (177,178). Equally rare, small, discrete gliomas in the subarachnoid space can arise also from such foci (180, 186). Meningeal gliomatosis is discussed under astrocytic tumors since most are astrocytic, although occasional cases are oligodendroglial (183).

Clinical and Radiographic Features. As might be expected, given the practical and nosologic difficulties in defining this entity, there is no specific clinicopathologic setting. Patients of all ages have been affected. Intracranial, intraspinal, and diffuse tumors have been described (179,181–183,185–188).

Macroscopic Findings. The tumors thicken and opacify the leptomeninges, encasing nerve roots and vessels in transit (figs. 3-58, 3-59).

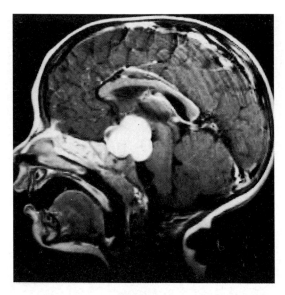

Figure 3-63
PILOCYTIC ASTROCYTOMA
OF THE HYPOTHALAMIC REGION
At this commonly affected site, the contrast-enhancing neoplasm often appears to lie within the third ventricle.

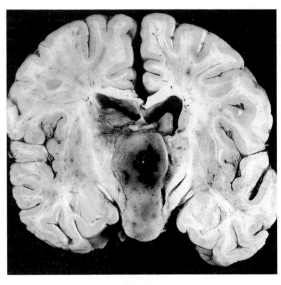

Figure 3-64
PILOCYTIC ASTROCYTOMA
OF THE HYPOTHALAMIC REGION
Pilocytic astrocytomas are soft, fleshy, and somewhat discrete. This example largely occupies the third ventricle.

involved optic nerve. Since enlarging chiasmal lesions are not restrained by a dural sheath, tumors in this location usually evolve into globular or even eccentric, rather than fusiform, masses.

Pilocytic astrocytomas of the hypothalamus and third ventricular region primarily affect children and present as seemingly discrete tumors which, when extending into the third ventricle, may appear to be largely intraventricular (figs. 3-63, 3-64) (see Appendix F). Since many tumors show an element of chiasmal involvement, their distinction from optic pilocytic tumors is somewhat artificial (213,219). As at other sites, the radiographic contrast enhancement of pilocytic astrocytoma distinguishes it from well-differentiated fibrillary or diffuse astrocytomas which generally do not enhance. On T1-weighted MRIs, some pilocytic tumors generate a very high signal intensity, appearing white or "bright." This is a diagnostically useful feature since it reflects the tumor's frequent content of proteinaceous (mucinous) material, and aids in the distinction of this lesion from other forms of astrocytoma.

Pilocytic astrocytomas of the cerebral hemispheres generally occur in patients older than those with visual system or hypothalamic involvement (194,196). Since young adults are most

often affected, hemispheric pilocytic tumors can arise in the same age group as the far more common (for this site and age group) diffuse or fibrillary astrocytoma, the lesion with which pilocytic tumors must not be confused. Radiographically, pilocytic astrocytoma of the cerebral hemispheres is an enhancing mass, one sometimes presenting as a mural nodule within a cyst (fig. 3-65) (196,215) (see Appendix D). Such an image would be highly atypical for a fibrillary astrocytoma. The lesions occur throughout the cerebral hemispheres. Some are superficial while others are largely intraventricular (see Appendix F). Calcification, occasionally dense, is present in some pilocytic lesions (see Appendix E).

Pilocytic astrocytomas of the cerebellum, long referred to by the confusingly nonspecific term cerebellar astrocytoma, are similar to cerebral examples in their somewhat discrete appearance and frequent cyst/mural nodule configuration (figs. 3-66, 3-67) (199,218). Despite gross circumscription, such tumors often permeate surrounding tissue, particularly white matter, for some distance and involve the overlying leptomeninges. Eccentric growth into the cerebellopontine angle may mimic an acoustic tumor. Cerebellar pilocytic astrocytomas usually present during the second

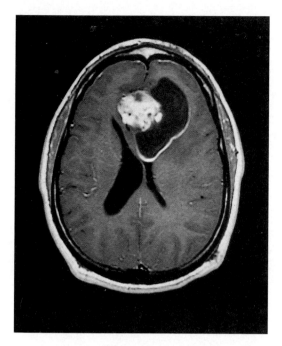

Figure 3-65
PILOCYTIC ASTROCYTOMA
OF THE CEREBRAL HEMISPHERES

Pilocytic astrocytomas in this site are often contrast-enhancing nodules associated with a large cyst. This radiographic appearance differs markedly from that of diffuse or fibrillary astrocytomas with which pilocytic astrocytomas can be confused.

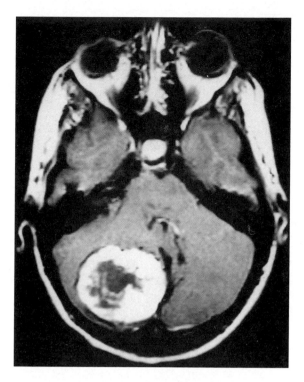

Figure 3-66
PILOCYTIC ASTROCYTOMA
OF THE CEREBELLUM

This, the most common glioma of the cerebellum, is an enhancing lesion which may be solid but is often cystic.

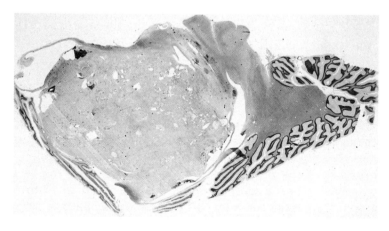

Figure 3-67
PILOCYTIC ASTROCYTOMA
OF THE CEREBELLUM

As is seen in this whole mount histologic section, cerebellar pilocytic astrocytomas are generally well-circumscribed masses.

decade of life and produce either symptoms referable to obstruction to the flow of cerebrospinal fluid or cerebellar dysfunction (197,223).

Astrocytomas of the brain stem are, in large part, infiltrative tumors of fibrillary type that produce diffuse enlargement or hypertrophy of the brain stem; only a small proportion are pilocytic. The latter constitute a part, and probably most, of a prognostically favorable group of brain stem astrocytomas described as "dorsally exophytic" (200,203,216a,226). Such tumors can be quite bulky and, since much of their mass lies outside the brain stem, are subject to at least partial resection. Radiographically, pilocytic tumors at this site are characterized by discreteness, contrast enhancement, and a tendency to

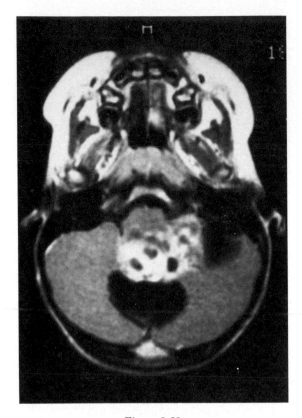

Figure 3-68
PILOCYTIC ASTROCYTOMA OF THE BRAIN STEM
As is typical, this pilocytic astrocytoma of the brain stem is contrast enhancing and multicystic. Its exophytic pattern of growth, in this case from the dorsal aspect of the brain stem, is also a common feature. This somewhat extrinsic location, coupled with contrast enhancement, sharply differs from that of the more common diffuse or fibrillary astrocytoma of the brain stem illustrated in figure 3-8, bottom. (Courtesy of Dr. James W. Langston, Memphis, TN.)

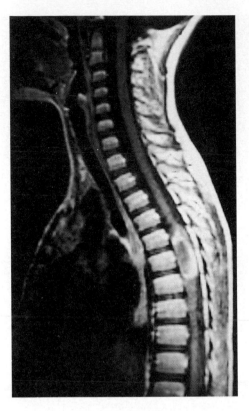

Figure 3-69
PILOCYTIC ASTROCYTOMA OF THE SPINAL CORD
Pilocytic astrocytomas of the spinal cord are relatively discrete and may be contrast enhancing. This radiographic appearance contrasts with that of diffusely infiltrative, and essentially nonresectable, fibrillary astrocytoma as shown in figure 3-9. (Courtesy of Dr. James W. Langston, Memphis, TN.)

multicystic architecture (fig. 3-68). They may be largely intraventricular (see Appendix F).

The clinical and radiographic features of pilocytic astrocytomas of the spinal cord are not well established and the percentage of pilocytic versus diffuse or fibrillary lesions remains to be defined (217,220) (see Appendix G). Pilocytic lesions are more common in young patients and are usually associated with a long history of symptoms. They are radiographically circumscribed, but may involve a considerable length of spinal cord (217). Some are contrast enhancing (fig. 3-69). Externally, the lesion produces a fusiform enlargement similar to that of other intramedullary tumors, including the fibrillary infiltrating astrocytoma with which the pilocytic neoplasm is most likely to be confused (fig. 3-70).

Microscopic Findings. The classic juvenile pilocytic astrocytoma is formed of loosely knit tissue composed of stellate astrocytes in microcystic regions alternating with compact tissue consisting of elongated and highly fibrillated cells (fig. 3-71). The former pattern typically contains brightly eosinophilic granular bodies whereas the piloid elements are associated with Rosenthal fiber formation. In addition to this prototypical type, there are many variants which must be recognized if this important entity is not to be overlooked (figs. 3-72–3-74).

The ratio of the loose to the more compact tissue varies greatly. Some tumors consist largely of the microcystic pattern whereas in others the compact pilocytic pattern predominates. Still

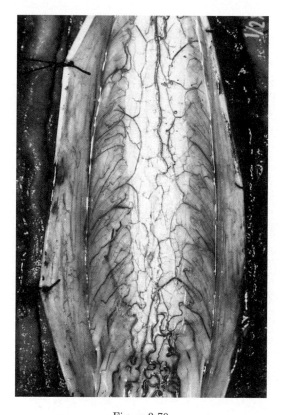

Figure 3-70
PILOCYTIC ASTROCYTOMA OF THE SPINAL CORD
The fusiform expansion of the spinal cord produced by this pilocytic astrocytoma is not, on external examination alone, distinguishable from that produced by a nonresectable diffuse glioma. (Courtesy of Dr. E. Michael Scott, Boston, MA.)

other tumors have an intermediate appearance. A superimposed microscopic pattern, often seen in the optic and hypothalamic varieties, consists of lobulation of neoplastic cells by delicate fibrovascular septa. Pilocytic astrocytomas of the optic nerve characteristically enlarge the compartment of the nerve and extend into the leptomeninges (fig. 3-75). Some pilocytic lesions lacking microcysts are rather myxoid due to stellate cells and abundant extracellular mucoid material.

Pilocytic astrocytomas at any site are noted for the ease with which they break through the pia to fill the overlying subarachnoid space (fig. 3-76). This should not be misinterpreted as malignant behavior or an indication that the tumor is about to disseminate within cerebrospinal pathways. As the tumors enter the leptomeninges, their cells become bundled into small lobules within a sometimes considerable fibroblastic reaction. In the optic nerve, this extension appears to be more common in patients with neurofibromatosis (226a).

In most instances, the nuclei of pilocytic astrocytomas are rather uniform, with delicate "open" chromatin and little variation in size and shape. Conspicuous pleomorphism is encountered in some cases, particularly in longstanding tumors, and is considered to be degenerative in nature and of no prognostic significance (fig. 3-77). Nuclear

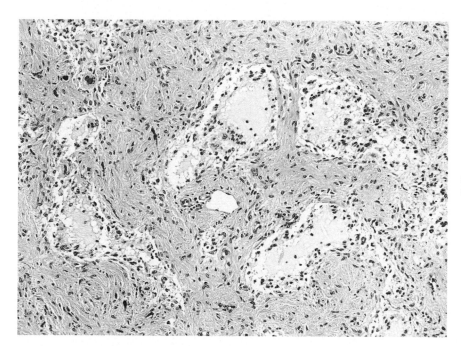

Figure 3-71
PILOCYTIC ASTROCYTOMA
The biphasic combination of microcystic and compact areas creates the classic picture.

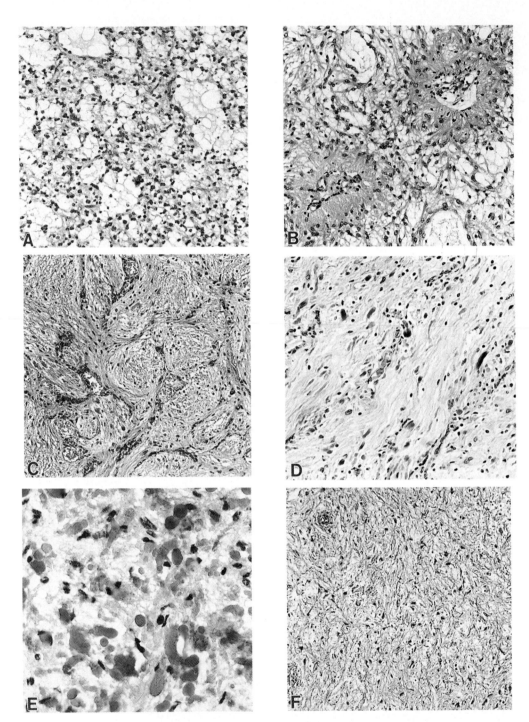

Figure 3-72
PILOCYTIC ASTROCYTOMA: VARIATIONS IN HISTOLOGIC APPEARANCE

As illustrated in A, many lesions are composed largely of spongy tissue rich in microcysts. Characteristic of pilocytic astrocytomas in general, the lesion is largely a solid mass of neoplastic cells without an obvious background of infiltrated brain. The perivascular radiating processes in some lesions can create a likeness to an ependymoma (B). Note the spongy background unusual for ependymomas. Other pilocytic astrocytomas are solid, rather than microcystic, and may be lobular (C). Rosenthal fibers, usually confined to the solid rather than spongy regions are found in many pilocytic astrocytomas, but are not requisite for the diagnosis (D). Rosenthal fibers are extremely abundant in some lesions (E). Particularly in the cerebellum, it can be difficult to distinguish such solid, paucicellular, highly fibrillar pilocytic astrocytomas from reactive gliosis with abundant Rosenthal fiber formation. A loose array of polar cells creates an additional variant of pilocytic astrocytoma (F).

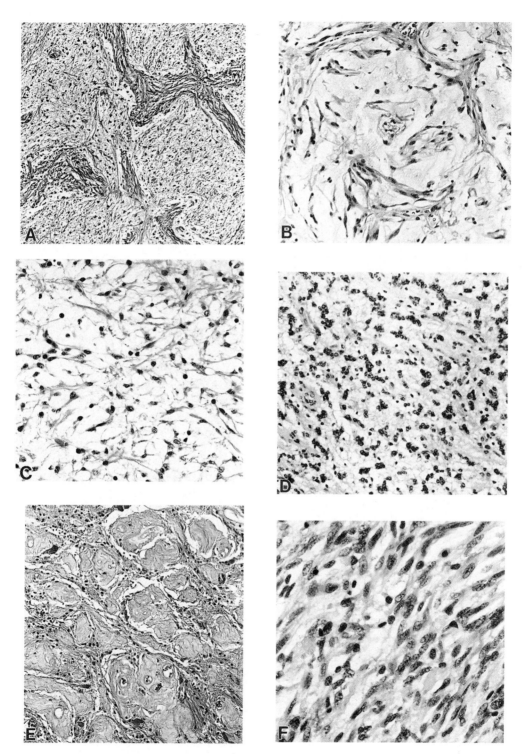

Figure 3-73
PILOCYTIC ASTROCYTOMA: VARIATIONS IN HISTOLOGIC APPEARANCE

Some pilocytic astrocytomas are traversed by prominent collagenous septa (A). Unusual pilocytic astrocytomas have an extensive mucinous background without microcysts (B). Elongated yet somewhat stellate cells separated by a mucoid matrix are seen in other cases (C). A distinctive clustering of nuclei marks some pilocytic astrocytomas (D). Prominent and sometimes markedly hyalinized vessels create the impression of a vascular malformation (E). The high cellularity of some pilocytic astrocytomas (F) can misrepresent the lesion as a malignant neoplasm.

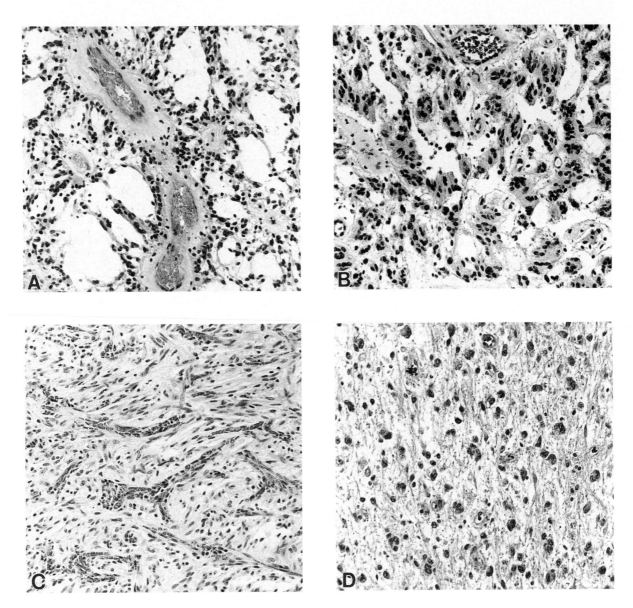

Figure 3-74
PILOCYTIC ASTROCYTOMA: VARIATIONS IN HISTOLOGIC APPEARANCE
The microcysts and clustering of nuclei can produce a likeness to a subependymoma (A). Other pilocytic astrocytomas combine microcysts with tight clusters of cells (B). Solid neoplastic tissue with polar cells between prominent vessels creates a distinctive pattern in other lesions (C). Widely spaced cells with pleomorphic, often multilobulated nuclei should not be interpreted as evidence of a high-grade infiltrative or "diffuse" astrocytic neoplasm (D).

roundness is typical in microcystic areas rich in protoplasmic astrocytes whereas elongation is a feature of piloid cells. Multinucleated giant cells with peripherally disposed nuclei are also common in pilocytic tumors, particularly those of the cerebellum and cerebrum. Mitoses are usually rare but may be found readily in some cases, particularly in infants.

Vascular proliferation is common within pilocytic astrocytomas and may be prominent in the walls of cysts where glomeruli are most likely to be found (fig. 3-78). As an eye-catching feature, it may prompt consideration of glioblastoma. In some tumors, presumably longstanding ones, blood vessels may be markedly hyalinized; spontaneous hemorrhage is rare. Occasional lesions

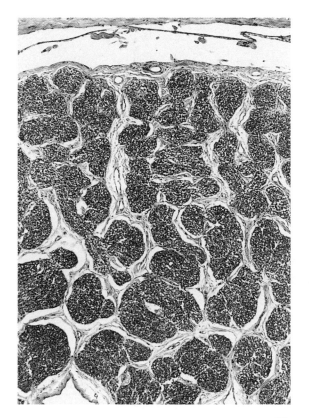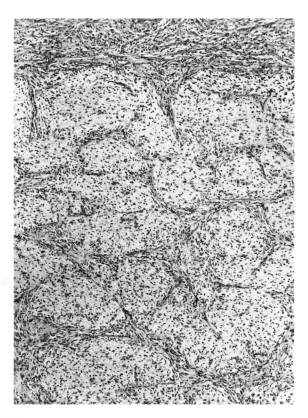

Figure 3-75
COMPARISON OF NORMAL OPTIC NERVE AND PILOCYTIC ASTROCYTOMA OF THE OPTIC NERVE
These two figures compare, at the same magnification, the normal optic nerve (left) with one containing a pilocytic astrocytoma (right). The neoplasm enlarges the compartments of the nerve and extends in collar-like fashion into the subarachnoid space.

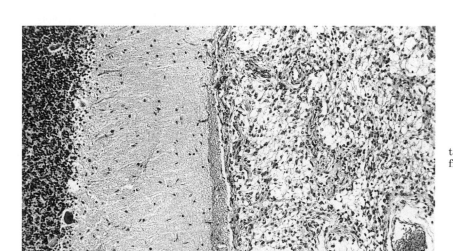

Figure 3-76
PILOCYTIC ASTROCYTOMA
As is apparent in this cerebellar tumor, pilocytic astrocytomas often fill the adjacent subarachnoid space.

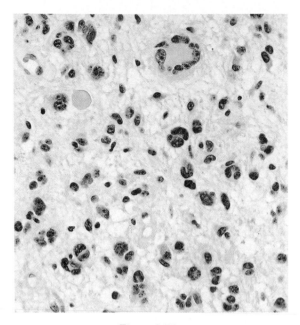

Figure 3-77
PILOCYTIC ASTROCYTOMA
Nuclear pleomorphism and multinucleation are not uncommon in pilocytic astrocytomas, particularly ones of long duration.

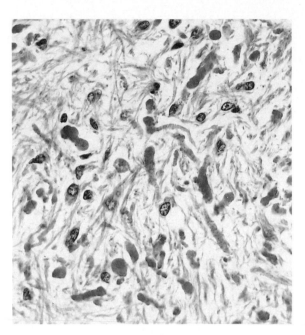

Figure 3-79
PILOCYTIC ASTROCYTOMA
Eosinophilic, refractile, somewhat corkscrew shaped structures termed Rosenthal fibers are found in many pilocytic astrocytomas. The bodies are particularly numerous in those tumors composed of compact, fibrillated, bipolar cells.

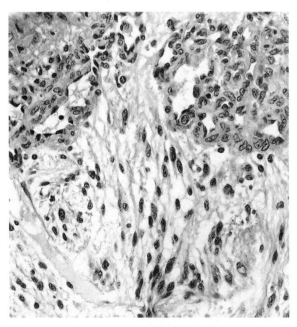

Figure 3-78
PILOCYTIC ASTROCYTOMA
Glomeruloid microvascular proliferation is a common feature of pilocytic astrocytoma and should not be misinterpreted as evidence of a high-grade glioma.

are especially rich in hyalinized vessels. The term *angioglioma* has been applied to tumors so remarkably vascular as to suggest the presence of a vascular malformation. Such lesions behave as ordinary pilocytic astrocytomas (207). Calcification may be seen but is rarely extensive. Necrosis is decidedly uncommon but, when seen, is unaccompanied by palisading.

Histologic features greatly facilitating the diagnosis of pilocytic astrocytoma include Rosenthal fibers and cells containing protein droplets or granular bodies. Rosenthal fibers are sausage or corkscrew shaped bodies with a brightly eosinophilic hyaline quality and are bright red on Masson trichrome stained smears. Many have one blunt and one tapered end (fig. 3-79). As seen in cytologic preparations, they represent impactions of lumpy material within the processes of neoplastic cells. Rosenthal fibers vary in number in pilocytic astrocytomas: they are absent in some cases and abundant in others. As discussed below, they are not diagnostic of neoplasia. Indeed, the greatest density of these structures is seen in pilocytic gliosis surrounding

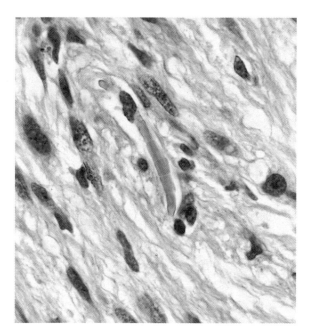

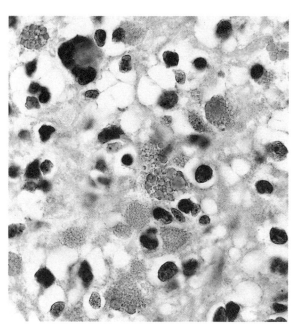

Figure 3-80
STACKED ERYTHROCYTES SIMULATING
A ROSENTHAL FIBER
A stack of compacted erythrocytes in a small vessel can resemble a Rosenthal fiber.

Figure 3-81
PILOCYTIC ASTROCYTOMA
Cells with eosinophilic granular bodies are common in pilocytic astrocytomas, particularly in those with loose-knit architecture.

craniopharyngiomas and other chronic lesions such as hemangioblastomas and vascular malformations. It may be difficult in some pilocytic lesions, particularly those in the cerebellum, to determine whether Rosenthal fibers are in neoplastic or reactive cells.

Since erythrocytes have a hyaline quality and stain positively with methods for connective tissue (Masson trichrome) and myelin (Luxol fast blue), Rosenthal fibers may be mimicked by erythrocytes tightly stacked in small vessels (fig. 3-80). Rosenthal fibers also must be distinguished from astrocytic processes so packed with glial filaments that they appear brightly eosinophilic and assume a hyaline quality. Such coarse processes are common in pilocytic astrocytomas and are a helpful but nonspecific finding without the diagnostic significance of Rosenthal fibers.

The two other diagnostically helpful features of pilocytic astrocytomas are cells with PAS-positive protein droplets and granular bodies (fig. 3-81) (202,210). Protein droplets is the descriptively accurate designation for clustered intracellular eosinophilic hyaline globules. Granular bodies are eosinophilic structures which are gen-

erally rounder and more finely granular than protein droplets. These two structures may represent variations of the same abnormality and are sometimes combined under the term eosinophilic granular body. Both granular bodies and protein droplets may also be seen in pleomorphic xanthoastrocytoma and ganglion cell tumors. They are especially common in the latter. In any lesion, they usually mark a slowly growing, well-differentiated neoplasm, and the diagnosis of a high-grade tumor should be made with caution in their presence (see Appendix C).

An interesting finding in some pilocytic astrocytomas, particularly those in the cerebellum, is tissue with a superficial resemblance to oligodendroglioma (fig. 3-82). Although the resemblance is usually vague, it can be remarkable. The significance of this phenotypic pattern, which is usually accompanied by other, more obvious features of pilocytic astrocytoma, is unclear.

Although pilocytic astrocytomas are macroscopically discrete, they do exhibit infiltration, ranging from several millimeters in most cases to centimeters, particularly in cerebellar examples.

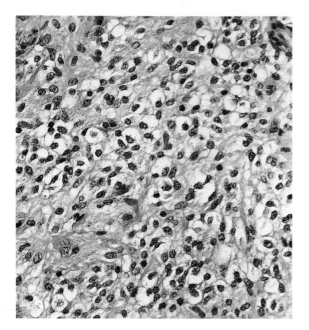

Figure 3-82
PILOCYTIC ASTROCYTOMA
As in this cerebellar example, foci closely resembling oligodendroglioma are sometimes seen.

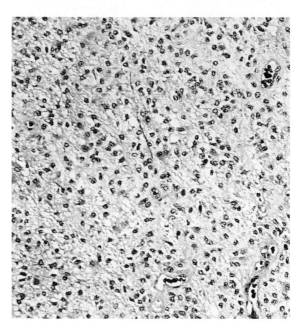

Figure 3-83
PILOCYTIC ASTROCYTOMA
Unlike diffuse or fibrillary astrocytomas, pilocytic astrocytomas exhibit a narrow peripheral zone of brain infiltration. Given the fibrillar background and the varying cytologic appearance of the tumor cells, however, a small specimen from this zone may easily be mistaken as a fibrillary astrocytoma.

As a result, what appears to the surgeon as circumscription is often not evident to the microscopist examining fragments of the tumor. One pattern of infiltration is best seen in sections taken through the equator of the mass, where peripheral incorporation of preexisting cells is readily seen as the tumor enlarges by a process known descriptively as "creeping substitution." An area of the brain is thus gradually taken over without the overt distant invasion that carries fibrillary neoplasms far from the site of origin. It is not surprising, therefore, that axis cylinders and even scattered neuron cell bodies are found trapped within the depth of some pilocytic lesions. Overrun neurons often raise the differential problem of a ganglion cell tumor, but in most instances these cells are few and normally formed. Ordinary infiltration, albeit limited when compared to that of fibrillary tumors, may be seen in pilocytic astrocytoma (fig. 3-83). It occurs more readily in white matter than in gray matter, a feature illustrated by the remarkably circumscribed thalamic tumors and the more ill-defined cerebellar ones. There is generally a very low degree of cellular atypia in such zones of infiltration.

Another form of infiltration is extension into perivascular spaces, common in pilocytic astrocytoma (fig. 3-84).

A rare glioma with cellular elongation alone has been referred to as the *adult variant of pilocytic astrocytoma*. Such monomorphic, somewhat fascicular tumors are, however, prone to malignant degeneration (222). There is little available information about these lesions and no consensus exists as to whether they represent a defined clinicopathologic entity.

The clinical and therapeutic significance of malignant or anaplastic transformation to pilocytic astrocytomas has not been resolved (199). Fortunately, pilocytic tumors with such features are rare and can remain radiologically and histologically stable for decades. Considerable cellular and nuclear pleomorphism, without mitotic activity, is acceptable in otherwise typical lesions, particularly in cerebellar examples. Pleomorphism, infrequent mitoses, and vascular proliferation are of no prognostic significance since such lesions behave in the same slowly growing,

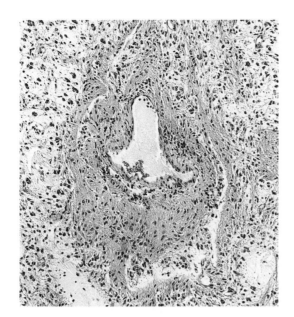

Figure 3-84
PILOCYTIC ASTROCYTOMA
Filling of perivascular spaces is common.

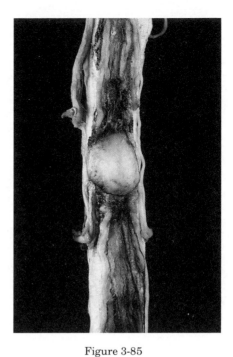

Figure 3-85
MALIGNANT PILOCYTIC ASTROCYTOMA
A 29-year-old woman died 2 years after a diagnosis of "atypical pilocytic astrocytoma" of the pineal region. At autopsy, multiple tumor implants were present in the craniospinal subarachnoid spaces.

indolent manner as tumors without these features. On occasion, pilocytic astrocytomas do recur rapidly and, in rare instances, disseminate in the subarachnoid space (figs. 3-85–3-87). Such lesions demonstrate increased cellularity, brisk mitotic activity, significant vascular proliferation, and occasional necrosis (fig. 3-87). They are also generally solid, lacking or losing the obvious sponginess so much a part of the classic juvenile pilocytic pattern. When a tumor with histologic features of malignancy also exhibits the basic features of pilocytic astrocytoma, the designation, *malignant pilocytic astrocytoma*, is appropriate (fig. 3-88). One must bear in mind, and relay to clinicians, the fact that many tumors with such features do not invariably exhibit biologically malignant behavior (227).

Astrocytomas showing only cellular elongation but none of the other pathognomonic features of pilocytic astrocytomas, such as Rosenthal fibers, are difficult to classify and grade (208). This is particularly the case when they occur at sites classic for pilocytic lesions, such as the hypothalamus.

The tissue pattern of primitive polar spongioblastoma is occasionally encountered in pilocytic astrocytoma. Its prognostic significance in this setting is unclear.

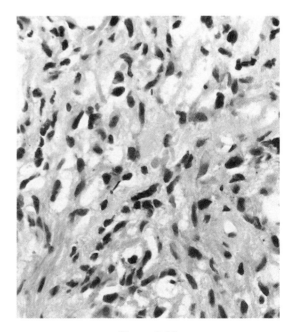

Figure 3-86
MALIGNANT PILOCYTIC ASTROCYTOMA
The initial surgical specimen of the case illustrated in figure 3-85 demonstrates a somewhat atypical pilocytic astrocytoma with Rosenthal fibers. Mitotic figures were scarce.

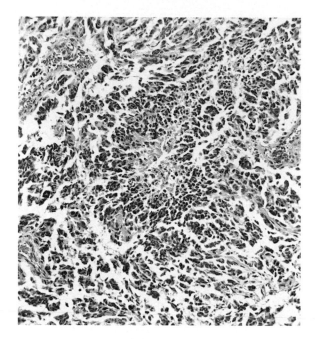

Figure 3-87
MALIGNANT PILOCYTIC ASTROCYTOMA

A photomicrograph of the spinal tumor implant shown in figure 3-85 illustrates both a fascicular pattern typical of pilocytic astrocytoma and necrosis with pseudopalisading, a feature generally alien to this tumor. Mitotic figures were abundant. Rosenthal fibers were seen throughout the lesion, both in the recurrent primary tumor and at distant sites.

Cytology. The benign cytologic features of classic pilocytic astrocytoma are best seen in squash or smear preparations in which uniformity and "blandness" of nuclei is especially evident. Cellular elongation is evident as fine hairlike bipolar processes which may often be followed across several high-power microscopic fields (pl. IIIA). Granular bodies (pl. IIIB) and Rosenthal fibers (pl. IIIC) may also be seen. Nuclear abnormalities are common in longstanding tumors and consist of pleomorphism (pl. IIIB), lobulation, intranuclear inclusions of cytoplasm, and smudged chromatin.

Immunohistochemical Findings. Pilocytic astrocytomas are immunoreactive for GFAP, with compact piloid cells staining more strongly than those in the microcystic spongy tissue. In Rosenthal fibers, immunoreactivity for GFAP is generally positive only on the surface; the body itself is reactive for alpha-β-crystallin (206,210). Eosinophilic granular bodies are reactive for GFAP, alpha-β-crystallin, ubiquitin, alpha-1-antichymotrypsin, and alpha-1-antitrypsin (202).

Ultrastructural Findings. Not surprisingly, the elongated piloid cells are packed with intermediate filaments, while cells from loose

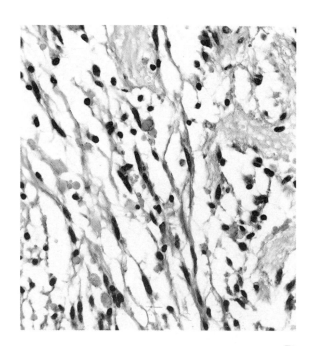

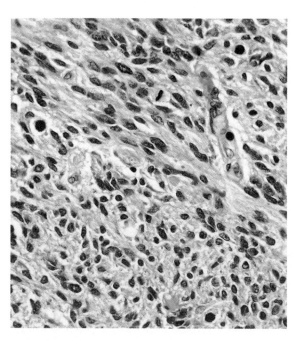

Figure 3-88
PILOCYTIC ASTROCYTOMA WITH MALIGNANT DEGENERATION
Only rarely is an otherwise typical pilocytic astrocytoma (left) associated with a malignant component (right).

PLATE III
PILOCYTIC ASTROCYTOMA

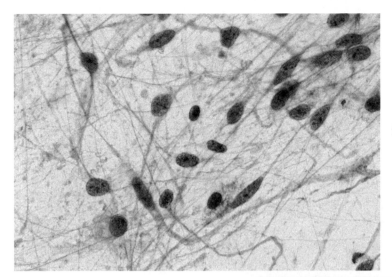

A. The "hair cells" for which this lesion is named are readily seen.

B. Nuclear hyperchromasia and pleomorphism are common. Note the typical cellular elongation, and, at the center of the illustration, the eosinophilic granular body that populates pilocytic astrocytomas and certain other slowly growing gliomas.

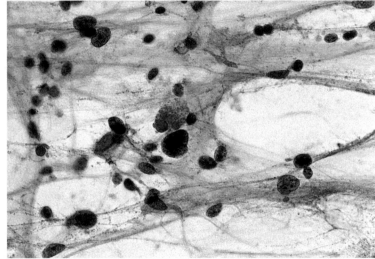

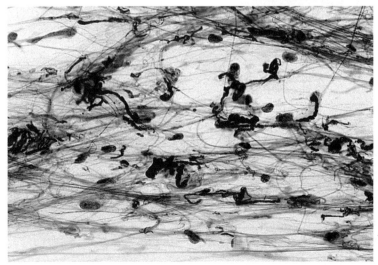

C. Intracytoplasmic Rosenthal fibers are prominent in some pilocytic neoplasms.

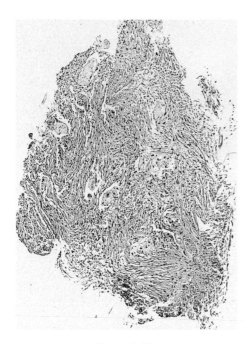

Figure 3-89
PILOCYTIC ASTROCYTOMA: FROZEN SECTION
In this needle biopsy specimen, microcysts, paucicellularity, and cellular elongation are visible even at low magnification.

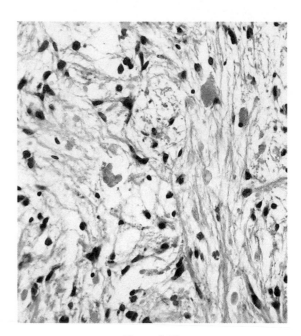

Figure 3-90
PILOCYTIC ASTROCYTOMA: FROZEN SECTION
Cellular elongation and Rosenthal fibers (center and top right) are apparent at high magnification.

textured microcystic zones are fibril poor. The Rosenthal fibers are nonfilamentous electron-dense masses surrounded by intermediate or glial filaments. Granular bodies represent cells, some of which contain intermediate, presumably glial, filaments. In addition, both the granules and droplets within these cells are osmophilic and contain lipid droplets, myelin figures, and granular debris (210). Whether these structures are a form of lysosome is unclear.

Frozen Section. Artifacts produced by freezing pilocytic tumors often distort architectural and cytologic features to such an extent as to mimic fibrillary or diffuse astrocytoma. Fortunately, microcysts usually persist but must be distinguished from the angular clefts formed by ice crystals (fig. 3-89). The slightly basophilic or eosinophilic proteinaceous content of microcysts, if present, is a helpful feature but not a specific finding since it can be seen in some well-differentiated infiltrating gliomas such as fibrillary astrocytoma or oligodendroglioma. The same is true of vacuolar scalloping on the periphery of the proteinaceous fluid. Rosenthal fibers and cells with protein drop-

lets are easily seen in frozen preparations and may be more obvious than in permanent sections (fig. 3-90). Hyaline cell processes, packed with intermediate filaments, are also conspicuous and aid in the identification of pilocytic tumors. Nuclear atypia in the face of virtually no mitotic activity should suggest a pilocytic astrocytoma.

Differential Diagnosis. Since most pilocytic astrocytomas are solid masses, the distinction of tumor from normal brain, often an issue in fibrillary astrocytomas, is not a problem. The principal differential diagnostic challenge is therefore to identify the lesion as a pilocytic tumor rather than a fibrillary astrocytoma, a pleomorphic xanthoastrocytoma, a ganglion cell tumor, or dense chronic pilocytic gliosis. The distinction from a diffuse or infiltrating astrocytoma is especially important since prognosis and treatment are so different (see Appendix B). Familiarity with the radiographic images thus assumes an importance that cannot be over-emphasized. The discreteness, contrast enhancement, and frequent cystic appearance of pilocytic astrocytoma all suggest the correct diagnosis. These features are strong presumptive

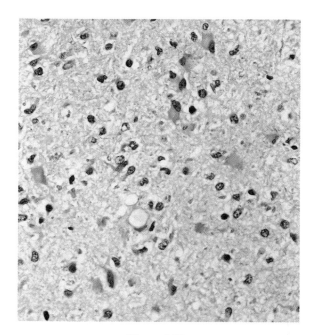

Figure 3-91
PILOCYTIC ASTROCYTOMA
Biopsies from the zone of infiltration surrounding pilocytic astrocytomas typically show a paucicellular, somewhat fibrillar lesion which can closely resemble the diffusely infiltrative fibrillary astrocytoma.

evidence that the lesion is not a diffuse fibrillary astrocytoma and raise the possibility of pilocytic astrocytoma and other similarly configured lesions (Appendix D).

Distinguishing pilocytic astrocytoma from well-differentiated fibrillary astrocytoma is usually straightforward given the relative demarcation of pilocytic tumors and their solid rather than diffusely infiltrative character; their spongy or focally cystic quality; and the presence of cellular elongation, Rosenthal fibers, and eosinophilic granular bodies. In some specimens, however, particularly those obtained by needle biopsy, these helpful architectural features may not be obvious and the pathologist is faced with little but a highly fibrillar, but not particularly pilocytic, tumor (fig. 3-91). If the search for microcysts, Rosenthal fibers, etc. is unfruitful, these two lesions may not be distinguishable. In such instances, the treatment plan must be based largely upon radiographic images and clinical features. Since surgical specimens from the brain stem are necessarily small, it is in this setting that it may be especially difficult to distinguish pilocytic from fibrillary or diffuse as-

trocytoma. In the latter, elongation of cells is not inherent but imposed by orientation, along with compact fiber tracts. Attention to clinical and radiographic features and the findings of looser textured areas, solid tumor composed of elongated cells, and particularly Rosenthal fibers permits identification of pilocytic lesions.

The resemblance of some pilocytic tumors to high-grade infiltrating fibrillary astrocytomas can be a significant problem, since some pilocytic lesions have fibrillar, but only somewhat polar, cells (figs. 3-78, 3-92). In the absence of distinctive architecture, and in the presence of mitotic activity, vascular proliferation, and, occasionally, foci of necrosis, a fibrillary astrocytic neoplasm may be suggested. This situation puts the pathologist in the unusual and uncomfortable position of trying to decide whether the lesion is a World Health Organization grade I tumor of pilocytic type, an anaplastic astrocytoma (grade III), or even glioblastoma multiforme (grade IV). Rosenthal fibers, cells with protein droplets, microcystic change, a solid rather than infiltrating character, and hyalinized vasculature become important points of distinction.

Differentiating between pilocytic astrocytoma and ganglion cell tumors can also be difficult because pilocytic astrocytomas can trap neurons while the astrocytic components of, or the chronic reactive elements surrounding, some ganglion cell tumors are patently pilocytic. Ganglion cell tumors, like pilocytic astrocytomas, share common clinical and radiographic features and both may extend into the subarachnoid space. Also, many neurons of ganglion cell tumors are not obviously neuronal, but are rather pleomorphic and therefore astrocytic in appearance. Nevertheless, ganglion cell tumors are distinctive in their greater compactness, clustering of abnormal neurons, abundance of cells with protein droplets, content of a reticulin- and collagen-containing stroma, and perivascular chronic inflammatory cells. Immunohistochemistry can be used to identify ganglion cells with their surface granular reactivity for synaptophysin. Neurofilament, tubulin, and chromogranin staining may also be seen.

The pleomorphic xanthoastrocytoma shares several features with pilocytic astrocytoma. These include young patient age, association with seizures, and frequent cyst/mural nodule

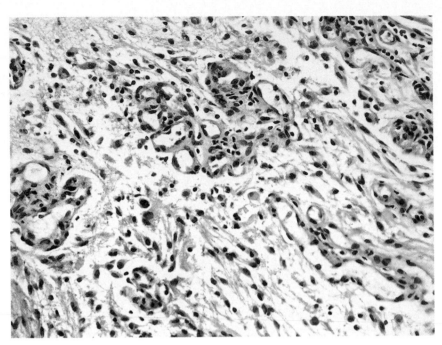

Figure 3-92
PILOCYTIC ASTROCYTOMA
RESEMBLING
MALIGNANT GLIOMA
The combination of vascular proliferation and a not particularly
piloid background can create a resemblance to a malignant glioma.
Distinguishing features in this case
were absence of mitoses and, elsewhere in the specimen, the presence
of microcysts, protein droplets, and
eosinophilic granular bodies.

configuration. A helpful distinguishing feature of the xanthoastrocytoma is the superficial, often largely leptomeningeal position of the mural nodule. Microscopically, this portion of xantho-astrocytoma exceeds the pilocytic tumor in its degree of cellularity and pleomorphism. Xanthic astrocytes are not a feature of pilocytic tumors, but are common in xanthoastrocytomas, as is occasionally a diffuse infiltrative component in the underlying brain. A very significant distin-guishing feature is the presence in xantho-astrocytomas of pericellular reticulin staining, a feature attributable in part to basal lamina pro-duction by tumor cells. This feature is often not evident throughout.

The classic juvenile pilocytic astrocytoma of the cerebellum is a distinctive entity, with its macroscopic cystic architecture and microscopic spongy quality. The diagnosis is readily apparent in such lesions. A vexing issue is the presence, in some pilocytic tumors, of tissue in which compact and microcystic patterns are only focally repre-sented, and Rosenthal fibers and granular bod-ies are scarce. These tumors, which behave like pilocytic astrocytomas (199), can closely resem-ble fibrillary or diffuse astrocytomas, but gener-ally exhibit remarkable nuclear uniformity and blandness, features that suggest the correct di-agnosis. Nonetheless, a minority of astro-

cytomas of the cerebellum are not pilocytic but are fibrillary or diffuse lesions of the type com-monly affecting the cerebral hemispheres. These uncommon tumors are more infiltrative and ex-hibit a greater degree of nuclear atypia than do diffuse pilocytic astrocytomas (fig. 3-93) (199). In some instances, despite sampling and a careful search for telltale pilocytic features, it may be impossible on histologic grounds alone to distin-guish the predominantly diffuse form of pilocytic astrocytoma from an infiltrating fibrillary astro-cytoma. In such cases clinical and radiographic features become decisive.

In the spinal cord, the differential diagnosis focuses first upon exclusion of reactive gliosis and second on distinguishing pilocytic astrocytoma from other tumors, especially the common dif-fusely infiltrating fibrillary astrocytoma. Distin-guishing between pilocytic astrocytoma and glio-sis can be especially difficult given the tendency of spinal cord tissue to exhibit a pilocytic form of gliosis, and the minute specimens often obtained from this slender and function-rich site. Pilocytic astrocytomas here are similar histologically to those in other locations, although the compact bipolar pattern often predominates and it may be difficult to find spongy tissue with microcysts. In the face of such minute specimens, pathologic confirmation that the process is neoplastic rather

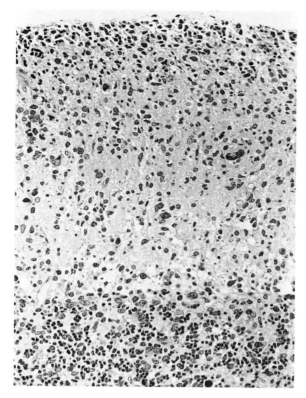

Figure 3-93
ANAPLASTIC FIBRILLARY OR "DIFFUSE"
ASTROCYTOMA OF THE CEREBELLUM

In addition to the common pilocytic astrocytoma, diffuse fibrillary astrocytic tumors also occasionally arise within the cerebellum. As in this section of cerebellar cortex, such tumors are noted for significant nuclear atypia, invasiveness, and, in most instances, mitotic activity.

than reactive may not be possible and appropriate treatment may depend on the assurance that the specimen comes from the center of a radiographically abnormal expansile lesion. A small proportion of specimens, therefore, are not, in and of themselves, diagnostic of tumor.

Distinguishing a pilocytic astrocytoma of the spinal cord from a fibrillary astrocytoma is often difficult but is associated with significant therapeutic ramifications (see Appendix B). Surgery is often terminated upon receipt of a diagnosis of diffuse fibrillary astrocytoma or the generic diagnosis "astrocytoma," but may continue with the goal of complete resection if a diagnosis of pilocytic astrocytoma is rendered. As emphasized in the discussion of infiltrating spinal cord astrocytomas, cautious analysis of clinical and radiographic data, as well as the pathologic specimen, is required in order to avoid misinterpretation.

Distinguishing a pilocytic astrocytoma from pilocytic gliosis, particularly in the hypothalamus and spinal cord, is important given the exuberant gliosis of this type that accompanies local infiltration of craniopharyngioma into the floor of the third ventricle (see fig. 15-7), the cyst wall of a cerebellar hemangioblastoma (see fig. 7-6), pineal cyst (see fig. 6-18), or syrinx in the spinal cord (see Appendix A). In contrast to most pilocytic tumors, such gliosis results in a compacted rather than microcystic pattern and is especially rich in Rosenthal fibers.

Treatment and Prognosis. The natural history of pilocytic astrocytoma at any site is one of slow growth. Many incompletely resected tumors enlarge little, if at all, over periods of 5, 10, or even 20 years. Overall survival of patients with anterior optic, cerebral (194–196,215), and cerebellar tumors is excellent. The favorable prognosis reflects the indolent nature of the tumor, young patient age, and resectability of these lesions in most anatomic sites (197–199,223). In one series of supratentorial tumors, the 10-year survival rate was 100 percent for 16 patients with gross total resection or radical subtotal removal and 74 percent for 35 patients undergoing subtotal resection or biopsy (196). Histologic factors such as mitoses or vascular proliferations and flow cytofluorometric findings, including S-phase index, were not prognostically significant (196). One detailed study suggested that the bromodeoxyuridine labeling index varied considerably but did not appear to have prognostic significance (201). Interestingly, the index was often higher in younger patients, suggesting to the authors that the growth rate of the tumors decreased with age.

The prognosis is especially favorable for optic nerve tumors where complete excision and cure are possible in many cases (191,221). Recurrences with a fatal outcome are more likely in chiasmatic/hypothalamic tumors, in which resection is precluded by neuroanatomic realities (213,219). Due to the relatively discrete nature of many pilocytic astrocytomas, stereotactic excision has been advocated for deep-seated lesions of the basal ganglia and thalamus (209).

The prognosis of patients with cerebellar lesions is also excellent, since total excision is possible in many cases and even residual tumor remains dormant or grows only slowly (197–199, 214). This is in sharp contrast to the less common but more infiltrative and aggressive fibrillary or diffuse astrocytomas occurring at this site (199). Of patients with "diffuse cerebellar astrocytomas" who do well, the vast majority actually have pilocytic tumors with a predominantly diffuse pattern of growth (215,216).

It remains to be seen whether the same aggressive radiotherapy administered for diffuse infiltrating astrocytic neoplasms of the brain stem is necessary, or effective, in the treatment of brain stem pilocytic astrocytoma. Longer survival periods have been noted for Rosenthal fiber–containing astrocytomas in this region (190,203,226,226a).

Only limited data are available regarding the clinical outcome and prognosis of patients with spinal cord pilocytic astrocytomas. Many lesions are reportedly discrete and amenable to gross total removal, although complete resection may not be possible for some lesions, particularly those that extend over many spinal levels (209a,217,220).

Identifying the rare clinically malignant pilocytic astrocytoma can be difficult, particularly if there is no clear pathologic evidence of anaplasia. The prognosis of patients with pilocytic versus fibrillary or diffuse cerebellar astrocytomas (199,216) is discussed above under Differential Diagnosis.

Malignant degeneration of pilocytic tumors, often after many years, has been reported. Although this event can occur without radiation (192,227), radiotherapy had been administered in many cases (204,211,224,227,228). As a result, it is difficult to exclude radiation as an oncogenic influence, particularly when the "recurrent" tumor is more fibrillary, i.e., anaplastic astrocytoma or glioblastoma, than pilocytic (195a). This was shown to be the case in some patients successfully treated for medulloblastoma and is discussed in chapter 5. There is little information on the course of patients presenting initially with histologically malignant pilocytic astrocytomas. In our limited experience, local recurrence and leptomeningeal dissemination may occur. In some cases, rapid "recurrence" of pilocytic astrocytoma is actually due to the reformation of cysts, ones that can be drained with impressive clinical improvement. Only rarely do well-differentiated, entirely typical pilocytic astrocytomas exhibit diffuse spinal spread (193,205,212).

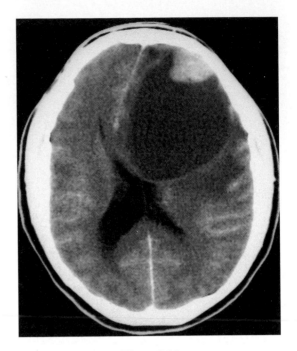

Figure 3-94
PLEOMORPHIC XANTHOASTROCYTOMA
As in this computerized tomographic scan, the classic radiographic appearance is one of a superficially situated tumor, here a mural nodule, associated with an underlying cyst.

Pleomorphic Xanthoastrocytoma

Definition. A superficially situated astrocytic neoplasm characterized by marked cellular pleomorphism and frequent xanthomatous change.

Clinical and Radiographic Features. The patients, usually adolescents or young adults, typically present with a long history of seizures and, less frequently, an expanding mass in the temporal or, less often, the parietal region (232a,234, 241). Radiographically, the lesion is usually superficial in location, forming a meningocerebral mass or nodule often underlain by a cyst (fig. 3-94) (236a,242) (see Appendix D). Some lesions are calcified (see Appendix E).

Macroscopic Findings. At surgery, the pleomorphic xanthoastrocytoma (PXA) appears as a firm circumscribed nodule or plaque, which often overlies a cyst filled with clear fluid. Some tumors appear to lie almost entirely outside the brain. Despite the perception of circumscription, particularly of the superficial component, no uniform cleavage plane may underlie the entire tumor: deep portions often exhibit some degree of parenchymal infiltration.

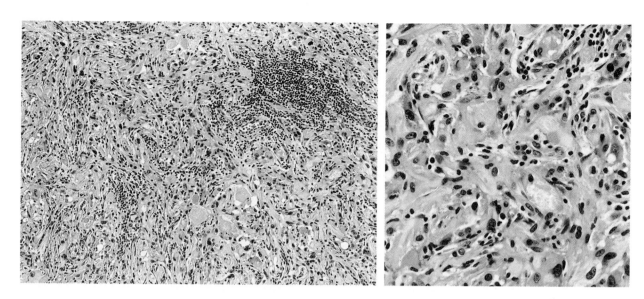

Figure 3-95
PLEOMORPHIC XANTHOASTROCYTOMA
The tumor nodule consists of closely packed pleomorphic cells with abundant pink cytoplasm. Foci of perivascular lymphocytes are frequently present in this entity. The cellular pleomorphism and overall astrocytic appearance of this uncommon, and often seizure-associated, tumor of young patients are readily apparent at high magnification.

Microscopic Findings. Seen in its entirety, the tumor consists of a pleomorphic, reticulin-positive superficial component (figs. 3-95–3-97) and, in some cases, of an underlying infiltrating front relative to the brain (fig. 3-98). Tissue from the often more prominent superficial portion may be all that is submitted for pathologic examination. This component both mushrooms as a mass from the cortical surface and extends horizontally within the subarachnoid space, forcing its way wedge-like to the periphery while surrounding cortical vessels in the perivascular (Virchow-Robin) spaces. Features of the tumor apparent at low magnification include cellular pleomorphism, patchy to widespread pericellular reticulin positivity, variable vascular sclerosis, and scattered perivascular lymphocytic infiltrates. The pleomorphic cells vary in shape from round to elongated and possess large, multilobed or multiple hyperchromatic nuclei. The cytoplasm of some cells has a glassy or fibrillar "astrocytic" appearance. Cytoplasmic vacuolization due to the accumulation of lipid droplets is variable and is not seen in all cases.

Also a feature of cells within superficial portions of the tumor are eosinophilic granular bodies such as are encountered in other slowly growing

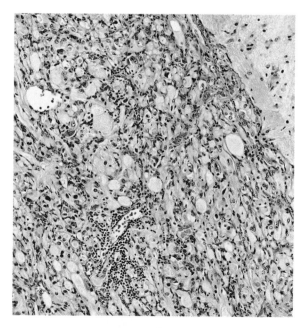

Figure 3-96
PLEOMORPHIC XANTHOASTROCYTOMA
The superficial nature of this example is apparent at low magnification. The cortical surface is seen at the upper right.

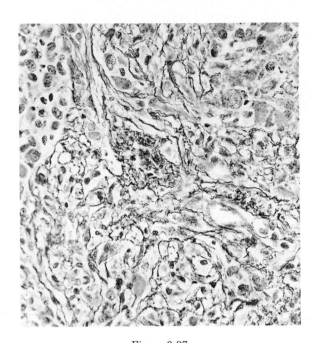

Figure 3-97
PLEOMORPHIC XANTHOASTROCYTOMA
An intercellular pattern of reticulin staining typifies the nodular portion of the lesion.

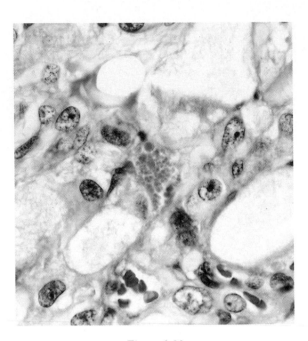

Figure 3-99
PLEOMORPHIC XANTHOASTROCYTOMA
Neoplastic cells containing brightly eosinophilic protein droplets are a common, albeit often focal, feature of these tumors.

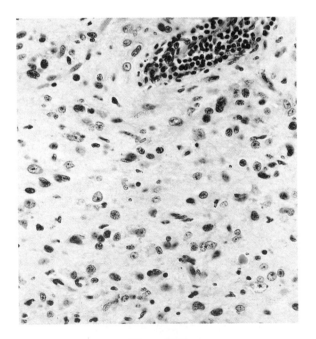

Figure 3-98
PLEOMORPHIC XANTHOASTROCYTOMA
In addition to a discrete, solid, superficially situated component, many pleomorphic xanthoastrocytomas show an element of invasion in the underlying brain.

glial lesions including pilocytic astrocytoma and ganglion cell tumors (fig. 3-99). Since protein droplets, as well as smaller more uniform granular bodies (fig. 3-100), are generally indicators of chronicity, a diagnosis of malignancy should be made with great caution in their presence.

Although the overall histologic appearance is that of a pleomorphic astrocytic neoplasm, in some cases the fascicular swirling, lipidization, and accompanying focal lymphocytic infiltrate can resemble histiocytic neoplasms such as malignant fibrous histiocytoma (238). In other lesions the giant cells are plumper and sufficiently compacted to produce an appearance resembling giant cell glioblastoma. Lesions that are highly vascular may resemble hemangiomas (239). An association with a ganglion cell tumor has even been described (230,236).

Despite the marked pleomorphism that characterizes PXA, mitotic figures are few and necrosis is absent. In fact, necrosis, especially when associated with accelerated mitotic activity, is considered prima facie evidence of malignant transformation. In such instances, diagnostic consideration should also be given to the possibility that the lesion is not PXA but rather an

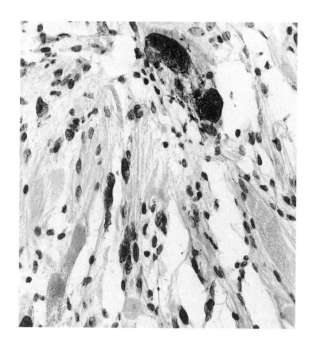

Figure 3-100
PLEOMORPHIC XANTHOASTROCYTOMA:
FROZEN SECTION

As seen in this frozen section, marked cellular pleomorphism and focal granular enlargement of cell processes are common. The term eosinophilic granular body is applied when the latter are seen in cross section.

anaplastic fibrillary astrocytoma or glioblastoma. Since the original description of PXA as an entity, it has become apparent that some lesions do exhibit mitotic figures and even foci of small mitotically active cells (fig. 3-101); the biologic behavior of such lesions remains to be defined. One must assume that the latter is a sign of imminent malignant degeneration (237a), one requiring at least gross total resection and very close observation, if not aggressive therapy.

Cells within the infiltrative portion of the tumor are often considerably less pleomorphic than are those in more superficial components. As a result, a specimen from this region suggests a diffuse or fibrillary astrocytoma, both in its cytologic appearance and infiltrative quality. Such astrocytic cells exhibit significant atypia and permeate the surrounding brain in a gradient fashion.

Frozen Section. Familiarity with clinical and radiographic data is of particular importance in cases of PXA. Without an awareness of the entity, its typical radiographic findings, and its protracted evolution, the cellular pleomorphism can be mistaken readily for that of glioblastoma

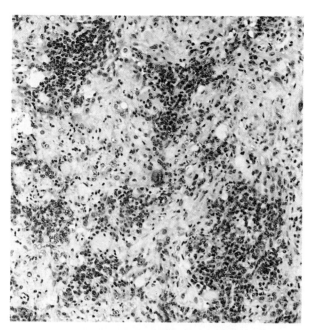

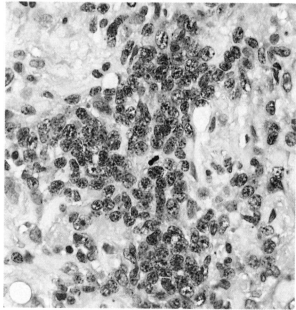

Figure 3-101
PLEOMORPHIC XANTHOASTROCYTOMA
WITH MALIGNANT DEGENERATION

This tumor exhibits both features of classic pleomorphic xanthoastrocytoma (top) as well as regions of small, mitotically active, less differentiated cells (bottom).

(fig. 3-100). The process of freezing may only compound the problem since the cells tend to separate, thus creating a loose-knit appearance resembling that of an ordinary high-grade astrocytoma of the giant cell type. Lacking, however,

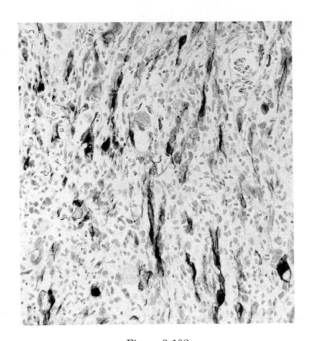

Figure 3-102
PLEOMORPHIC XANTHOASTROCYTOMA
Some of the astrocyte-appearing cells in the nodular portion of this tumor were immunoreactive for GFAP.

are brisk mitotic activity, vascular proliferation, and necrosis. Other diagnostically helpful features include fragments with evident sharp tumor-brain demarcation, xanthomatous change, perivascular lymphocytic aggregates, and cells with protein droplets (fig. 3-100).

Cytology. Marked nuclear pleomorphism and hyperchromasia are easily seen in cytologic preparations (pl. IVA). Absent are the readily identified mitoses, proliferated vasculature, and necrotic debris so typical of malignant gliomas.

Immunohistochemical Findings. Immunoreactivity for GFAP as well as S-100 protein is noted in both superficial and infiltrating components (fig. 3-102). At least some of the cells in the superficial component are immunoreactive for GFAP, albeit patchy or weak (231,234,235). Reactivity for S-100 protein is stronger. Many lesions also exhibit immunoreactivity for other markers, including alpha-1-antitrypsin and nonspecific esterase (235,238). Although the latter suggest the presence of a histiocytic component, the nonspecific nature of these antigens, as well as of vimentin, is well known. In contrast, lysozyme reactivity, a far more specific marker of histiocytes, is lacking. The evolution of some lesions to

typical GFAP-positive glioblastomas also supports the clearly glial nature of PXA (233).

Ultrastructural Findings. Some of the neoplastic cells contain intermediate filaments while others demonstrate predominantly rough endoplasmic reticulum, occasional lysosomes, or lipid droplets. Complex lysosomes corresponding to light microscopic granular bodies may be seen as well. Collagen is typically scant. Cellular investment by basal lamina is variable but has been used to suggest an origin of PXA from subpial astrocytes (232,234), the surfaces of which are normally covered by basement lamina as they fan out over the surface of the brain.

Differential Diagnosis. In light of the important therapeutic consequences, the principal challenge to the pathologist faced with a PXA is to avoid overgrading by confusing it with glioblastoma or malignant fibrous histiocytoma (231, 235) (see Appendix B). This procedure begins with recognition of the clinical and radiographic features which, when classic, are highly suggestive of the diagnosis and most atypical for glioblastoma. As previously noted, microscopic features distinguishing these lesions center upon a discrepancy between the extent of cellularity and pleomorphism and the absence of frequent mitoses, vascular proliferation, and necrosis. Scattered, brightly eosinophilic protein droplets are alien to most glioblastomas. Specimens taken exclusively from the deep-seated infiltrating component of PXA pose a particular problem since they are identical in appearance to ordinary infiltrating astrocytomas.

The discrete nature of PXA, especially when exhibiting a cyst/mural nodule architecture, raises the possibility of a pilocytic astrocytoma or ganglion cell tumor. The cellularity, compactness, and pleomorphism of PXA typically exceeds that of the pilocytic lesion. In addition, pilocytic astrocytomas often exhibit a biphasic pattern wherein compacted, fibrillar, and elongated cells associated with Rosenthal fibers alternate with a spongy microcystic component containing protoplasmic hypofibrillar astrocytes associated with granular bodies. When pleomorphic cells are present, they are usually not as prominent and numerous as in PXA. The pleomorphism of some ganglion cell tumors clearly overlaps with that of PXA and creates a diagnostic challenge since both tumors favor younger patients and

PLATE IV

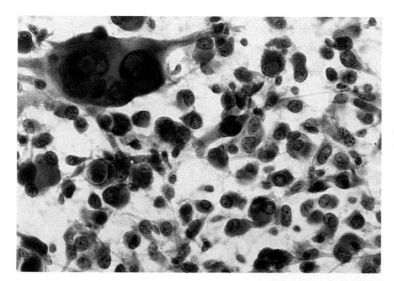

A. PLEOMORPHIC
XANTHOASTROCYTOMA
An astrocytic phenotype, marked nuclear pleomorphism, and absence of mitotic activity are typical cytologic features.

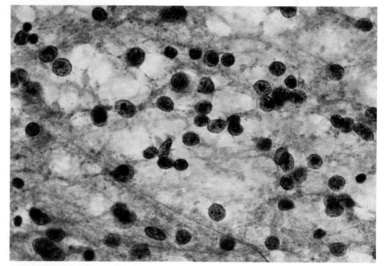

B. OLIGODENDROGLIOMA
Uniform round nuclei with small nucleoli are characteristic. Note the scant cytoplasm and only slight fibrillar background.

C. MALIGNANT
OLIGODENDROGLIOMA
Dense cellularity, high nuclear cytoplasmic ratios, and relative hyperchromatism characterize the malignant oligodendroglioma. The brightly eosinophilic "microgemistocytes" are common in such lesions.

have abundant reticulin and patchy lymphocytic infiltrates. Although PXAs often contain cells resembling bizarre neurons, such cells lack Nissl substance and usually show some degree of GFAP immunoreactivity rather than the synaptophysin and neurofilament protein positivity observed in ganglioglioma. When ganglion cells are encountered in PXA, they generally represent trapped neurons within underlying brain, but a variant with a ganglion cell component has been reported as described above. The neurons in the infiltrating portion of a conventional PXA are somewhat jostled by the passing of infiltrative tumor cells, but are otherwise morphologically normal.

Malignant histiocytic tumors are excluded by the demonstration of GFAP immunoreactivity (231), which, admittedly, may be sparse in otherwise typical PXAs.

Treatment and Prognosis. The rarity and relatively recent recognition of PXA as an entity have made it difficult to draw a close parallel between histologic features and biologic behavior. It is particularly difficult to prognosticate in individual cases in which mitoses are more than rare and only focal necrosis is present. There is also uncertainty regarding the prognostic significance of deep parenchymal infiltration as well as the minimal criteria for the identification of anaplastic or malignant transformation.

Despite our incomplete understanding of the pathobiology of PXA, it is clear that it is a considerably less aggressive lesion than is suggested by its microscopic appearance. There is, nonetheless, increasing recognition that not all lesions are truly benign. Although it was initially hoped that PXAs might be cured by excision alone (234), a significant proportion recur, sometimes with increased cellularity and mitotic activity. Only somewhat less often does the lesion undergo transformation to an overtly anaplastic tumor composed of small, more uniform cells exhibiting brisk mitotic activity, conspicuous necrosis, and loss of intercellular reticulin staining (229,233,237,237a,240,241). Vascular proliferation may also become apparent.

Although most patients with PXA survive for many years, some die quickly following one or more recurrences. Recurrent tumors often exhibit malignant transformation. The frequency of the latter is estimated to be 10 to 25 percent. Nevertheless, the initial approach to the treatment of PXA should be conservative: gross total removal is generally followed by radiologic observation. At present, there is no consensus regarding the role of radiotherapy.

Subependymal Giant Cell Astrocytoma (Tuberous Sclerosis)

Definition. A demarcated, largely intraventricular tumor of large astrocyte-like cells which usually arises in the setting of tuberous sclerosis.

Clinical and Radiographic Features. Subependymal giant cell astrocytomas (SEGAs) are geographically limited to the region of the foramen of Monro, the near-midline channels by which cerebrospinal fluid passes from the lateral ventricles to the third ventricle (figs. 3-103, 3-104) (see Appendix F for other intraventricular tumors). The lesions are detected either in the clinical setting of increased intracranial pressure or during radiographic evaluation of a neurologically asymptomatic patient with tuberous sclerosis. Since the syndrome may be incompletely expressed (formes frustes) and since manifestations may, on rare occasion, be limited to the central nervous system, some patients come to surgery for an intraventricular mass before the underlying abnormality is recognized (244). Tuberous sclerosis is described in chapter 18.

Although SEGAs appear to evolve from enlargement of hamartomatous subependymal nodules (see figs. 18-17–18-19), symptomatic tumors are restricted to the anterior region near the foramen of Monro, whereas nodules are found more widely in the walls of the lateral ventricle.

Rarely, malignant gliomas appear in the setting of tuberous sclerosis (251). It is not clear whether these are pathogenetically related to the syndrome or are simply chance occurrences. Occasional giant cell tumors in patients with tuberous sclerosis are paraventricular in location, arising largely within the substance of the brain.

Radiographically, the typical intraventricular lesions are often large, bulky, and variably calcified (see Appendix E). Smaller coexistent subependymal hamartomas are often calcified as well. The association of a large symptomatic lesion with smaller periventricular "precursors" is virtually diagnostic of tuberous sclerosis (248).

Macroscopic Findings. The dome-like, broadly based lesions are smooth surfaced, soft to firm, and gray (fig. 3-104). A gritty consistency accompanies calcification.

Microscopic Findings. Despite their stereotypic clinical associations and radiologic features, SEGAs show considerable microscopic variation. Most exhibit vague perivascular pseudorosettes but in some cases the large eosinophilic cells are disposed in clusters demarcated by perivascular fibrillarity (figs. 3-105–3-107). Orderly ependymoma-like pseudorosettes are a less frequent, and often only focal, feature. Organoid patterns are exceptional.

Most SEGAs are demarcated or minimally infiltrative relative to neighboring brain parenchyma (fig. 3-105). As a consequence of their discreteness, the masses are composed only of tumor cells and a vascular stroma without the incorporated brain parenchyma so characteristic of astrocytomas of the diffuse or fibrillary type. Uniform cellularity and vasocentric cell patterns are the rule. Although the neoplastic cells are spindle to epithelioid in shape and are larger than those of gemistocytic astrocytoma, most are, nevertheless, phenotypically very astrocytic. Occasional cells possess such vesicular nuclei and prominent nucleoli as to resemble neurons. Despite the tumor's name, its constituent cells usually do not reach the truly "giant" proportions seen occasionally in glioblastoma or pleomorphic xanthoastrocytoma.

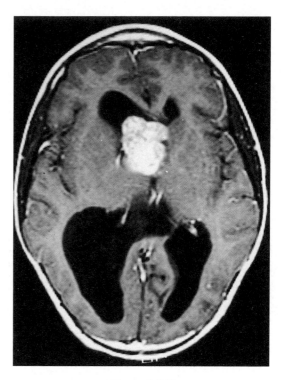

Figure 3-103
SUBEPENDYMAL GIANT CELL ASTROCYTOMA
(TUBEROUS SCLEROSIS)

Subependymal giant cell astrocytomas of the type associated with tuberous sclerosis are typically bulky, contrast-enhancing masses in the region of the foramen of Monro. Most overlie the head of the caudate nucleus. Foramen obstruction has produced hydrocephalus.

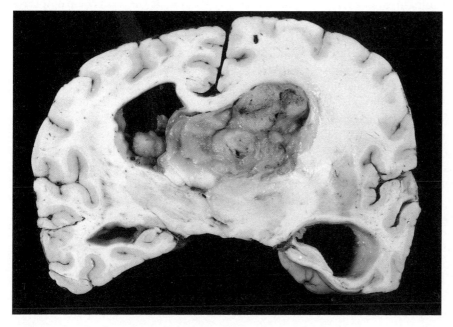

Figure 3-104
SUBEPENDYMAL GIANT
CELL ASTROCYTOMA
(TUBEROUS SCLEROSIS)

This large fleshy mass straddles the midline and produces marked dilatation of the lateral ventricles.

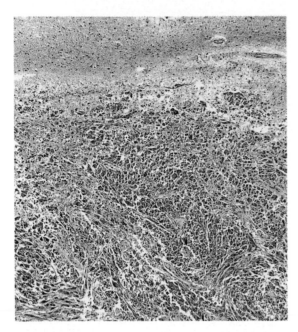

Figure 3-105
SUBEPENDYMAL GIANT CELL ASTROCYTOMA
(TUBEROUS SCLEROSIS)
In contrast to ordinary fibrillary astrocytomas, subependymal giant cell astrocytomas are discrete masses which abut the ventricular wall. Infiltration of underlying or partly surrounding brain parenchyma is minimal.

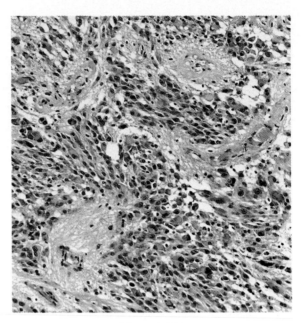

Figure 3-106
SUBEPENDYMAL GIANT CELL ASTROCYTOMA
(TUBEROUS SCLEROSIS)
At low magnification, the large cells have a somewhat fascicular or swirled appearance. In most cases, cells appear to sweep from vessels in a perivascular pseudorosette-like fashion.

Despite the distinctive astrocytic quality of the abundant pink cytoplasm and a fibrillar background, the cells of SEGA differ from more stellate reactive astrocytes in that their eccentric nuclei lie within copious cytoplasm and their asymmetric processes emanate from the cell surface opposite the nucleus rather than uniformly from the entire circumference of the cell.

The cells, either multipolar or bipolar, possess distinctly eosinophilic and, in a minority of cases, "brick red" cytoplasm. Somewhat vesicular chromatin, distinct nucleoli, and intranuclear cytoplasmic inclusions are common features. Mitoses vary in number from case to case: they are infrequent in half the cases and are only rarely readily apparent. Calcospherites and vascular calcification are frequently observed. Scattered mast cells are a regular feature. Vascular proliferation and necrosis are uncommon and should prompt consideration of a high-grade fibrillary or diffuse astrocytoma.

Immunohistochemical Findings. Despite their overtly astrocytic appearance, the cells are variably, and often only focally or weakly, immu-noreactive for GFAP (fig. 3-108). In contrast, S-100 protein reactivity is more widespread and stronger. Some cells are reactive for neuronal markers such as neurofilament protein and class III beta-tubulin (245). This mixed immunophenotype suggests that the tumors are heterogeneous or hybrid in nature, expressing structural proteins of both glial and neuronal cells (243,245). As is the case for large cells within the tubers, the giant cell astrocytes are immunoreactive for alpha-β-crystallin (247).

Ultrastructural Findings. Intermediate filaments vary greatly in number and disposition within neoplastic cells and their processes (243, 244,253). Some cells are relatively lacking in fibrils and possess more in the way of electron-dense lysosomes and small Nissl-like stacks of rough endoplasmic reticulum. Unlike some of the large cells in tubers, those of SEGA lack the bona fide features of neuronal differentiation, secretory granules, vesicles, and synapses, but may exhibit microtubules within their processes (250).

Differential Diagnosis. Given the variation in morphologic pattern and cytology, the differential diagnosis of SEGA includes a number of lesions,

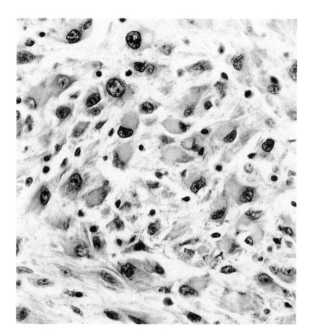

Figure 3-107
SUBEPENDYMAL GIANT CELL ASTROCYTOMA
(TUBEROUS SCLEROSIS)
Most tumors possess full-bodied, somewhat epithelioid cells. Given their glassy cytoplasm, eccentric nuclei, and prominent nucleoli, they have a neuronal appearance.

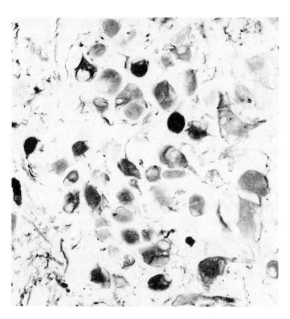

Figure 3-108
SUBEPENDYMAL GIANT CELL ASTROCYTOMA
(TUBEROUS SCLEROSIS)
Immunoreactivity for GFAP is highly variable, both within and between tumors. This lesion shows gradations of reactivity from negative to strongly positive.

which are generally eliminated by attention to histologic as well as clinical and radiographic features. The presence of pink cytoplasm, cell processes, and cytoplasmic GFAP positivity combine to mimic the histologic appearance of gemistocytic astrocytoma. The latter is an intraparenchymal lesion rather than a well-demarcated, exophytic, intraventricular mass. Furthermore, gemistocytic astrocytomas are infiltrative and therefore contain remnants of overrun parenchyma, such as myelinated axons, neurons, and reactive astrocytes. Cytologically, neoplastic gemistocytic astrocytes are usually somewhat smaller than those of SEGA, are diffusely distributed rather than patterned, and possess a uniform pericellular corona of short processes, whereas those of the SEGA emanate from one pole of the cell. Gemistocytic tumors typically lack intranuclear cytoplasmic inclusions as well as mast cells and calcifications. Despite the finding of some atypia and occasional mitoses in SEGA, malignant transformation to glioblastoma, a frequent occurrence in gemistocytic astrocytomas, is not a common feature.

Treatment and Prognosis. Serial radiographic studies have established beyond question that subependymal lesions are capable of progressive growth (249). The postoperative course is uniformly favorable, however, since even large lesions can be excised or debulked and enlargement of residual tissue is slow. The same favorable outlook accompanies lesions with mitoses, microvascular proliferation, and even foci of necrosis (246,252). Treatment is usually limited to surgical excision. Long-term survival is excellent, although, recurrence or death is possible (252).

Infantile Desmoplastic Astrocytoma

Definition. A highly desmoplastic, superficially situated, supratentorial glioma of the young.

General Comments. Infantile desmoplastic tumors (IDAs) often contain a ganglion cell component (see Desmoplastic Infantile Gangliocytoma). If, despite a careful search, these neurons are not identified in otherwise identical tumors, the designation infantile desmoplastic astrocytoma is applied (254,254a,255). It remains to be seen whether these two types of neoplasm are distinct entities or variations of one.

Clinical and Radiographic Features. These rare, superficially situated, often hemispheric masses are generally detected during the first year of life.

Macroscopic Findings. Intraoperatively, the lesions appear as large, firm, pancake-like or globular masses often densely adherent to the surface of the brain and, on occasion, the meninges including the dura (255). Reported cases have been supratentorial.

Microscopic Findings. The most distinctive feature of IDA is its intense desmoplasia which lends a reactive fibrotic, rather than neoplastic, low-power appearance. Many consist of a mass of paucicellular collagen-rich tissue sharply demarcated from underlying brain, intruding only along the perivascular (Virchow-Robin) spaces. Scattered elongated glial cells, which at first appear as fibroblasts, are strongly positive for GFAP. Elsewhere, even in H&E stained sections, nodules or lobules of cells more obviously astrocytic are seen. Occasionally, the glial foci exhibit perivascular pseudorosette formation, a pattern suggesting ependymoma.

Focally, IDAs often show patchy or extensive areas of high cellularity in which hyperchromasia, cellular elongation, and mitotic activity are apparent. In combination, these create the impression of a malignant tumor. Indeed, it is sometimes difficult to accept that such worrisome cellular tissue can be part of a neoplasm with a favorable prognosis.

Immunohistochemical Findings. Intense immunoreactivity for GFAP is a prominent feature, both in areas that are obviously glial as well as in the densely desmoplastic component containing only isolated immunopositive cells.

Differential Diagnosis. IDA should be high on the list of superficially situated desmoplastic tumors in patients less than 1 year of age. A diagnosis of sarcoma, malignant glioma, or gliosarcoma may be erroneously entertained if attention is focused solely upon markedly cellular areas.

Treatment and Prognosis. Despite this lesion's large size and the presence of focal mitotic activity, even subtotally resected IDAs have been associated with longstanding postoperative stabilization. The superficial location has made total excision possible in some cases.

Gliofibroma

Definition. A tumor containing both glia and abundant fibrous connective tissue.

General Comments. The gliofibroma is an extremely rare and as yet incompletely characterized tumor. A variety of benign and malignant lesions have been loosely included under this designation. By one analysis, gliofibromas are those tumors in which collagen is formed directly by astrocytes, and can range from well differentiated to anaplastic. Such lesions need to be distinguished from tumors with both glial and mesenchymal elements. The latter includes the common gliosarcoma, where vessels are the presumed source of the sarcoma and the rare mixed glioma/fibroma (257).

Clinical and Radiographic Features. The rarity of gliofibroma precludes comments regarding its typical clinical and radiographic features. Most of the few published cases have occurred in children (258,259,261,262,), but the tumor also appears in adulthood (260). Both the brain (258,260–262) and the spinal cord (256, 259,262) have been affected.

Macroscopic Findings. The lesions are relatively well-circumscribed firm masses.

Microscopic Findings. Gliofibromas exhibit an intimate admixture of fibrous connective tissue and glia (fig. 3-109). The former often predominates and is composed of bundles or dense hyaline zones. Collagen and reticulin staining is abundant. The glial component appears as islands, cords, or single cells enmeshed in the mesenchymal stroma (256,259,260). Mitoses are rare.

Other reported cases expand this generic description by the addition of pattern variations or other tissue components including densely compact spindle cell areas (262), foci of pleomorphic multinucleated cells (260), foci of high mitotic activity (261), overt histologic malignancy (258), and the presence of a possible Schwann cell component (262).

Immunohistochemical Findings. The glial element is positive for GFAP (fig. 3-110) and S-100 protein. "Schwannian" components are strongly reactive for S-100 protein.

Ultrastructural Findings. Ultrastructural studies have established the presence of fibroblasts, glial cells, and occasional trapped axons. Individual cells wrapped in basement membranes

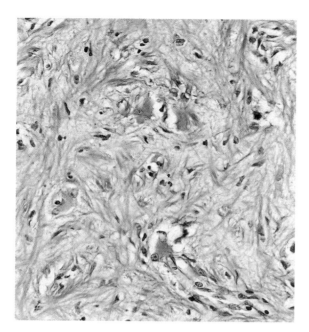

Figure 3-109
GLIOFIBROMA
The gliofibroma is a paucicellular mass in which cells or small lobules of neoplastic glia are enmeshed in a dense connective tissue stroma.

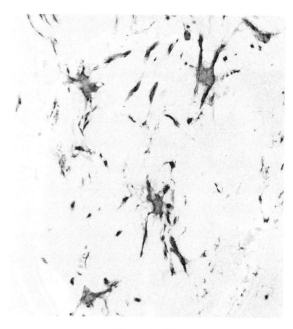

Figure 3-110
GLIOFIBROMA
The glial nature of the aggregated, often fibrillar cells is readily apparent on immunostaining for GFAP.

may be noted in gliofibromas (258,259,261) and have been considered Schwann cells by some (262). The juxtaposition of collagen fibers with glial processes suggests that the glial cells of this lesion are collagen forming (257,258).

Differential Diagnosis. Since, as a clinicopathologic entity, gliofibroma is poorly understood, it is difficult in concept and practice to differentiate it from various other collagen-rich glial lesions. It remains unclear whether those with Schwann cell features (glioneurofibroma) represent the same entity as that historically described as a gliofibroma.

Treatment and Prognosis. The paucity of reported cases and their histologic variation precludes definitive comments regarding prognosis. Some examples represent incidental collagen-rich lesional foci with little, if any, potential for progression, whereas others have contained anaplastic glial elements that seeded the subarachnoid space (258). It is a subject of debate whether anaplastic, mitotically active tumors should be included among gliofibromas since this lesion is considered by some to be an indolent, benign, or even reactive process.

OLIGODENDROGLIAL NEOPLASMS

Oligodendroglioma and Anaplastic (Malignant) Oligodendroglioma

Definition. Infiltrative gliomas composed of oligodendrocytes.

Clinical and Radiographic Features. Oligodendrogliomas arise throughout the neuraxis, but primarily affect the cerebral hemispheres, especially the frontal lobes. Examples in the spinal cord are rare. Although there is a general perception that these tumors are uncommon, they are nearly as frequent as well-differentiated astrocytomas of the diffuse or fibrillary type. Patients with oligodendrogliomas usually present in adulthood with any of the usual consequences of an infiltrating expanding intracranial neoplasm (278). Many patients experience a long history of seizures, sometimes of a decade or more. MRI can now detect oligodendrogliomas earlier in life, even in childhood, and at an earlier stage of evolution (283,287a).

The diagnosis of oligodendrogliomas is suggested preoperatively when intratumoral or peritumoral calcification is noted on neuroimaging studies (see Appendix E). The diagnosis is

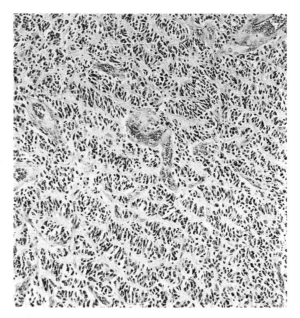

Figure 3-116
OLIGODENDROGLIOMA
Alignment of tumor cells into ribbons or palisades is seen in a minority of cases.

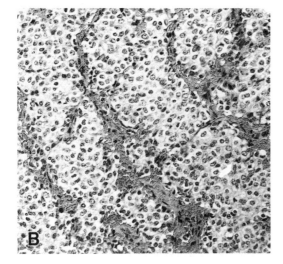

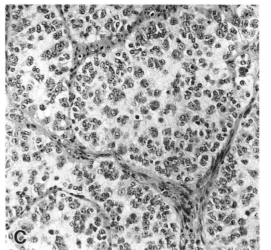

Figure 3-117
PATTERNS IN OLIGODENDROGLIOMA
Distinctive tissue patterns in oligodendroglioma include compact architecture with prominent microcysts (A), islands of neoplastic cells separated by vascular septa (B), and lobules in which clusters of cells lend an epithelioid or somewhat cartilaginous quality (C).

The "fried egg" artifact is a distinctive feature of many oligodendrogliomas, created by autolytic imbibition of water accompanying delayed fixation (figs. 3-112, 3-113). This process forms clear perinuclear halos, which at low power produce the "honeycomb" appearance characteristic of the tumor. While this artifact is diagnostically valuable, it is not always present (fig. 3-118). When fixation is prompt and halos are absent, the diagnosis must be reached on the basis of other criteria. Perinuclear clearing is often lacking in specimens frozen prior to paraffin embedding as is discussed below. Furthermore, in oligodendrogliomas previously frozen, nuclei are often condensed and angulated, and cytoplasm becomes indistinct from surrounding normal tissue (fig. 3-119). The features of such biopsies mimic those of ordinary fibrillary astrocytomas. The cytoplasm of neoplastic astrocytes is most prominent in previously frozen tissue.

Most oligodendroglial neoplasms are associated with calcification, either within the tumor or in surrounding brain. This is particularly true in the cerebral cortex.

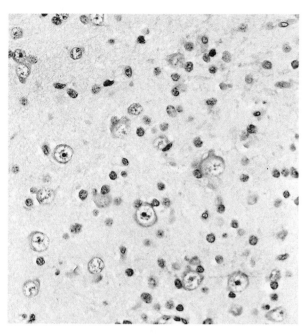

Figure 3-118
OLIGODENDROGLIOMA

In the absence of perinuclear halos, the diagnosis of oligodendroglioma depends upon other features such as uniformity and roundness of nuclei, as well as extensive cortical infiltration.

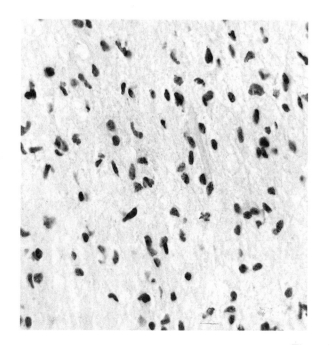

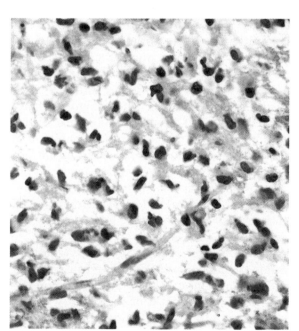

Figure 3-119
OLIGODENDROGLIOMA IN PREVIOUSLY FROZEN TISSUE

Left: Prior freezing can have a profound effect on the cytologic characteristics of neoplastic oligodendrocytes. The appearance of a high-grade astrocytic neoplasm is created by artifactual nuclear hyperchromatism and angulation.

Right: In other settings, a lower-grade astrocytoma appears evident when the amount of the oligodendrocytic cytoplasm is exaggerated.

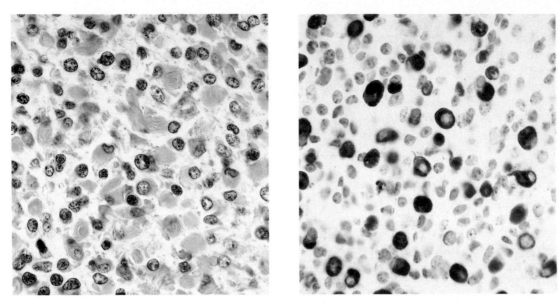

Figure 3-120
OLIGODENDROGLIOMA
Left: Microgemistocytic cells with an eccentric body of glassy or finely fibrillar cytoplasm are commonly encountered in oligodendrogliomas, particularly those of intermediate or higher grade.
Right: The filament-rich cytoplasm of such cells is intensely reactive for GFAP.

At medium and high magnification, the nuclei of optimally processed oligodendroglioma cells come into focus as round and generally uniform. Scattered larger hyperchromatic cells are noted more often than overt nuclear pleomorphism. Not surprisingly, the density and distribution of chromatin varies with histologic grade. In well-differentiated lesions, nuclei are only slightly larger than normal oligodendroglia and exhibit a minor increase in chromatin density and coarseness, and in nucleolar size. As a rule, mitoses are absent or sparse. In higher-grade tumors, chromatin density increases, as does anisonucleocytosis, nucleolar prominence, and mitotic activity. In all grades, however, the majority of nuclei are round.

Another helpful feature in the diagnosis of oligodendroglioma is the character and distribution of its vasculature (fig. 3-112). Blood vessels in better differentiated tumors typically consist of short capillary segments arranged geometrically to resemble the patterned angulation of "chicken wire." In anaplastic lesions, thickening of vessels due to hypertrophy and hyperplasia of vascular cells is common, but the prominent glomerular tufts so characteristic of glioblastoma are not usually prominent.

Reactive astrocytes are, to some extent, a regular accompaniment of all infiltrative gliomas, but are particularly obvious in oligodendrogliomas, where they appear as evenly distributed stellate cells with delicate nuclei, a moderate amount of eosinophilic cytoplasm, and long uniform radiating processes. They are strikingly positive for GFAP. Such cells should not engender a diagnosis of mixed oligodendroglioma-astrocytoma (oligoastrocytoma).

In any oligodendroglioma, with the possible exception of highly differentiated examples, neoplastic cells with eccentric, hyaline eosinophilic intracytoplasmic bodies are found (fig. 3-120) (268, 271,272,285). Alternatively, the cytoplasm may be filled with brightly eosinophilic bands of fibrillar material which form paranuclear whorls or encircle nuclei (pl. IVC, p. 101). The resemblance to an inclusion body is most apparent when the whorls displace the nucleus. Some especially highly fibrillated cells also contain small eosinophilic bodies resembling Rosenthal fibers (figs. 3-121, 3-122). Collectively, such rotund GFAP-positive cells tend to be most prominent in perivascular regions. Variously referred to as signet ring cells, gliofibrillary oligodendrocytes, or microgemistocytes or minigemistocytes, they have a decided astrocytic

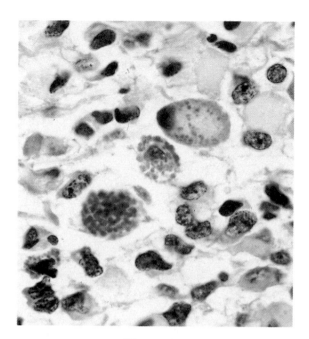

Figure 3-121
OLIGODENDROGLIOMA
Occasional oligodendrogliomas contain cells with minute, refractile eosinophilic bodies representing miniature Rosenthal fibers.

quality, despite their clearly oligodendroglial nuclear features and coexistence with obvious oligodendrocytes devoid of these cytoplasmic changes (268,271,272,274). Short processes may emanate from these cells, although they lack the angulated or elongated nuclei and the polarity of neoplastic astrocytes. We consider these cells oligodendrocytes rather than astrocytes and do not classify neoplasms with such elements as mixed gliomas.

More cellular high-grade oligodendrogliomas often contain tumor cells more astrocytic in appearance in terms of their cell profile, cytoplasmic fibrillarity, and process formation, yet retain their round to oval nuclei as if reluctant to relinquish their oligodendroglial heritage (fig. 3-123). In other cases, a portion of the tumor is inescapably and genuinely astrocytic. We consider these tumors to be mixed glioma or oligoastrocytoma.

Grading. A number of studies have confirmed the prognostic significance of certain histologic features, although not all investigations identified the same factors as being relevant.

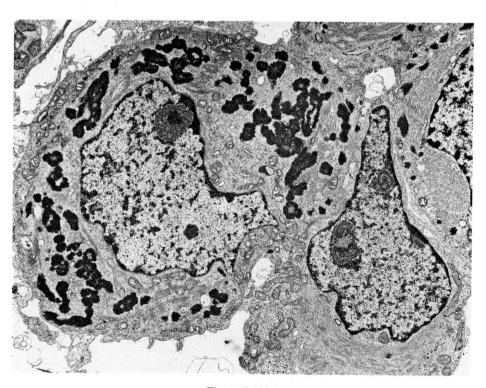

Figure 3-122
OLIGODENDROGLIOMA
Ultrastructurally, the small cytoplasmic bodies seen in figure 3-121 have the marked electron density seen in classic larger Rosenthal fibers. Note the abundance of intermediate filaments.

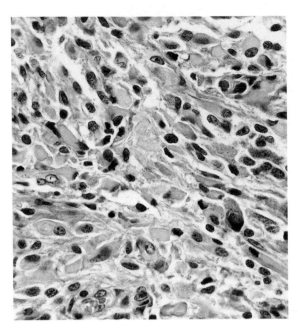

Figure 3-123
OLIGODENDROGLIOMA
The cells of some oligodendrogliomas acquire sufficient cytoplasm and process formation to become decidedly astrocytic, but their nuclei retain the roundness, uniformity, and chromatin distribution typical of oligodendroglioma.

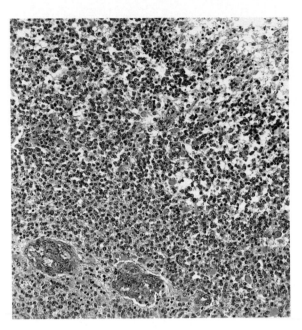

Figure 3-124
ANAPLASTIC OLIGODENDROGLIOMA
At low magnification, this markedly cellular neoplasm exhibits both vascular proliferation and necrosis.

These features include: increased cellularity, microcysts, cytologic atypia, mitotic activity, vascular hypertrophy, vascular proliferation, pleomorphism, and necrosis (263,273,275,279,287). Despite statistical data clearly demonstrating that microcysts and low cellularity are favorable factors, and that the others are unfavorable, there is presently no consensus on the definition of histologic grades or whether a two-, three-, or four-tiered scheme is optimal. The significance of focal nodules of higher-grade tumor in an otherwise well-differentiated oligodendroglioma is uncertain. There is a relationship between patient age and degree of anaplasia on one hand, and the length of survival on the other, but the association is not as pronounced as in patients with diffuse or fibrillary astrocytomas (263,272,275).

Our own experience suggests that the tumors can be subdivided profitably into well-differentiated oligodendrogliomas and malignant or anaplastic lesions. The well-differentiated category contains both paucicellular lesions with minimal cytologic atypia as well as the more cellular classic oligodendroglioma. We do not, however, make a distinction between these for diagnostic purposes. Well-differentiated tumors correspond roughly to the combined grades A and B of the system proposed by Smith et al. (273,275,287). Better differentiated lesions include the often small, occasionally only microscopic, tumors consisting of cells with little more than increased cell density and nuclear size and chromasia to distinguish them from normal oligodendrocytes (fig. 3-118). A faint basophilic mucoid matrix may be apparent in some. Such "grade A" lesions should prompt consideration of an important differential diagnostic entity, dysembryoplastic neuroepithelial tumor.

The classic oligodendroglioma is hypercellular and deviates from normal nuclear size, chromatin density, and nucleolar prominence (fig. 3-112). Mitoses, if any, are few and blood vessels, though increased in number, are delicate. The malignant or anaplastic oligodendroglioma is a frankly cellular tumor with considerable nuclear hyperchromasia, conspicuous mitotic activity, and often vascular hypertrophy or proliferation (figs. 3-124, 3-125). Necrosis may be present. Limited perinecrotic pseudopalisading is seen in some

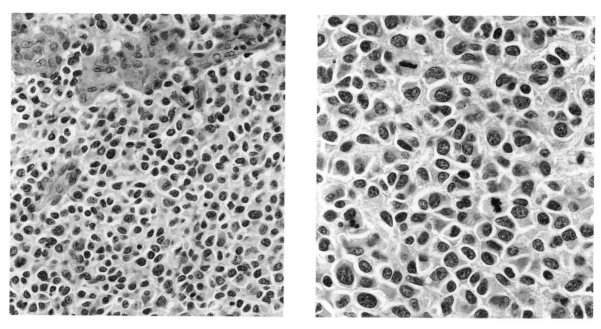

Figure 3-125
ANAPLASTIC OLIGODENDROGLIOMA
Left: Anaplastic oligodendrogliomas are highly cellular and associated with vascular proliferation.
Right: The high mitotic activity and cytologic atypia are seen at high magnification. Note the skirts of eosinophilic cytoplasm not uncommon in malignant oligodendrogliomas.

cases but is often absent. Despite cytologic malignancy and considerable cellularity, anaplastic lesions retain the nuclear uniformity so characteristic of oligodendrogliomas. The chicken wire vasculature of the well-differentiated oligodendroglioma tends also to be preserved, often frequently with hypertrophy or hyperplasia of vascular cells and adventitial elements. In some cases a prominent lobularity is seen. As discussed above, a number of malignant oligodendrogliomas contain large numbers of neoplastic cells with astrocyte-like cytoplasm but the nuclei of oligodendrocytes.

The relationship of oligodendroglioma to glioblastoma multiforme remains problematic. While most malignant oligodendrogliomas do not, by our criteria, evolve into glioblastomas, occasional cases seem to make this transition (fig. 3-126). There is no sharp line of distinction between an anaplastic glioma which is unequivocally oligodendroglial and one with cellular anaplasia, marked vascular proliferation, and palisading necrosis resembling ordinary glioblastoma, an essentially astrocytic tumor. This issue is discussed below under Differential Diagnosis.

Frozen Section and Cytology. The frozen section process often robs oligodendroglial tumors of one of their most characteristic features: perinuclear halos (fig. 3-127). Nevertheless, the correct diagnosis is suspected if extensive cortical infiltration with perineuronal satellitosis and subpial accumulation are seen. The general roundness of nuclei, although altered by the freezing process, is largely retained and is more pronounced than in astrocytomas of comparable grade.

The adverse effects and diagnostic pitfalls introduced by the freezing process can be circumvented by the concurrent use of cytologic methods. These emphasize nuclear roundness, some prominence of nucleoli, and the presence of an eccentric skirt of cytoplasm (pl. IVB, p. 101). Paucity of cytoplasmic processes is another important feature, although there is often more background fibrillarity on smears than one would expect looking at the histologic sections alone. The presence of signet ring cells, which are easily seen in frozen sections, should also prompt consideration of oligodendroglioma (pl. IVC).

Anaplastic oligodendroglial neoplasms, although highly cellular and replete with malignant

astrocytic neoplasms of comparable grades (286). The fate of patients with small lesions detected early by MRI is unclear and the outlook may be considerably more favorable (287a). In some series, shorter survival periods have been reported in older patients (273,289); this is not seen in other studies (280). Historically, postoperative therapy centered upon radiation with or without chemotherapy. There is evidence, however, that many oligodendrogliomas respond favorably to chemotherapy (264,265,267) and this may be the treatment of choice for some patients. The efficacy of radiotherapy appears maximal in at least partially resected tumors (276,288). As is the case in other gliomas, extracranial metastasis is rare (269,270).

The need for postoperative radiotherapy and chemotherapy in small, very well-differentiated lesions remains to be justified. Similarly, the extent to which aggressive surgery should be undertaken is also unclear. Although surgical cure would seem most likely for focal well-differentiated tumors, enthusiasm for extirpative surgery is counterbalanced by uncertainty regarding the natural history of such small lesions as well as the neurologic deficits that accompany large volume resections.

Oligodendrogliomas exhibit a propensity for tumor progression or malignant degeneration similar to fibrillary astrocytic neoplasms, but the process evolves more slowly. The prognostic significance of an astrocytoma component (oligoastrocytoma) is discussed in the section, Mixed Gliomas.

EPENDYMAL NEOPLASMS

Ependymoma and Anaplastic (Malignant) Ependymoma

Definition. Neoplasms of ependymal cells.

General Features. Ependymomas arise throughout the neuraxis in intimate relationship to the ependyma or its remnants. Exceptions include rare ectopic examples involving the presacral or postsacral soft tissue as well as intracranial tumors far removed from the ventricular system. Truly exceptional examples have been reported in such improbable sites as the mediastinum, lung, ovary, or broad ligament (312). Intracranial lesions occur most often in childhood, although adults are also affected (295, 298,304,309). Most spinal ependymomas occur in adults (309,318–320).

From a geographic point of view both clinically and radiographically, ependymomas are considered to be intracranial, intraspinal, or sacral, lying either in bone or soft tissue. Intracranial lesions are further categorized as supratentorial or infratentorial (fourth ventricular) (see Appendix F). Intraspinal examples lie either within the spinal cord proper or the filum terminale (see Appendix G). Ependymomas of the filum, as well as rare ectopic examples in soft tissues about the sacrum, usually have a distinctive myxopapillary appearance as discussed below. Only a rare myxopapillary variant is intracranial (306).

Clinical and Radiographic Features. Supratentorial ependymomas typically produce symptoms of increased intracranial pressure or local mass effects, whereas those in the posterior fossa more readily elevate intracranial pressure by obstructing the flow of cerebrospinal fluid. In the latter site, ependymomas are more likely than medulloblastomas to produce cranial nerve deficits. Ependymomas of the spinal cord induce patterns of motor and sensory deficit reflecting their segmental level. Myxopapillary lesions in the filum terminale compress nerve roots, with most patients experiencing pain, lower extremity weakness, and sphincter dysfunction (318,320).

Radiographically, the frequent calcification of intracranial ependymomas is a key factor in the differential diagnosis of posterior fossa tumors since there is usually no calcification in medulloblastomas (see Appendix E). On MRI, ependymomas are largely intraventricular or paraventricular masses (fig. 3-130) (322). Supratentorial examples are often associated with a cyst (see Appendix D). Intraspinal ependymomas are readily identified on MRI with gadolinium contrast agent and seen as discrete, sausage-shaped, enhancing masses. In contrast to intracranial lesions, they are rarely calcified, but frequently include a cyst or induce a fluid-filled cavity (syrinx) in the adjacent cord, either above or below the lesion.

Macroscopic Findings. Supratentorial ependymomas intrude upon the ventricular system but also enlarge centrifugally into the surrounding brain where they present to the surgeon as fleshy gray and, most importantly, relatively discrete masses. Since the epicenter in the ventricular zone may not be apparent, the diagnosis may not be suspected when approached laterally. The ventricular relationship is more evident in

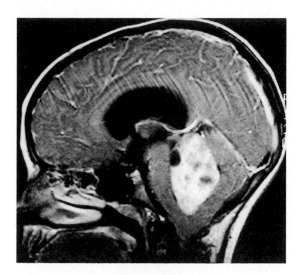

Figure 3-130
EPENDYMOMA
Ependymomas such as this fourth ventricle tumor are discrete and contrast enhancing. (Courtesy of Dr. Frederick B. Askin, Baltimore, MD.)

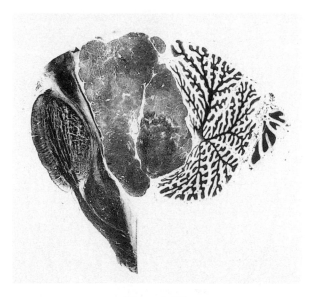

Figure 3-131
EPENDYMOMA
The discrete nature of ependymomas, as well as their tendency to involve the ventricular system, is well illustrated in this whole mount histologic section of a fourth ventricle lesion.

posterior fossa ependymomas since they are typically accessed from within the fourth ventricle which they fill from their origin on its floor (fig. 3-131). These same lesions may also extend into the lateral recesses from which they gain access to the subarachnoid space at the cerebellopontine angle via the foramen of Luschka or into the cisterna magna (fig. 3-132). They may also develop primarily outside the ventricle from the dorsal surface of the lateral medullary velum. Rare examples occur within the leptomeninges.

Intraspinal ependymomas are discrete, gray, soft, noncalcified, and often associated with a syrinx in the adjacent cord (see Appendices D, G). Occasional tumors are intrinsically cystic. The myxopapillary tumors arise from the filum terminale but may extend to involve the conus medullaris as well (fig. 3-133). Intraoperatively it may be difficult to distinguish the filum, the delicate fibrovascular extension of the spinal cord, from adjacent nerve roots, which are similar in caliber and to which ependymomas as well as other regional tumors may be secondarily attached. Many myxopapillary neoplasms resemble delicately encapsulated "bags" of soft tan tissue. The tumor may spontaneously break out of the delicate capsule and seed the subarachnoid space prior to surgery.

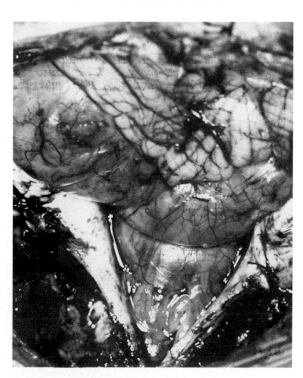

Figure 3-132
EPENDYMOMA
Fourth ventricle ependymomas frequently extend out of the ventricle into the subarachnoid space. (Courtesy of Dr. E. Michael Scott, Boston, MA.)

121

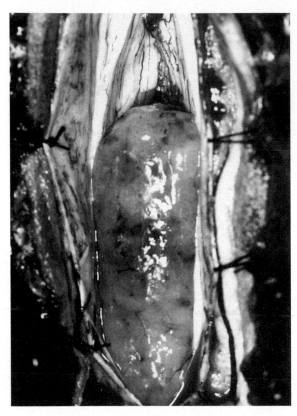

Figure 3-133
MYXOPAPILLARY EPENDYMOMA
Myxopapillary ependymomas are soft, gray, discrete masses which almost always arise from the filum terminale. (Courtesy of Dr. E. Michael Scott, Boston, MA.)

Microscopic Findings. As a rule, ependymomas are well-circumscribed masses that displace rather than infiltrate brain parenchyma (fig. 3-131). Somewhat greater infiltration may be seen in overtly malignant examples and in rare mixed gliomas in which foci of ependymal differentiation accompany a more infiltrative form of glioma, most often astrocytoma. The nuclei of ependymomas are generally uniform, moderately hyperchromatic, and vary from round to elongated. Nucleoli, though small, are generally distinct. Increased nuclear-cytoplasmic ratios and brisk mitotic activity are features of malignant examples but, in contrast to other malignant gliomas, such lesions usually lack significant nuclear pleomorphism.

The *classic ependymoma*, whether of the brain or spinal cord proper, demonstrates the so-called cellular pattern (fig. 3-134). Its cells lie close to one another, forming a moderately cellular lobular tumor often punctuated by areas of diminished cellularity or of nuclear free zones. The latter appear fibrillar and usually form perivascular zones in which tumor cell processes converge upon vessel walls, an arrangement known as the perivascular pseudorosette (fig. 3-135). The diameter of such pseudorosettes varies considerably, but nearly all ependymomas exhibit this diagnostically helpful feature. It is

Figure 3-134
EPENDYMOMA
The dense cellularity of the cellular ependymoma is interrupted by anuclear perivascular fibrillar zones termed perivascular pseudorosettes.

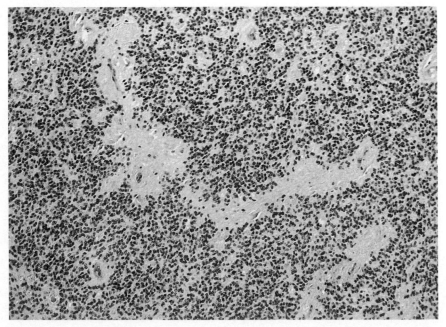

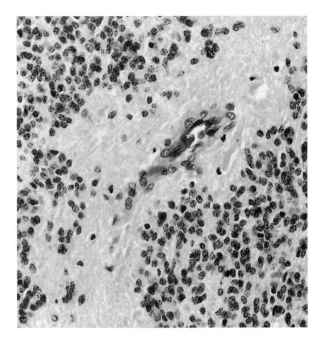

Figure 3-135
EPENDYMOMA
The fibrillarity within perivascular pseudorosettes is apparent at high magnification.

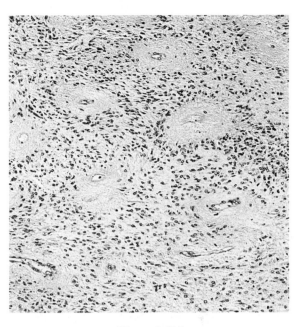

Figure 3-136
EPENDYMOMA
Perivascular pseudorosettes may be inconspicuous in paucicellular tumors.

difficult, if not ill-advised, to render a diagnosis of ependymoma in their absence. Pseudorosettes can be distinguished from nonspecific perivascular collagenous deposition, a feature found in many brain tumors, either by application of collagen stains or by demonstrating immunoreactivity for GFAP. The distinction of perivascular pseudorosettes from the perivascular fibrillar zones of neuroblastic tumors is discussed below under Differential Diagnosis. In some ependymomas of low cellularity, the difference in nuclear density between the parenchyma of the tumor and the perivascular regions is not great and the rosettes are less obvious (fig. 3-136). In such tumors there are often fibrillar areas which, though they include vessels, are so large that they cannot be considered strictly perivascular (fig. 3-137). The impression of an astrocytoma is created when these regions make up the majority of a tumor. As is discussed in the section on Mixed Gliomas, we consider such tumors as ependymal rather than mixed in composition. Demarcation of such lesions on CT or MRI scan supports this contention.

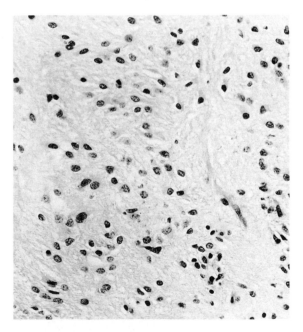

Figure 3-137
EPENDYMOMA
At high magnification, some fibrillar zones of ependymomas, particularly large or poorly organized ones, may be misinterpreted as astrocytoma.

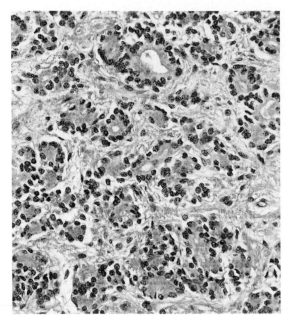

Figure 3-138
EPENDYMOMA
Only in occasional ependymomas are small gland-like structures with clearly defined central lumina, ependymal rosettes, the predominant feature.

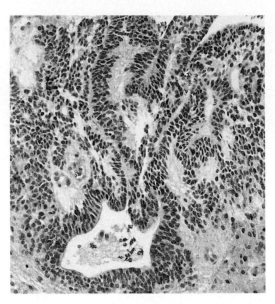

Figure 3-140
EPENDYMOMA
Only infrequently do ependymomas have epithelial surfaces so extensive and complex as to justify the term papillary. Even in these instances, the papillae have a perivascular glial stroma rather than broad fibrovascular cores.

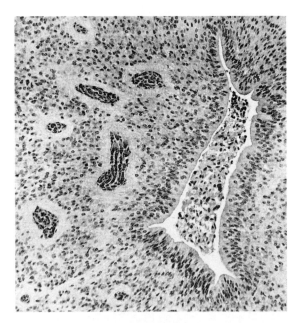

Figure 3-139
EPENDYMOMA
The epithelial phenotype of ependymoma is expressed as ependymal canals at the right of the illustration. Note the perivascular pseudorosettes at the left.

Some ependymomas express obvious epithelial features in the form of round rosettes with central lumina (true ependymal rosettes) (fig. 3-138), canals, or simple or elaborate expanses of epithelial surface (fig. 3-139). The true ependymal rosette consists of columnar epithelium surrounding a distinct lumen, an arrangement not to be confused with the less structured perivascular pseudorosette with its vascular core surrounded by radiating, often tapering, cell processes. True rosettes range from microscopic clusters of cells within which lumina may be easily overlooked, to large tubules or canals which are inescapably epithelial. As a rule, there is a mixture of rosettes and canals of varying size and configuration. Interestingly, these structures are usually seen in ependymomas with considerable background fibrillarity rather than emerging within densely cellular tumors. *Papillary ependymomas* or tumors exhibiting extensive surface epithelium are rare in our experience and do not assume the frond-like, overtly papillary quality of choroid plexus papilloma (fig. 3-140). They also lack the smooth contoured, light microscopically apparent basement membranes found in choroid plexus tumors.

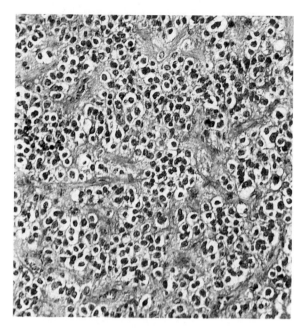

Figure 3-141
CLEAR CELL EPENDYMOMA
Perinuclear clearing similar to that seen in oligodendrogliomas is a prominent feature of the clear cell variant. Note the vague perivascular pseudorosettes. The lesion was a discrete occipital intraventricular mass.

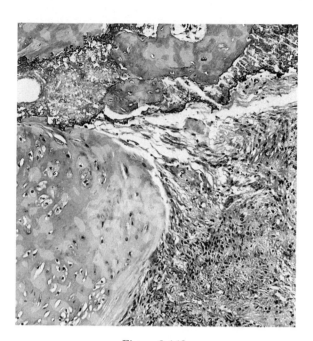

Figure 3-142
EPENDYMOMA
Osseous and cartilaginous metaplasia are rare.

In many otherwise typical ependymomas, focal perinuclear halos and nuclear uniformity create a distinct oligodendroglial appearance. Despite the histologic similarity of these clear cells to oligodendrocytes, such lesions do not warrant a diagnosis of a mixed glioma (ependymoma-oligodendroglioma). Some intracranial tumors composed almost entirely of such cells form an incompletely studied subtype of ependymoma, the so-called *clear cell ependymoma*, which has many of the microscopic characteristics of oligodendroglioma (fig. 3-141) (302). These features include striking nuclear uniformity, perinuclear halos, and angulated capillaries. In contrast to the oligodendroglioma, however, this ependymoma is discrete, largely noninfiltrating, and at least focally exhibits perivascular pseudorosette formation. In addition, the tumor's ultrastructural features are clearly ependymal.

Particularly in fourth ventricular ependymomas, a focal subependymoma pattern is created by the clustering of nuclei within a circumferentially sweeping matrix. This pattern is exclusive in the subependymoma. Little prognostic significance is attached to the finding of a subependymoma pattern in an otherwise typical ependymoma. Occasional ependymomas contain bone or cartilage (fig. 3-142) (307).

An unusual variant of ependymoma is the *tanycytic type* which expresses the cellular elongation typical of a specialized form of ependymal cell (297). This tumor differs from classic ependymoma in its composition of markedly elongated cells, with highly fibrillar processes that produce an appearance somewhat resembling pilocytic astrocytoma (fig. 3-143). An ill-defined pattern of perivascular pseudorosetting is best seen at low power. By and large, tanycytic lesions are well differentiated and mitoses are rare. Given its low cellularity and somewhat haphazard architecture, the pathologist may misinterpret the lesion as astrocytic and not attempt resection.

Although occasional examples of *myxopapillary ependymoma* arise intracranially or within the spinal cord, the variant is restricted to the filum terminale and, rarely, to presacral or postsacral tissues where an origin from ependymal rests is presumed (313).

Myxopapillary lesions are noteworthy for their pseudopapillary architecture, perivascular and

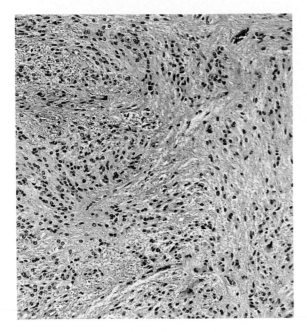

Figure 3-143
TANYCYTIC EPENDYMOMA
Paucicellularity, inconspicuous perivascular pseudorosettes, and a somewhat fascicular architecture are typical of the tanycytic variant.

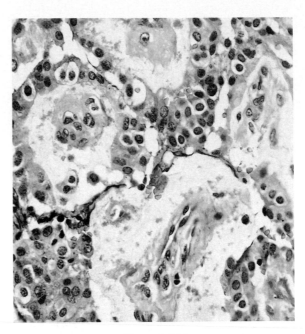

Figure 3-145
MYXOPAPILLARY EPENDYMOMA
Broad collars of mucin about blood vessels are diagnostically useful features of this lesion.

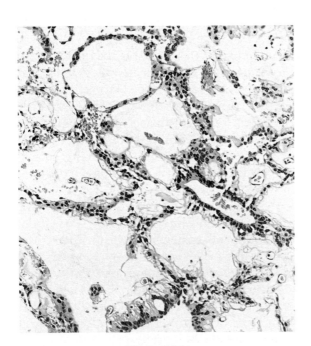

Figure 3-144
MYXOPAPILLARY EPENDYMOMA
Epithelial surfaces and abundant perivascular collars of mucin are classic features of this distinctive ependymoma variant.

intercellular mucin deposition, and a tendency to cellular elongation (fig. 3-144). Mucin, which is readily highlighted by the PAS or Alcian blue stains, is the lesion's most conspicuous diagnostic feature. It can occur as large extravascular pools but is typically and characteristically confined to the walls of blood vessels (fig. 3-145). In the conventional lesion, neoplastic cells are either columnar (epithelial) or elongated (glial) and show only minor variation in nuclear shape, size, and chromasia. Adherence of the cells to the vessels produces a somewhat papillary appearance, but the tumor only infrequently possesses true papillae. In some cases, the mucin is so extensive as to separate the neoplastic cells and produce a mucoid lesion that mimics chordoma or carcinoma. In other cases the glial cytology predominates so that a fibrillary background is present and mucin, if any, is confined to small vascular deposits. Such tumors may resemble neurilemmoma (fig. 3-146). Additional features of myxopapillary lesions are round PAS-positive bodies which, in spite of their prickly profile on reticulin staining, have been referred to as "balloons" (fig. 3-147).

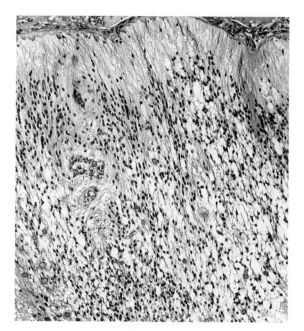

Figure 3-146
MYXOPAPILLARY EPENDYMOMA
Marked cellular elongation and background fibrillarity in some myxopapillary lesions bring schwannoma into the differential diagnosis.

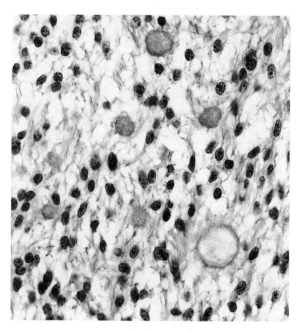

Figure 3-147
MYXOPAPILLARY EPENDYMOMA
Circular zones of collagen-rich tumor stroma known as "balloons" are a distinctive feature of some myxopapillary ependymomas.

Ependymomas share with a close relative, the choroid plexus papilloma, a rarely expressed capacity for melanosis. In most *pigmented* or *"melanotic" ependymomas* the pigment is not melanin but a dark, coarsely granular, lipochrome-like pigment (lipofuscin) which, though argyrophilic, stains strongly with PAS (316).

Grading. Histologic grading of ependymomas continues to be a contentious issue and little consensus has been reached on the prognostic value of specific histologic features (290, 295,296,300,304,314,317,319). Since for practical purposes, myxopapillary ependymomas are not known to undergo anaplastic change, attempts at grading ependymomas have centered upon lesions of the brain and spinal cord proper. The whole issue is confounded by a number of geographic and clinical factors, including the need to consider supratentorial and infratentorial lesions separately, the variable definition of grades in published series, the considerable prognostic effect of patient age, the extent of tumor resection, and the relatively long followup period necessary to adequately assess the biologic behavior of the ependymomas under study. It is our opinion, albeit one that can be both supported and refuted by selected references from the abundant literature on the subject, that highly cellular lesions with brisk mitotic activity, often in association with vascular proliferation, are more likely to recur and do so more quickly (290,295,296,311,317,319). Cytologic atypia in the absence of these features appear to be of no significance. Necrosis, particularly in large areas, has been identified as a possible indicator of more rapid recurrence. In our experience, however, necrosis is so common, even in very welldifferentiated lesions, that we have difficulty relying upon it as a prognostic indicator. Proliferation markers may have utility as a prognostic aid (310), but there is, as yet, little information regarding their application to ependymomas.

Any discussion of the grading of ependymomas must confront the issue of tumor heterogeneity. Commonly encountered in many otherwise welldifferentiated ependymomas are blue, circular regions of hypercellularity in which perivascular pseudorosettes are less noticeable, nuclei are coarser, nuclear-cytoplasmic ratios are increased, and mitotic figures are more abundant

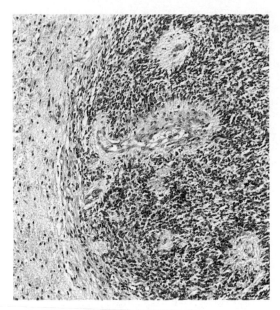

Figure 3-148
EPENDYMOMA WITH NODULES OF
HYPERCELLULARITY

Arising in the background of many otherwise well-differentiated ependymomas are lobules of increased cell density. In limited number this finding does not justify a diagnosis of anaplastic ependymoma.

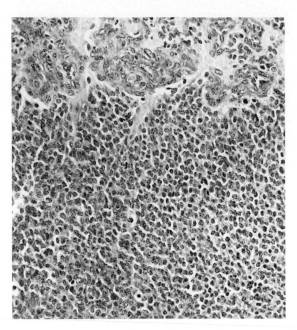

Figure 3-150
ANAPLASTIC EPENDYMOMA

The diagnosis of anaplastic ependymoma is based upon high cell density, brisk mitotic activity, and vascular proliferation. Cytologic atypia or necrosis is often seen, but may be observed also in low-grade ependymomas.

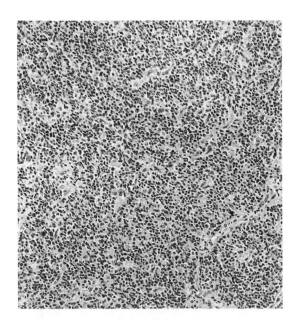

Figure 3-149
ANAPLASTIC EPENDYMOMA

Some intraventricular or paraventricular neoplasms exhibit the cellular monotony of ependymoma, but inconspicuous, if any, perivascular pseudorosettes. In such cases, the diagnosis of anaplastic ependymoma may be difficult to establish without extensive sampling, immunostaining for GFAP, and perhaps electron microscopy.

(fig. 3-148). Arcades of proliferating vessels with plump, often multilayered, vascular elements may be seen just outside of the nodules. Ependymomas can readily be assigned to the anaplastic or malignant category if such cellular foci predominate. The significance of only occasional or small foci is unclear, although their presence has been found to contribute somewhat to a poorer prognosis (311). We accept occasional cellular and atypical foci within the spectrum of well-differentiated ependymomas, but can suggest no clear end point at which their abundance is a criterion for malignancy. To us, an anaplastic ependymoma is a markedly cellular, mitotically active tumor with perivascular pseudorosettes and, usually, vascular proliferation and necrosis (fig. 3-149). Some intraventricular neoplasms carry this malignant degeneration a step farther and lose the perivascular pseudorosettes (fig. 3-150). In this situation, the diagnosis of an ependymal neoplasm may be presumptive, and the lesion must be distinguished from other densely cellular neoplasms such as medulloblastoma.

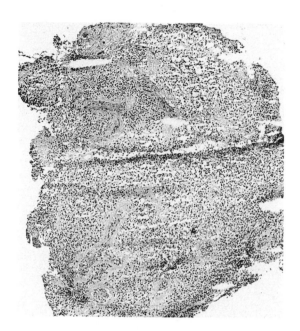 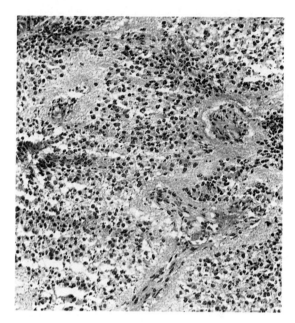

Figure 3-151
EPENDYMOMA: FROZEN SECTION
On frozen section, ependymomas may be difficult to recognize unless the preparations are viewed at low magnification (left), with attention directed to lobulation and perivascular pseudorosettes (right).

Only an occasional ependymoma continues on to a malignancy replete with necrosis and pseudo-palisading, features common to highly anaplastic oligodendroglial tumors and to glioblastoma. Since such ependymal tumors are often circumscribed rather than diffusely invasive, and since their prognosis is less predictable than that of astrocytic tumors with vascular proliferation and necrosis with pseudopalisading, we consider them to be highly anaplastic or grade 4 ependymomas rather than glioblastomas. We reserve the latter designation for patently astrocytic neoplasms of the diffuse type.

Frozen Section and Cytology. Ependymomas with epithelial surfaces are readily recognized in frozen section and require no specific comment, other than to reiterate the need to be aware of clinical and radiographic features of a given case and to begin the microscopic examination at low magnification. Radiographic features are especially important in intramedullary tumors since they establish whether the lesion is well circumscribed or diffuse. Discrete lesions include ependymomas, pilocytic astrocytomas, hemangioblastomas, and the rare intramedullary schwannoma (see Appendix G). Ill-defined infiltrating tumors are largely astrocytomas of the diffuse or fibrillary type, although rare oligodendrogliomas do arise in the spinal cord.

For less cellular and more fibrillar tumors without epithelial features, the possibility of an astrocytoma must be considered. Resolution of this differential diagnostic issue is important since the diagnosis of an ependymoma will start the surgeon on a tedious and exacting course of complete resection. In contrast, surgery is usually terminated in favor of radiotherapy if a diagnosis of an infiltrative fibrillary astrocytic neoplasm is received. An attempt at resection may be appropriate for pilocytic astrocytomas, most of which are somewhat discrete.

Erroneous diagnoses can generally be avoided by using low magnification to define the generally high cellularity and homogeneous noninfiltrating nature of ependymomas and to identify their sometimes subtle perivascular pseudorosettes (fig. 3-151). Higher magnification is useful in documenting the generally uniform nuclei and lack of overrun, preexisting neurons and glia. Care must be taken not to focus too closely on cytologic characteristics at the time of frozen section, since neoplastic ependymal cells often look remarkably astrocytic with this technique (fig. 3-152).

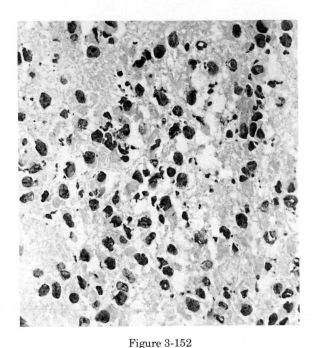

Figure 3-152
EPENDYMOMA: FROZEN SECTION
On frozen section, neoplastic ependymal cells frequently assume an astrocyte-like appearance. The presence of distinct nucleoli may suggest the correct diagnosis.

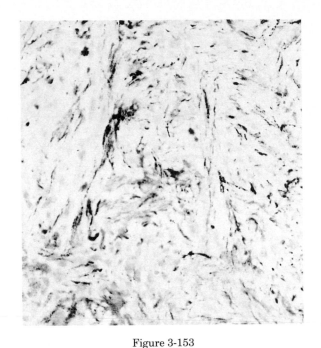

Figure 3-153
EPENDYMOMA
The presence of cell processes immunoreactive for GFAP eliminates many other histologically similar neoplasms.

Smear or touch preparations demonstrate small cells with generally uniform, dark, somewhat elongated nuclei and a small amount of cytoplasm (pl. VA). There is often cohesion and a tendency to perivascular arrangement. The latter is prominent in the myxopapillary type (pl. VB).

Immunohistochemical Findings. All differentiated ependymomas, including those of the myxopapillary type, are characterized by immunoreactivity for GFAP (fig. 3-153) (293,296,305,320, 321). Reactivity is present in all histologic types but is prominent in perivascular pseudorosettes; here at least some cell processes are almost invariably positive. True rosettes, on the other hand, are largely nonreactive. Immunoreactivities for epithelial markers such as epithelial membrane antigen and cytokeratins are apparent on the epithelial surfaces of some ependymomas, particularly well-differentiated ones (292,296,301,305,323), but ependymomas do not exhibit the diffuse cytoplasmic positivity for cytokeratin noted in choroid plexus papillomas (291).

Ultrastructural Findings. Apposed membranes of ependymoma cells adhere to one another by multipart "zipper-like" junctions lacking inserting tonofilaments. Well-formed terminal bars are evident at apical or luminal portions of cells where ependymal rosettes or canals are formed. Luminal surfaces bristle with microvilli and scattered cilia. Minute lumina, some filled by these apical specializations, may be small enough to escape detection by light microscopy.

The oligodendroglial-like cells in the clear cell ependymoma clearly express ependymal differentiation in the form of complex desmosomal junctions, microvilli, and cilia (302). The myxopapillary lesions are noted for cellular elongation, paucity of cilia, extensive basement laminae, microtubular aggregates, and flocculent intercellular and perivascular mucin (299,315,321).

Differential Diagnosis. Classic ependymomas with prominent perivascular or, especially, true ependymal rosettes seem unlikely to be confused with any other lesion. In practice, however, the ependymoma remains a frequent diagnostic problem because epithelial features are often absent and the high degree of fibrillarity frequently raises the possibility of an astrocytoma or a mixed glioma. This is especially true in small specimens from the spinal cord. Other

PLATE V

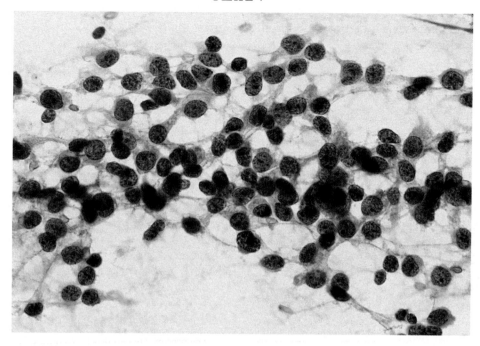

A. EPENDYMOMA

The glial nature of ependymomas is seen well in cytologic preparations which resolve the fine processes emanating from neoplastic cells. The rather dark, somewhat elongated nuclei are typical. Although the eosinophilic cytoplasm lends an astrocytic quality, there is greater nuclear uniformity than in most astrocytomas.

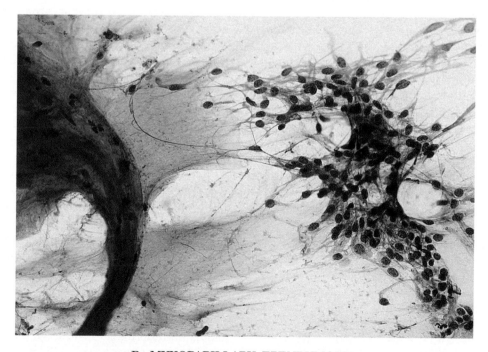

B. MYXOPAPILLARY EPENDYMOMA

The cells relate to the vessel at the left of the illustration through a perivascular collar of mucin.

ependymomas may be so cellular as to generate concern about medulloblastoma, other small cell embryonal neoplasms, or central neurocytoma. In tumors at unusual locations, even carcinoma, pituitary adenoma, or meningioma may enter into the differential diagnosis.

Many ependymomas unquestionably resemble astrocytoma if attention is focused only upon fibrillar areas (see fig. 3-137). In the posterior fossa, for example, a fibrillary-appearing ependymoma may resemble astrocytoma of the brain stem or cerebellum. Even the most fibrillar ependymomas, however, exhibit cellular foci and some perivascular pseudorosettes. In contrast to most astrocytomas, ependymomas are exophytic masses unassociated with enlargement of the pons. The presence of a subependymoma pattern further confirms the diagnosis.

The cerebellar astrocytoma, although usually hemispheric, can extend inferiorly from the vermis to occupy the fourth ventricle. Such tumors, however, lack the broad-based origin from the ventricular floor that characterizes ependymoma at that site. Most cerebellar astrocytomas exhibit, at least in part, a microcystic component, Rosenthal fibers, or granular bodies, structures not generally encountered even in astrocytic-appearing areas of ependymoma.

Given their high degree of fibrillarity, tanycytic ependymomas can be confused with astrocytoma, particularly pilocytic astrocytoma, unless the observer is familiar with the fibrillarity and fascicular architecture of this unusual ependymoma variant. Perivascular pseudorosettes, albeit ill-defined, provide conclusive support for the diagnosis. At low magnification tanycytic ependymomas are solid and lack parenchymal invasion. The fascicular architecture of tanycytic tumors is not seen in ordinary infiltrating astrocytomas of the fibrillary type.

Markedly cellular ependymomas can resemble such aggressive neoplasms as embryonal tumors, especially when their nuclei are hyperchromatic and mitotically active (fig. 3-150). The documentation of perivascular pseudorosettes, therefore, becomes extremely important. Without such rosettes, the diagnosis of ependymoma, even a malignant variant, should be made with great caution. Immunohistochemistry for GFAP is potentially useful when a ventricle-based mass with high cellularity, elevated mitotic rate, and nuclear regularity lacks more diagnostic features (fig. 3-150). Small cell embryonal tumors, particularly medulloblastomas and cerebral neuroblastomas, as well as central neurocytoma, exhibit perivascular fibrillar zones that at first glance resemble the perivascular pseudorosettes of ependymoma. In contrast to ependymoma, the cell processes contributing to the fibrillar zones of all these neuronal tumors are more delicate and are synaptophysin rather than GFAP positive. The central neurocytoma is especially likely to be confused with ependymoma since both are largely intraventricular. The neurocytoma's fibrillar zones tend to be larger, somewhat stellate, and less symmetric relative to vessels. Foci with an oligodendroglial appearance are also common in this tumor, as well as in neuroblastic lesions, and contribute to the difficulty in distinguishing them from the ependymoma of clear cell type. Ultrastructurally, ependymomas are recognized by their extensive intermediate junctions, microvilli, and cilia. Neurocytomas are poor in cell junctions and noted for processes containing microtubules and neurosecretory granules.

Most myxopapillary ependymomas of the cauda equina region are highly distinctive. Some examples, however, have a solid fascicular and less mucinous pattern that prompts consideration of a schwannoma (neurilemmoma) (fig. 3-146). The presence of perivascular mucin and pseudorosettes and lack of pericellular reticulin in ependymomas permits a ready distinction.

A regional lesion that may closely resemble myxopapillary ependymoma is the paraganglioma of the filum terminale, which, as a soft discrete mass, can radiographically and macroscopically mimic myxopapillary ependymoma (fig. 3-154). Although the radiation of neoplastic cells from vessels simulates that seen in ependymoma (see fig. 11-9), paraganglioma cells are more obviously epithelial and may exhibit delicate cytoplasmic granularity. Nesting and festooning of cells are also distinguishing features of neuroendocrine cells. Argyrophilic and, to a lesser extent, argentaffin-positive granules typify paragangliomas but are lacking in ependymoma. Lastly, paragangliomas are chromogranin, and often somatostatin or serotonin, immunoreactive. Although the chief cells of paraganglioma are largely GFAP negative, their sustentacular cells may be reactive. Ganglion cells are noted in about half of paragangliomas.

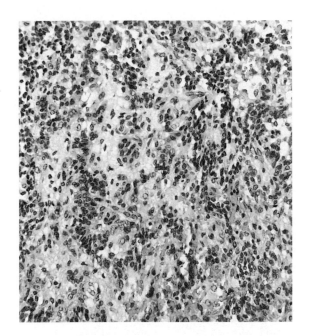

Figure 3-154
PARAGANGLIOMA RESEMBLING
MYXOPAPILLARY EPENDYMOMA
Compact regions of paragangliomas can resemble myxopapillary ependymoma.

Treatment and Prognosis. In the past, most intracranial ependymomas recurred in the tumor bed and were ultimately lethal. Since advances in neurosurgical techniques now make macroscopically complete resections possible in some cases, considerably longer survival periods are noted. How often these result in cure remains to be established. A small percentage of ependymomas, certainly less than 5 percent, undergo cerebrospinal dissemination to form implants which may become symptomatic. These usually occur in concert with local recurrence at the original tumor site; only rarely are spinal metastases an isolated finding. Although there is an association between rate of tumor recurrence and cerebrospinal spread on the one hand and histologic features on the other, the relationship is not precise. For instance, cerebrospinal fluid dissemination appears to be an uncommon occurrence, even in ependymomas with significant cytologic atypia and mitotic activity (298,304).

The outlook for patients with spinal ependymomas is considerably more favorable since these often small tumors lend themselves to gross total removal (309,318–320). This is especially true for myxopapillary ependymomas, particularly the smaller examples, many of which can be totally resected by severing the filum terminale from its origin and dissecting the lesion free from adherent nerve roots. Local and even widespread dissemination in the spinal subarachnoid space may follow incomplete removal of myxopapillary tumors (fig. 3-155) (294, 318,320,324) or, as indicated above, occur prior to surgery. Distant metastases, particularly to the lungs, are rarely observed; such behavior appears limited to tumors invading or arising within lumbosacral soft tissue (303,308,325).

Subependymoma

Definition. A highly differentiated, slow-growing glioma composed of ependymal and astrocyte-like cells, arising in the walls of the ventricular system (see Appendix F) or, rarely, the parenchyma of the spinal cord (see Appendix G).

Clinical and Radiographic Features. Subependymomas are most often encountered as incidental postmortem findings. Only occasional examples come to surgical attention (334). Children are rarely affected (338).

Symptomatic tumors in the posterior fossa compress the brain stem and elicit cranial nerve symptoms or produce dysfunction of subjacent respiratory centers. Cerebrospinal fluid obstruction with hydrocephalus is another consequence. Tumors in the lateral ventricles are usually asymptomatic, but may be large enough to produce hydrocephalus, or may undergo intratumoral or intraventricular hemorrhage, precipitating a neurosurgical emergency (328). Subependymomas in the spinal cord cause the generic symptoms of a slow-growing intramedullary mass.

Radiographically, supratentorial subependymomas are large spherical tumors in and around the region of the foramen of Monro (fig. 3-156) (334). Many, particularly those in the posterior fossa, are calcified (see Appendix E). Like the related ependymoma, they may extend from the lateral recess of the fourth ventricle through a foramen of Luschka to reach the cerebellopontine angle (fig. 3-157).

Macroscopic Findings. Small subependymomas in the lateral ventricles typically appear as smooth surfaced, dome-shaped sessile or polypoid excrescences, often in the general region of the foramen of Monro (329). They arise either from the

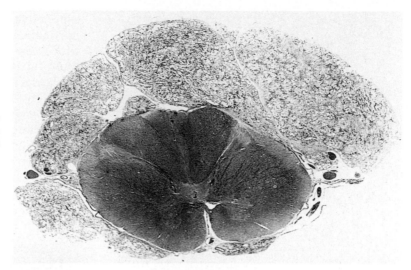

Figure 3-155
DISSEMINATED
MYXOPAPILLARY EPENDYMOMA
Subtotally resected myxopapillary ependymomas may seed the spinal meninges and, on rare occasion, the intracranial meninges.

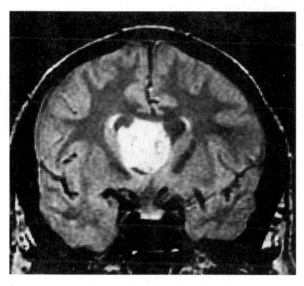

Figure 3-156
SUBEPENDYMOMA
The uncommon symptomatic subependymoma, such as this example seen on a proton density magnetic resonance image, is a discrete intraventricular mass near the foramen of Monro. (Courtesy of Dr. Stephen A. Goscin, Hollywood, FL.)

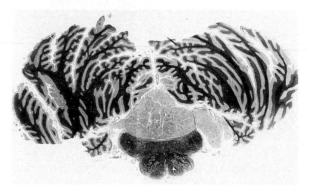

Figure 3-157
SUBEPENDYMOMA
Subependymomas of the fourth ventricle arise from the floor or roof of the ventricle to obstruct cerebrospinal fluid flow and to compress the underlying medulla. Such tumors may extend into the cerebellopontine angle via the foramen of Luschka, as is seen at the right of the illustration.

anterolateral walls of the ventricle or from the septum pellucidum. Those in the posterior fossa arise from the floor of the fourth ventricle and are frequently multinodular and gritty (331,341). Extension into a lateral recess is common. Spinal tumors form discrete intramedullary masses (333,337,339,340,343). Occasional intracranial or intraspinal examples arise away from the ventricular system or central canal (327,332,336).

Microscopic Findings. Subependymomas of the lateral ventricles are distinctive not only for the sweeping of highly fibrillar processes about clustered nuclei, but also for the frequent prominent microcystic changes (fig. 3-158). Nuclear pleomorphism is not uncommon and occasional mitoses are seen in fully half of these slowly growing tumors. Necrosis is rare and results from degenerative fibrosis and thrombosis of vessels rather than from rapid tumor growth. Hemosiderin deposits are often present in large lesions. The interface between tumor and brain is typically sharp. Foci of plump, gemistocytic or elongated fibrillar cells may also be evident.

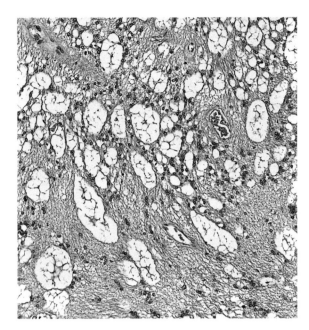

Figure 3-158
SUBEPENDYMOMA
Subependymomas of the lateral ventricles are noted for their high degree of fibrillarity and prominent microcystic change. Moderate nuclear pleomorphism is not uncommon and even a rare mitotic figure may be seen.

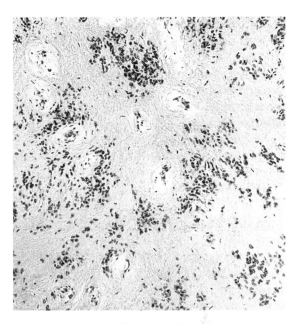

Figure 3-159
SUBEPENDYMOMA
Subependymomas of the posterior fossa are highly fibrillar lesions with prominent clustering of nuclei.

Fourth ventricle subependymomas are usually less microcystic and more fibrillar than their supratentorial counterparts, but retain the distinctive clustered pattern of nuclei (figs. 3-159, 3-160). The cells often appear more uniform, and therefore more ependymal, than those of lateral ventricular lesions. Mitotic figures are less common and pleomorphism is scant. Foci of cells with Rosenthal fibers are not common.

The relationship of subependymoma to classic ependymoma is highlighted by the occurrence of a subependymoma pattern in a minority of ependymomas. The rare spinal subependymoma, although confined within cord parenchyma rather than jutting into a space, is identical in appearance to intracranial examples.

Anaplastic transformation of subependymomas remains to be reported, but sarcomatous change in their vasculature (335) and rhabdomyosarcomatous differentiation (342) have both been encountered.

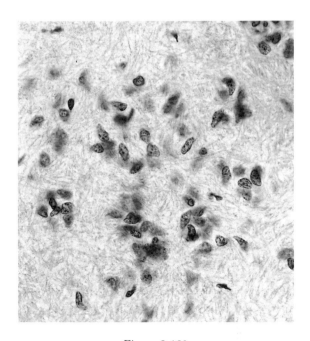

Figure 3-160
SUBEPENDYMOMA
The cytologic benignity of most subependymomas is apparent at high magnification of this fourth ventricular lesion. Note the markedly uniform delicate nuclei, relative lack of perinuclear cytoplasm, and the finely fibrillar background produced by aggregates of long cell processes.

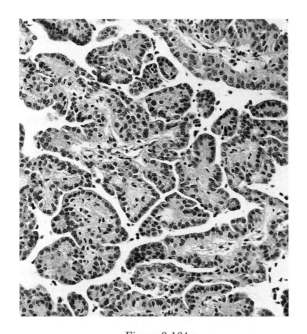

Figure 3-164
CHOROID PLEXUS PAPILLOMA
Regimented columnar cells rest upon distinct fibrovascular stalks.

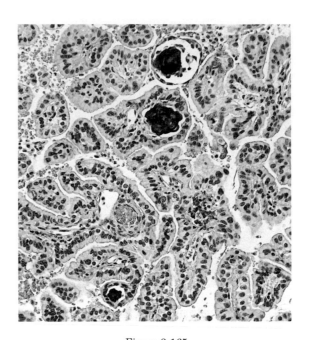

Figure 3-165
CHOROID PLEXUS PAPILLOMA
Stromal concretions are not uncommon, particularly in papillomas of the posterior fossa.

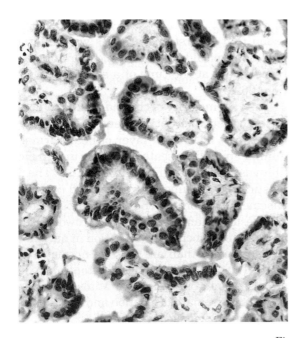

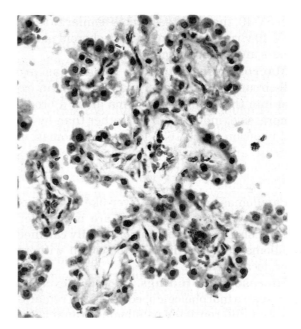

Figure 3-166
COMPARISON OF NEOPLASTIC AND NORMAL CHOROID PLEXUS EPITHELIUM
The epithelial surface of the choroid plexus papilloma (left) is flatter than the cobblestoned profile of the normal choroid plexus (right).

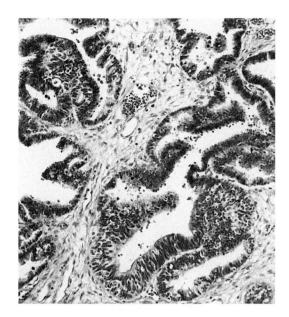 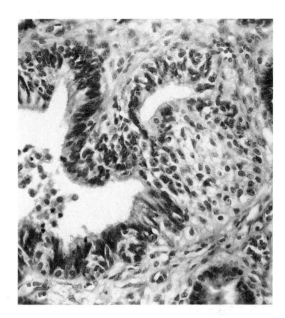

Figure 3-167
CHOROID PLEXUS PAPILLOMA WITH ATYPICAL CHANGES
Some choroid plexus neoplasms exhibit significant cytoplasmic atypia, scattered mitoses, and nests of cells in the underlying stroma. In the absence of more overt changes of malignancy, such lesions are considered papillomas rather than carcinomas.

variants of choroid plexus tumors are those designated as acinar (357), tubular (346), pigmented (350,376), and oncocytic (365,378). Bone (352,358) and cartilage (377) are noted in rare cases.

Within the papilloma group are lesions with significant cytologic atypia, increased nuclear-cytoplasmic ratios, scattered mitotic figures, and nests of cells that have broken through the basement membrane into the stroma (fig. 3-167). Although concern is appropriate regarding the biologic behavior of such intermediate lesions, they are considered atypical papillomas and not carcinomas. More diagnostically troublesome lesions are those that are more atypical yet still lack poorly differentiated regions. When brisk mitotic activity occurs in such tumors, we place them into the carcinoma category.

Tumors that readily qualify as carcinoma demonstrate unequivocal cytologic and histologic malignancy (fig. 3-168). These tumors are usually highly cellular and show architectural disarray with complex glands, cribriform arrangements, and only poorly formed papillae. Nuclear malignancy is obvious and the mitotic index is typically high. At the extreme end of the spectrum are largely undifferentiated tumors with cells lying in patternless sheets with no

appreciable papillae. Some carcinomas are made up in part of uniform, medium-sized polygonal cells with perinuclear halos, an effect that lends a somewhat oligodendroglial appearance (fig. 3-168C). Still others possess both papillae with epithelial cells and patternless sheets of small anaplastic cells which at first glance resemble those of glioblastoma.

Immunohistochemical Findings. The immunophenotype of choroid plexus papillomas expresses the hybrid nature of choroid plexus epithelium, being both epithelial and glial. Accordingly, most neoplastic cells demonstrate not only immunoreactivity for cytokeratins (fig. 3-169), but also diffuse staining for S-100 protein, vimentin and, in some cases, GFAP (fig. 3-170) (347,355, 356,365a,367,372). The term ependymal or glial differentiation is sometimes applied to foci of elongated GFAP-positive cells (fig. 3-170), but no prognostic significance is attached to this finding (351). Choroid plexus carcinomas retain the high rate of cytokeratin positivity, but reduced staining for S-100 has been noted (375).

Several studies have indicated the diagnostic utility of immunoreactivity of choroid plexus for prealbumin (transthyretin) (363,369). Both normal and neoplastic tumors are reactive. Since

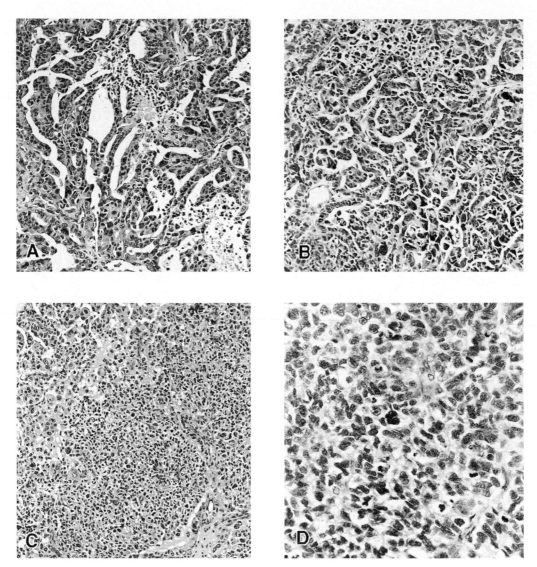

Figure 3-168
CHOROID PLEXUS CARCINOMA

As illustrated in these microscopic fields, all from the same neoplasm, differing degrees of differentiation may be found in the same specimen. In A, well-formed papillae are evident. Epithelial surfaces are less well structured in B. There is only focal papillary architecture at the top left of the illustration in C, and the majority of the tumor is largely solid and composed of undifferentiated cells. Perinuclear halos create somewhat of an oligodendroglioma appearance. Elsewhere (D) the small cell undifferentiated tumor resembles glioblastoma multiforme.

occasional metastatic carcinomas have been shown to be positive, staining for transthyretin cannot be considered as choroid plexus specific but nevertheless may be useful (345,347). Both normal and neoplastic choroid plexus epithelium are reactive for carbonic anhydrase C, but it has not been our experience that commercial immunostains are of diagnostic use when applied to paraffin-embedded sections. In one series, immunopositivity for

carcinoembryonic antigen was reported in carcinomas and, less often, in papillomas (354). Another study recommended the antibodies HEA 25 and Ber EP4 as useful in distinguishing choroid plexus tumors from metastatic papillary carcinomas. Only a rare plexus tumor was positive for either antibody (361a). Although its significance remains to be determined, SV-40 large T antigen has been found within nuclei in some tumors (348).

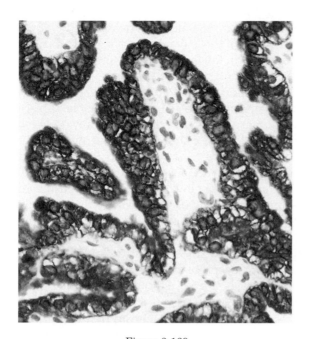

Figure 3-169
CHOROID PLEXUS PAPILLOMA
The epithelial character is reflected in the cells' immuno-reactivity for cytokeratins.

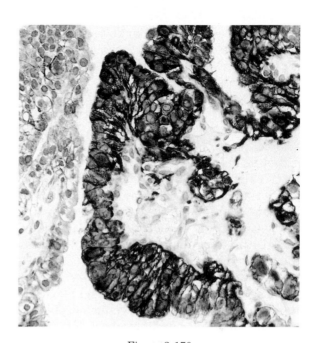

Figure 3-170
CHOROID PLEXUS PAPILLOMA
Cells with long tapering processes immunoreactive for GFAP constitute glial or ependymal differentiation.

Ultrastructural Findings. The papilloma closely resembles normal choroid plexus since the cells rest upon basal laminae, show interdigitation of their lateral cell membranes, contain occasional intermediate filament bundles, project apical microvilli and scattered cilia, and form lateral desmosomes as well as apical junction complexes (368,373). To some extent these features are also found in choroid plexus carcinoma (362,369,370).

Differential Diagnosis. The diagnosis of choroid plexus tumors usually focuses on four issues: 1) is the papillary tissue normal choroid plexus?; 2) is it a papillary ependymoma?; 3) if it is a plexus neoplasm, is it a papilloma or a carcinoma?; and 4) if it is a carcinoma, what other primary or metastatic neoplasms need to be considered?

In nearly all instances, architectural and cytologic features readily distinguish papilloma from normal choroid plexus epithelium (fig. 3-166). The neoplasm's epithelium is more complicated and more cellular than the normal plexus, often by a factor of two or more. As a consequence, the crowded cells are more columnar than the regularly spaced, domed, cobblestone-like cells of normal plexus. Nuclear-cytoplasmic ratios are increased, although only slightly in some cases.

Papillary ependymoma infrequently enters the differential of plexus papilloma since only a rare ependymoma is so truly papillary as to necessitate distinction. Even then, the ependymoma is characterized not only by epithelial-appearing elements but by nonepithelial glial cells, whose processes aggregate to form the fibrillar background so typical of gliomas (see fig. 3-140). Highly fibrillated areas are not a feature of papillomas. Ependymomas also lack the prominent basement membrane seen so well on PAS preparations or by immunohistochemistry for laminin (361). Ependymomas, in distinction to papillomas, are widely positive for GFAP and negative for cytokeratin.

The distinction between atypical papilloma and choroid plexus carcinoma is discussed above. Although no clearly defined criteria permit their ready separation, we render a diagnosis of papilloma in borderline cases, commenting upon the presence of atypia and suggesting close follow-up.

Choroid plexus carcinoma is readily distinguished from most other malignancies if the diagnosis is suspected on the basis of clinical or neuroradiologic findings. Simple awareness of its intraventricular location is key. In children, the principal differential diagnoses include embryonal tumors, malignant ependymoma, and germ cell tumors. In adults, metastatic carcinomas must be considered.

The distinction between choroid plexus carcinoma and embryonal tumors is not always easy, particularly if the carcinoma is largely undifferentiated. Among embryonal tumors, medulloepithelioma most closely resembles choroid plexus carcinoma, but the former features not only a PAS-positive basement membrane surrounding gland-like structures but a layer of reactivity atop the flat epithelium. Papillae are not a feature of medulloepithelioma, nor is immunoreactivity for keratin.

Malignant ependymomas share the intraventricular location of the choroid plexus tumors but are generally more monomorphic, expressing their epithelial features, if any, as ependymal rosettes rather than as papillae. Elsewhere, the typical choroid plexus carcinoma is to some extent a large cell undifferentiated or poorly differentiated epithelial neoplasm. Unlike ependymomas, choroid plexus carcinomas are GFAP negative.

Germ cell tumors that enter into the differential diagnosis are primarily those with an epithelial phenotype and include embryonal carcinoma, endodermal sinus tumor, and immature teratoma. These lesions usually have distinctive histologic patterns, are placental alkaline phosphatase immunoreactive, and, in the case of the endodermal sinus tumor, show reactivity for alpha-fetoprotein.

An entirely different diagnostic problem is presented by intraventricular epithelial malignancies occurring in adults. Metastatic carcinoma is the first to be excluded. Immunoreactivity for cytokeratins and even vimentin does not distinguish these two lesions, but positivity for S-100 protein favors a choroid plexus primary, as does the rare occurrence of GFAP staining in better differentiated examples. Positivity for pre-albumin (transthyretin), a regular feature of choroid plexus tumors, has been noted in metastatic carcinomas. The use of HEA 25 and Ber EP4 is discussed above. In some instances, only the diagnosis of high-grade papillary carcinoma can be rendered; resolution of the problem is left to the clinician and radiologist to find a systemic primary. Since choroid plexus carcinomas are rare in adults, the odds are heavily in favor of a metastasis if the lesion is overtly malignant, and somewhat in favor of a primary plexus neoplasm if it is well differentiated.

Treatment and Prognosis. Well-differentiated papillomas are generally amenable to resection and are cured without radiotherapy or chemotherapy (359,371). Despite their intraventricular location and the passing stream of cerebrospinal fluid, the incidence of craniospinal dissemination of papillomas is low (360). Most deposits are asymptomatic microscopic nodules, found only by meticulous autopsy examination. Most carcinomas are frankly infiltrative, nonresectable, and therefore likely to recur, often within months (375). Craniospinal dissemination is common but only occasional cases metastasize outside of the central nervous system (380).

It is difficult to comment on the prognosis of patients with atypical papillomas, although the ease of total gross resection in many cases would suggest that cure is possible in most instances. One study suggests that they behave like papillomas rather than carcinomas (371). Another noted that most of the atypical lesions recurred, either as atypical papillomas or as carcinomas (375). When all plexus neoplasms were considered, the latter study found that mitoses, brain invasion, and paucity of S-100 staining were poor prognostic indicators.

It remains to be seen whether radical removal and postoperative radiotherapy and chemotherapy can improve the outlook for patients with carcinomas (374). There seems no reason why curative total gross resection should not be possible in some instances.

GLIOMAS OF MIXED COMPOSITION

Mixed Gliomas

Definition. A glioma composed of more than a single type of glia.

General Comments. Criteria for a diagnosis of mixed glioma are difficult both to define and to apply. Many otherwise typical gliomas include cells that deviate phenotypically from those of the parent neoplasm. Oligodendrogliomas, for example, often contain neoplastic cells that appear astrocytic, whereas cells resembling both astrocytes and oligodendroglia are found in many ependymomas. Foci of oligodendroglioma

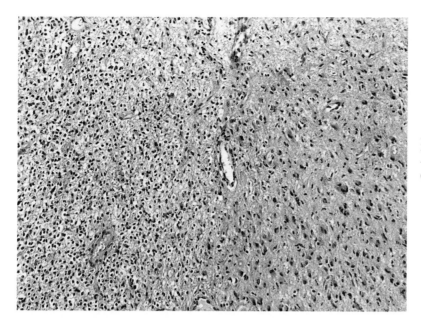

Figure 3-171
MIXED GLIOMA
(OLIGOASTROCYTOMA)
The term mixed glioma, most often applied to oligoastrocytomas, is appropriate when geographically distinct areas of astrocytoma (right) and oligodendroglioma (left) are seen.

are not uncommon in pilocytic astrocytomas. It has even been suggested that a percentage of cells in well-differentiated astrocytomas are undifferentiated or oligodendroglial (387).

Although a number of gliomas may be mixed in composition, overuse of the designation "mixed" blurs distinction between the classic glial entities and creates unnecessary confusion regarding prognosis and appropriate therapy. We accept considerable phenotypic heterogeneity in gliomas. True mixed gliomas, i.e., biphasic tumors composed of two clearly distinct cell types, are uncommon by our criteria. A related, more frequent problem is that of the well-differentiated infiltrating glioma which is not so much biphasic in pattern as hybrid in nature.

Oligoastrocytoma. Many oligodendrogliomas contain cells with an ample eccentric cell body which is eosinophilic and strongly positive for GFAP (see fig. 3-120). These cells often arise in transition from obvious oligodendrocytes and usually retain a round oligodendroglial nucleus. We, like others, consider them to be oligodendrocytes even if occasional short cytoplasmic processes are seen. The immunoreactivity of some of these for both GFAP and galactocerebroside supports this conclusion (382). This position becomes less tenable, perhaps, when the processes become longer, stouter, or more stellate, but we still generally consider such tumors to be oligodendroglial if the cells retain round nuclei and

demonstrate classic features of oligodendroglioma. As well-differentiated oligodendrogliomas become anaplastic, GFAP-positive astrocyte-like cells with epithelioid, spindled, or multipolar features often become more prominent and the background can take on an obvious fibrillar quality. In the presence of a clear oligodendroglioma component, we still consider such tumors to be oligodendrogliomas. Nonetheless, in some instances the astrocyte phenotype cannot be denied, and a diagnosis of malignant mixed glioma is appropriate.

There is general agreement that the term mixed oligodendroglioma/astrocytoma or oligoastrocytoma is appropriate for tumors in which geographically distinct areas of unequivocal oligodendroglioma and astrocytoma coexist (figs. 3-171–3-173). Controversy surrounds those with a more homogeneous composition in which cells with differing cytology are intimately admixed. In addition to their content of uniform oligodendrocytes, such tumors also exhibit cells with nuclear elongation or pleomorphism, relative abundance of cytoplasm, and elongate processes. There have been suggestions that in such tumors a diagnosis of mixed glioma is reached when the contribution of the minority cell type exceeds some arbitrary proportion, perhaps 20 percent. In practice, we find it difficult to arrive at such a figure, given the considerable morphologic overlap of such neoplastic glia. Consequently, we

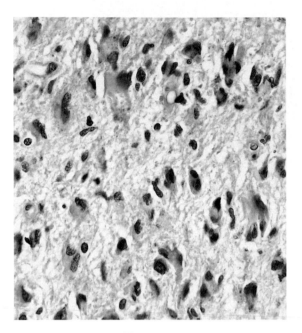

Figure 3-172
MIXED GLIOMA
The tumor on the right side of figure 3-171 has the process-forming cytoplasm and hyperchromatic, pleomorphic nuclei typical of a fibrillary astrocytic neoplasm.

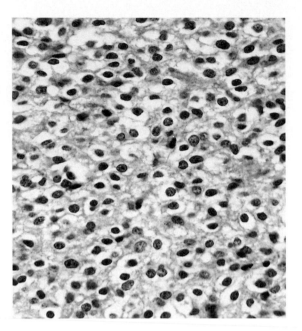

Figure 3-173
MIXED GLIOMA
The tumor on the left of figure 3-171 has the monotonous round nuclei and perinuclear halos of an oligodendroglioma.

suggest using the designation mixed glioma only in the presence of a distinct and unequivocal astrocytic component.

The diagnosis of oligoastrocytoma should be made with some hesitation if the specimen has previously been frozen. The frozen section process gives oligodendroglia a decidedly astrocytic appearance (fig. 3-119, right). Their nuclei become artifactually dark, irregular in shape, and the cytoplasm and underlying parenchyma are less distinct, lending an astrocytoma-like fibrillarity.

There is conflicting evidence about the prognostic significance of mixed lesions. The question arises whether patients with an oligodendroglioma with an astrocytic component or astrocytic-like cells do less well than those with pure oligodendroglioma. In view of the greater aggressiveness and increased likelihood of malignant degeneration of fibrillary astrocytoma, as opposed to oligodendrogliomas, the question is entirely reasonable. One study, however, found that both groups of patients responded equally well to chemotherapy (383). Another study found no relation between survival and the relative

percentages of oligodendrocytes and astrocytes (384). Still another investigation of oligodendroglioma found no prognostic significance in the presence of gliofibrillary oligodendrocytes or minigemistocytes (386). A more recent and larger study found that patients with pure oligodendrogliomas and oligoastrocytomas did better than those with pure astrocytomas (388).

Oligoependymoma. Use of the term mixed oligodendroglioma/ependymoma (oligoependymoma) is complicated by the presence of cells resembling oligodendroglia in many ependymomas. Such tumors are not mixed gliomas in our opinion. The oligoependymoma phenotype reaches its fullest expression in the so-called clear cell ependymoma (fig. 3-141) (385). Experience with the latter neoplasm is limited, but in its radiologic and macroscopic appearance, and biologic behavior it resembles ependymoma rather than oligodendroglioma. True oligoependymomas are rare. The diagnosis should only be made in the rare setting of an infiltrative oligodendroglioma in which a component exhibiting unequivocal ependymal differentiation, generally perivascular pseudorosettes, is seen.

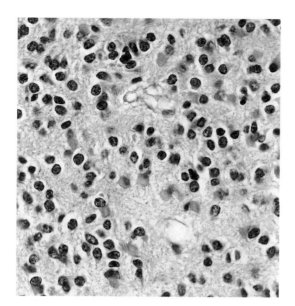 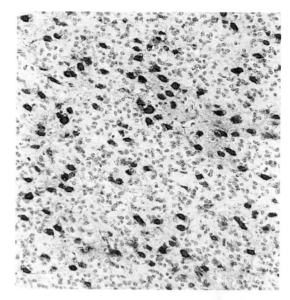

Figure 3-174
EPENDYMOMA/"MIXED" GLIOMA
Some ependymomas contain cells with ample eosinophilic cytoplasm with radiating processes (left) and strong immunoreactivity for GFAP (right). Such lesions appear more "mixed" in nature than the common ependymomas with only a high degree of background fibrillarity. Nevertheless, radiologic demarcation of these enhancing lesions is usually seen and the designation mixed glioma, while morphologically descriptive, may produce clinical confusion.

Ependymoastrocytoma. Many ependymomas, especially those in the posterior fossa, contain highly fibrillar areas devoid of perivascular rosettes. The neoplastic cells in these regions contribute processes to the fibrillar background but generally lack the array of radiating processes typical of astrocytoma. Since such paucicellular, fibrillar areas are common in otherwise typical ependymomas, the diagnosis of mixed glioma seems unnecessary and confusing. No prognostic significance has been attached to such astrocytoma-like areas.

In young children, intraventricular neoplasms with prominent cells with glassy cytoplasm are seen lying at the periphery of more cellular lobules with ependymal cytologic features and perivascular pseudorosettes (fig. 3-174). These stellate cells resemble astrocytes rather than ependymal cells of the fibrillar areas just described. Since other areas of such tumors are obviously ependymal, we classify them as ependymomas. By all microscopic criteria, the stellate, GFAP-positive cells are astrocytes. Nonetheless, such cells are few and deserve little more than a mention in the microscopic description of the surgical pathology report. It is not

clear whether such tumors represent a clinicopathologic entity.

Rarely, one encounters a tumor of the cerebral hemispheres which features prominent perivascular pseudorosettes in association with an infiltrating astrocytoma. The diagnosis of ependymoastrocytoma is appropriate in such instances.

Ependymal or Glial Differentiation in Choroid Plexus Papilloma. Some choroid plexus papillomas consist in part of tapered fibrillated cells with intense GFAP positivity, a feature termed ependymal or glial differentiation (fig. 3-170) (381). Since such foci are of no known prognostic significance, they do not affect the classification of these lesions. Because the issue is entirely semantic, we do not mention the finding in the diagnosis. A diagnosis of "choroid plexus papilloma with ependymal differentiation" may be confusing and prompt overaggressive treatment.

Hybrid Tumors. Although it is necessary to assign gliomas to principal categories whenever possible, a number of tumors resist this attempt since they are phenotypic hybrids. Such neoplasms are commonly encountered as tumors with a morphologic overlap between oligodendroglioma and astrocytoma (see fig. 3-129).

astroblastoma rest upon a basal lamina where they abut the vasculature. Given its ultrastructural phenotype, including both ependymal and astrocytic features, it has been suggested by some that astroblastomas may arise from tanycytes (392).

Differential Diagnosis. Without the presence of tumor demarcation, astroblastoma is difficult to distinguish from other gliomas exhibiting some degree of stout perivascular glial process formation, a feature loosely termed astroblastic. By utilizing a strict definition of astroblastoma, the diagnosis is simpler, since the tumor is well demarcated, distinctively constructed, and prone to vascular hyalinization.

Given the presence of radiating perivascular processes and the absence of brain invasion, the compact regions of astroblastoma distinctly resemble ependymoma. The differential diagnosis is further complicated by the fact that, like astroblastoma, occasional ependymomas occur away from the ventricle, sometimes even at the surface of the brain. As noted above, the perivascular cytoplasmic processes of astroblastoma are broad based and coarse, rather than narrow and tapering. As a result, the perivascular fibrillar zones of astroblastoma lack the fine fibrillarity that characterizes those of ependymoma, and assume more of an epithelial quality. Although marked vascular sclerosis is not unique to astroblastoma, it is sufficiently characteristic to bring this entity to mind. Ependymomas do not usually exhibit such sclerosis. Astroblastoma may also resemble papillary meningioma since both are demarcated, often superficially situated, cytologically uniform, rich in perivascular pseudorosettes, and potentially reactive for epithelial membrane antigen. Both also occur primarily in young patients. Most papillary meningiomas, however, are clearly dura based and show areas of clear-cut meningioma. Insofar as any negative result can be conclusive, the meningioma's lack of reactivity for GFAP distinguishes its papillary variant from the immunopositive astroblastoma.

Prognosis. Since few astroblastomas have been described, their behavior, relative to tumor grade, remains unsettled. One study suggested that long survivals and cures are possible in low-grade forms, whereas only short survival periods of 1 to 2 years could be expected with high-grade lesions (390).

Granular Cell Tumor of the Infundibulum

Definition. A tumor of cells with lysosome-rich granular cytoplasm arising in the infundibulum or neurohypophysis.

General Comments. Although the term granular cell tumor is applied to a more common lesion of peripheral nerves, including the intracranial segment of the trigeminal nerve, and to rare variants of astrocytoma, the infundibular or neurohypophysial lesion described here is, to us, a distinct entity. The term *pituicytoma* has also been applied to granular cell tumors but is nonspecific since it has been used to refer to other astrocytomas in this region, most of which are of the pilocytic type.

The most common granular cell proliferations are microscopic nodules in the infundibulum or neurohypophysis. Such lesions represent incidental findings known as tumorettes or choristomas (fig. 3-179) (396,398,401). Only rarely do they grow to sufficient size to form symptomatic masses (393,394).

The origin or nature of infundibular granular cell tumors has not been firmly established, but is reasonably assigned to regional specialized glia. At the periphery of granular cell lesions, the constituent cells merge via transition forms with infundibular astrocytes (396,401). Isolated and clustered granular cells, similar to those of granular cell tumors, may be seen in the normal neurohypophysis (400). In addition, scattered cells of granular cell tumor contain fine pigment granules resembling those in regional glial cells (395). Ultrastructural studies clearly show normal pituicytes containing varying numbers of electron-dense structures identical to those in granular cell tumors (400,402).

Clinical and Radiographic Features. Of the rare symptomatic examples of granular cell tumor, most are spherical contrast-enhancing masses associated with endocrine deficiency states or diminished visual acuity (fig. 3-180) (393,397).

Macroscopic Findings. The tumors are soft, discrete, vascular masses which become attached to, but generally not invasive of, the overlying optic chiasm or hypothalamus.

Microscopic Findings. The features of granular cell tumor are identical, in cytologic terms, to tumorettes, from which they are presumably derived. Large tumors, unlike the

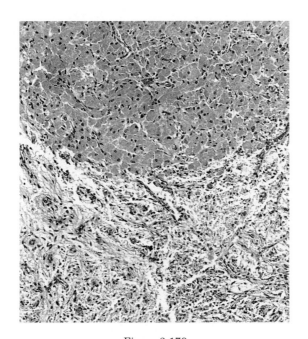

Figure 3-179
INFUNDIBULAR GRANULAR CELL NEST
Small nodules of granulated pituicytes, "choristomas," are common incidental findings in the infundibulum.

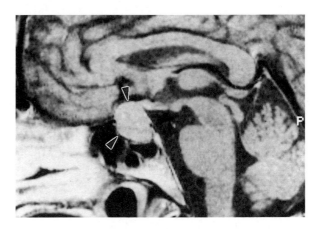

Figure 3-180
INFUNDIBULAR GRANULAR CELL TUMOR
The rare, symptomatic, infundibular granular cell tumor is a nonspecific mass in the sellar region. This example produced visual field changes in a 44-year-old man. (Courtesy of Dr. Stephen A. Goscin, Hollywood, FL.)

tumorettes, are often septated by delicate fibrovascular bands or exhibit a somewhat fascicular architecture (fig. 3-181). The granular cells possess ample pink cytoplasm of delicate granular texture which is strongly PAS positive. Nuclei are often eccentric, are uniformly round with delicate chromatin, and are free of mitotic activity. Perivascular lymphoid aggregates are common.

Immunohistochemical Findings. In light of the rarity of granular cell tumor, the essentials of its immunoprofile remain to be established. Investigations have variably reported positive or negative reactions for S-100 protein or vimentin (397,399). Several studies have found a lack of reactivity for GFAP (397,399), but its presence was demonstrated by both routine immunohistochemistry and immunoelectron microscopy in another study (403). The authors of the latter investigation suggested that GFAP is present in these tumors but that immunoreactivity is compromised or lost as the cells become increasingly granulated. A similar loss of reactivity is seen in the granular cell variant of astrocytomas at other sites. Variable reactivity for alpha-1-antitrypsin and alpha-1-antichymotrypsin has been noted (399).

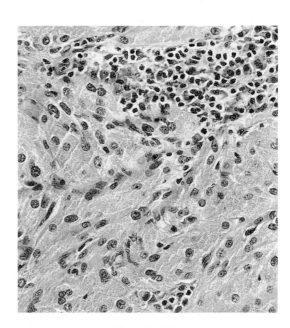

Figure 3-181
INFUNDIBULAR GRANULAR CELL TUMOR
This rare, symptomatic lesion is noted for its demarcation, granular cells, and perivascular lymphocytic infiltrates.

Ultrastructural Findings. The granular cells are filled with heterolysosomes but lack intermediate filaments. If present, basement membranes are scant (397,400,403).

Differential Diagnosis. Low-power examination of large tissue fragments reveals a distinctive appearance of clusters and fascicles of granular cells lying within the interstices of prominent, often geometrically arranged, capillaries. In small specimens, cellular elongation, whether real or imposed by artifact, can resemble that of pilocytic astrocytoma. Even the most spindled elements of a granular cell tumor do not, however, reach the degree of elongation regularly achieved by pilocytic astrocytoma cells. An additional distinguishing feature of the granular cell tumor is its distinctive granular cytoplasm which contrasts

with the markedly fibrillar cytoplasm of compacted portions of the pilocytic tumor and the loose-knit, often microcystic architecture of other portions. In addition, the astrocytoma features GFAP reactivity and typically exhibits Rosenthal fibers and eosinophilic granular bodies.

Prognosis. In some symptomatic lesions that were largely excised, residual tumor has been reported to grow slowly, if at all, during periods of observation (393,397).

REFERENCES

Astrocytoma/Anaplastic Astrocytoma/Glioblastoma Multiforme

1. Albers GW, Hoyt WF, Forno LS, Shratter LA. Treatment response in malignant optic glioma of adulthood. Neurology 1988;38:1071–4.

1a. Albert FK, Forsting M, Sartor K, Adams HP, Kunze S. Early postoperative magnetic resonance imaging after resection of malignant glioma: objective evaluation of residual tumor and its influence on regrowth and prognosis. Neurosurg 1994;34:45–61.

2. Albright AL, Guthkelch AN, Packer RJ, Price RA, Rourke LB. Prognostic factors in pediatric brain-stem gliomas. J Neurosurg 1986;65:751–5.

3. _____, Price RA, Guthkelch AN. Brain stem gliomas of children: a clinicopathological study. Cancer 1983;52:2313–9.

4. Anzil AP. Glioblastoma multiforme with extracranial metastases in the absence of previous craniotomy. Case Report. J Neurosurg 1970;33:88–94.

5. Barnard RO, Geddes JF. The incidence of multifocal cerebral gliomas: a histologic study of large hemisphere sections. Cancer 1987;60:1519–31.

6. Bigner SH, Burger PC, Wong AJ, et al. Gene amplification in malignant human gliomas: clinical and histopathologic aspects. J Neuropathol Exp Neurol 1988; 47:191–205.

7. Brooks WH, Markesbery WR, Gupta GD, Roszman TL. Relationship of lymphocyte invasion and survival of brain tumor patients. Ann Neurol 1978;4:219–24.

8. Bucciero A, Vizioli L, Giamundo A, Villano M, Quaglietta P, Cerillo A. Prognostic significance of lymphoid infiltration in cerebral malignant gliomas. J Neurosurg Sci 1990;34:145–8.

9. Burger PC. Classification, grading, and patterns of spread of malignant gliomas. In: Apuzzo ML, ed. Neurosurgical topics: malignant cerebral glioma. Park Ridge, Ill: American Association of Neurological Surgeons, 1990:3–17.

10. _____, Boyko OB. The pathology of central nervous system radiation injury. In: Gutin PH, Leibel SA, Sheline GE, eds. Radiation injury to the nervous system. New York: Raven Press, 1991:191–208.

11. _____, Green SB. Patient age, histologic features, and length of survival in patients with glioblastoma multiforme. Cancer 1987;59:1617–25.

12. _____, Heinz ER, Shibata T, Kleihues P. Topographic anatomy and CT correlations in the untreated glioblastoma multiforme. J Neurosurg 1988;68:698–704.

13. _____, Kleihues P. Cytologic composition of the untreated glioblastoma with implications for evaluation of needle biopsies. Cancer 1989;63:2014–23.

14. _____, Mahaley MS Jr, Dudka L, Vogel FS. The morphologic effects of radiation administered therapeutically for intracranial gliomas: a postmortem study of 25 cases. Cancer 1979;44:1256–72.

15. _____, Scheithauer BW, Vogel FS. Surgical pathology of the nervous system and its coverings. 3rd ed. New York: Churchill Livingstone, 1991.

16. _____, Shibata T, Kleihues P. The use of the monoclonal antibody Ki-67 in the identification of proliferating cells: application to surgical neuropathology. Am J Surg Pathol 1986;10:611–7.

17. _____, Vogel FS. Frozen section interpretation in surgical neuropathology. I. Intracranial lesions. Am J Surg Pathol 1977;1:323–47.

18. _____, Vogel FS, Green SB, Strike TA. Glioblastoma multiforme and anaplastic astrocytoma: pathologic criteria and prognostic implications. Cancer 1985;56:1106–11.

19. _____, Vollmer RT. Histologic factors of prognostic significance in the glioblastoma multiforme. Cancer 1980;46:1179–86.

20. Chamberlain MC, Silver P, Levin VA. Poorly differentiated gliomas of the cerebellum: a study of 18 patients. Cancer 1990;65:337–40.

21. Chowdhary UM, Boehme DH, Al-Jishi M. Turcot syndrome (glioma polyposis): case report. J Neurosurg 1985;63:804–7.

22. Ciappetta P, Salvati M, Capoccia G, Artico M, Raco A, Fortuna A. Spinal glioblastomas: report of seven cases and review of the literature. Neurosurgery 1991; 28:302–6.

23. Cohen AR, Wisoff JH, Allen JC, Epstein F. Malignant astrocytomas of the spinal cord. J Neurosurg 1989; 70:50–4.

23a. Coons SW, Johnson PC. Regional heterogeneity in the proliferative activity of human gliomas as measured by Ki-67 labeling index. J Neuropathol Exp Neurol 1993;52:609–18.

24. Cooper PR, Epstein F. Radical resection of intramedullary spinal cord tumors in adults: recent experience in 29 patients. J Neurosurg 1985;63:492–9.

25. Cosgrove M, Fitzgibbons PL, Sherrod A, Chandrasoma PT, Martin SE. Intermediate filament expression in astrocytic neoplasms. Am J Surg Pathol 1989;13:141–5.

26. Daumas-Duport C, Scheithauer BW, Kelly PJ. A histologic and cytologic method for the spatial definition of gliomas. Mayo Clin Proc 1987;62:435–49.

27. _____, Scheithauer BW, O'Fallon J, Kelly P. Grading of astrocytomas: a simple and reproducible method. Cancer 1988;62:2152–65.

28. Deckert M, Reifenberger G, Wechsler W. Determination of the proliferative potential of human brain tumors using the monoclonal antibody Ki-67. J Cancer Res Clin Oncol 1989;115:179–88.

29. Dohrmann GJ, Dunsmore RH. Glioblastoma multiforme of the cerebellum. Surg Neurol 1975;3:219–23.

30. _____, Farwell JR, Flannery JT. Glioblastoma multiforme in children. J Neurosurg 1976;44:442–8.

31. Dolman CL. Lymph node metastasis as first manifestation of glioblastoma: case report. J Neurosurg 1974;41:607–9.

32. El-Gindi S, Salama M, El-Henawy M, Farag S. Metastases of glioblastoma multiforme to cervical lymph nodes: report of two cases. J Neurosurg 1973;38:631–4.

33. Epstein FJ, Farmer JP, Freed D. Adult intramedullary astrocytomas of the spinal cord. J Neurosurg 1992;77:355–9.

34. Erlich SS, Davis RL. Spinal subarachnoid metastasis from primary intracranial glioblastoma multiforme. Cancer 1978;42:2854–4.

35. Francavilla TL, Miletich RS, Di Chiro G, Patronas NJ, Rizzoli HV, Wright DC. Positron emission tomography in the detection of malignant degeneration of low-grade gliomas. Neurosurgery 1989;24:1–5.

36. Freeman CR, Krischer J, Sanford RA, et al. Hyperfractionated radiotherapy in brain stem tumors: results of treatment at the 7020 cGy dose level of Pediatric Oncology Group study 8495. Cancer 1991;68:474–81.

37. Fulling KH, Garcia DM. Anaplastic astrocytoma of the adult cerebrum: prognostic value of histologic features. Cancer 1985;55:928–31.

38. Gamis AS, Egelhoff J, Roloson G, et al. Diffuse bony metastases at presentation in a child with glioblastoma multiforme: a case report. Cancer 1990;66:180–4.

39. Gerstner L, Jellinger K, Heiss WD, Wöber G. Morphological changes in anaplastic gliomas treated with radiation and chemotherapy. Acta Neurochir (Wein) 1977;36:117–38.

40. Giangaspero F, Burger PC. Correlations between cytologic composition and biological behavior in the glioblastoma multiforme. A postmortem study of 50 cases. Cancer 1983;52:2320–33.

41. Glantz MJ, Burger PC, Herndon JE II, et al. Influence of the type of surgery on the histologic diagnosis in patients with anaplastic gliomas. Neurology 1991;41:1741–4.

42. _____, Hoffman JM, Coleman RE, et al. Identification of early recurrence of primary central nervous system tumors by [18F] fluorodeoxyglucose positron emission tomography. Ann Neurol 1991;29:347–55.

43. Golden GS, Ghatak NR, Hirano A, French JH. Malignant glioma of the brain-stem: a clinicopathological analysis of 13 cases. J Neurol Neurosurg Psychiatry 1972;35:732–8.

44. Haddad SF, Moore SA, Schelper RL, Goeken JA. Smooth muscle can comprise the sarcomatous component of gliosarcomas. J Neuropathol Exp Neurol 1992;51:493–8.

45. _____, Moore SA, Schelper RL, Goeken JA. Vascular smooth muscle hyperplasia underlies the formation of glomeruloid vascular structures of glioblastoma multiforme. J Neuropathol Exp Neurol 1992;51:488–92.

46. Haggitt RC, Reid BJ. Hereditary gastrointestinal polyposis syndromes. Am J Surg Pathol 1986;10:871–87.

47. Hayostek C, Shaw EG, Scheithauer BW, et al. Astrocytomas of the cerebellum: a comparative clinicopathologic study of pilocytic and diffuse astrocytomas. Cancer 1993;72:856–69.

48. Herpers MJ, Ramaekers FC, Aldeweireldt J, Moesker O, Slooff J. Co-expression of glial fibrillary acidic protein- and vimentin-type intermediate filaments in human astrocytomas. Acta Neuropathol (Berl) 1986;70:333–9.

48a. Hirato J, Nakazato Y, Ogawa A. Expression of nonglial intermediate filament proteins in gliomas. Clin Neuropathol 1994;13:1–11.

49. Hochberg FH, Pruitt A. Assumptions in the radiotherapy of glioblastoma. Neurology 1980;30:907–11.

50. Hoshino T, Rodriguez LA, Cho KG, et al. Prognostic implications of the proliferative potential of low-grade astrocytomas. J Neurosurg 1988;69:839–42.

51. Hoyt WF, Meshel LG, Lessell S, Schatz NJ, Suckling RD. Malignant optic glioma of adulthood. Brain 1973;96:121–32.

52. Hulbanni S, Goodman PA. Glioblastoma multiforme with extraneural metastases in the absence of previous surgery. Cancer 1976;37:1577–83.

53. Hurtt MR, Moossy J, Donovan-Peluso M, Locker J. Amplification of epidermal growth factor receptor gene in gliomas: histopathology and prognosis. J Neuropathol Exp Neurol 1992;51:84–90.

54. Iwaki T, Iwaki A, Miyazono M, Goldman JE. Preferential expression of alpha-β-crystallin in astrocytic elements of neuroectodermal tumors. Cancer 1991;68:2230–40.

55. Iwama T, Yamada H, Sakai N, et al. Correlation between magnetic resonance imaging and histopathology of intracranial glioma. Neurol Res 1991;13:48–54.

56. Johnson PC, Hunt SJ, Drayer BP. Human cerebral gliomas: correlation of postmortem MR imaging and neuropathologic findings. Radiology 1989;170:211–7.

57. Kelly PJ, Daumas-Duport C, Scheithauer BW, Kall BA, Kispert DB. Stereotactic histologic correlations of computed tomography- and magnetic resonance imaging-defined abnormalities in patients with glial neoplasms. Mayo Clin Proc 1987;62:450–9.

57a. _____, Hunt C. The limited value of cytoreductive surgery in elderly patients with malignant gliomas. Neurosurg 1994;34:62–7.

58. Kepes JJ, Fulling KH, Garcia JH. The clinical significance of "adenoid" formations of neoplastic astrocytes, imitating metastatic carcinoma, in gliosarcomas. A review of five cases. Clin Neuropathol 1982; 1:139–50.

59. _____, Rubinstein LJ, Chiang H. The role of astrocytes in the formation of cartilage in gliomas: an immunohistochemical study of four cases. Am J Pathol 1984;117:471–83.

60. Kernohan JW, Mabon RF, Svien HJ, Adson AW. A simplified classification of the gliomas. Proc Staff Meet Mayo Clin 1949;24:71–5.

61. _____, Sayre GP. Tumors of the central nervous system. Atlas of tumor pathology, Section X—Fascicles 35 and 37. Washington DC: Armed Forces Institute of Pathology, 1952.

62. Kim TS, Halliday AL, Hedley-Whyte ET, Convery K. Correlates of survival and the Daumas-Duport grading system for astrocytomas. J Neurosurg 1991;74:27–37.

140. von Ammon K, von Deimling A, Seizinger BR, Wiestler OD, Yasargil MG. Molecular genetic evidence for two variants of glioblastoma multiforme. Clin Neuropathol 1991;10:244.

141. Wesseling P, Vandersteenhoven JJ, Downey BT, Ruiter DJ, Burger PC. Cellular components of microvascular proliferation in human glial and metastatic brain neoplasms. A light microscopic and immunohistochemical study of formalin-fixed, routinely processed material. Acta Neuropathol (Berl) 1993;85:508–14.

142. Winger MJ, MacDonald DR, Cairncross JG. Supratentorial anaplastic gliomas in adults: the prognostic importance of extent of resection and prior low-grade glioma. J Neurosurg 1989;71:487–93.

143. Wood JR, Green SB, Shapiro WR. The prognostic importance of tumor size in malignant gliomas: a computed tomographic scan study by the Brain Tumor Cooperative Group. J Clin Oncol 1988;6:338–43.

144. Yung WK, Luna M, Borit A. Vimentin and glial fibrillary acidic protein in human brain tumors. J Neurooncol 1985;3:35–8.

145. Zampieri P, Zorat PL, Mingrino S, Soattin GB. Radiation-associated cerebral gliomas: a report of two cases and review of the literature. J Neurosurg Sci 1989;33:271–9.

146. Zuber P, Hamou MF, de Tribolet N. Identification of proliferating cells in human gliomas using the monoclonal antibody Ki-67. Neurosurgery 1988;22:364–8.

Gliosarcoma

147. Barnard RO, Bradford R, Scott T, Thomas DG. Gliomyosarcoma: report of a case of rhabdomyosarcoma arising in a malignant glioma. Acta Neuropathol (Berl) 1986;69:23–7.

148. Feigin I, Allen LB, Lipkin L, Gross SW. The endothelial hyperplasia of the cerebral blood vessels with brain tumors, and its sarcomatous transformation. Cancer 1958;11:264–77.

149. Grant JW, Steart PV, Aguzzi A, Jones DB, Gallagher PJ. Gliosarcoma: an immunohistochemical study. Acta Neuropathol (Berl) 1989;79:305–9.

150. Haddad SF, Moore SA, Schelper RL, Goeken JA. Smooth muscle can comprise the sarcomatous component of gliosarcomas. J Neuropathol Exp Neurol 1992;51:493–8.

150a. Hayashi K, Ohara N, Jeon HJ, et al. Gliosarcoma with features of chondroblastic osteosarcoma. Cancer 1993;72:850–5.

151. Ho KL. Histogenesis of sarcomatous component of the gliosarcoma: an ultrastructural study. Acta Neuropathol (Berl) 1990;81:178–88.

152. Jones H, Steart PV, Weller RO. Spindle-cell glioblastoma or gliosarcoma? Neuropathol Appl Neurobiol 1991;17:177–87.

153. Kepes JJ, Fulling KH, Garcia JH. The clinical significance of "adenoid" formations of neoplastic astrocytes, imitating metastatic carcinoma, in gliosarcomas. A review of five cases. Clin Neuropathol 1982;1:139–50.

154. Lalitha VS, Rubinstein LJ. Reactive glioma in intracranial sarcoma: a form of mixed sarcoma and glioma ("sarcoglioma"). Report of eight cases. Cancer 1979;43:246–57.

155. Meis JM, Ho KL, Nelson JS. Gliosarcoma: a histologic and immunohistochemical reaffirmation. Mod Pathol 1990;3:19–24.

156. _____, Martz KL, Nelson JS. Mixed glioblastoma multiforme and sarcoma: a clinicopathologic study of 26 radiation therapy oncology group cases. Cancer 1991;67:2342–9.

157. Murphy MN, Korkis JA, Robson FC, Sima AA. Gliosarcoma with cranial penetration and extension to the maxillary sinus. J Otolaryngol 1985;14:313–6.

158. Ng HK, Poon WS. Gliosarcoma of the posterior fossa with features of a malignant fibrous histiocytoma. Cancer 1990;65:1161–6.

159. Richman AV, Balis GA, Maniscalco JE. Primary intracerebral tumor with mixed chondrosarcoma and glioblastoma—gliosarcoma or sarcoglioma? J Neuropathol Exp Neurol 1980;39:329–35.

160. Tada T, Katsuyama T, Aoki T, Kobayashi S, Shigematsu H. Mixed glioblastoma and sarcoma with osteoid-chondral tissue. Clin Neuropathol 1986;6:160–3.

Protoplasmic Astrocytoma

161. Russell DS, Rubinstein LJ. Pathology of tumours of the nervous system. 5th ed. Baltimore: Williams & Wilkins, 1989:100–1.

Granular Cell Astrocytic Neoplasms

162. Dickson DW, Suzuki KI, Kanner R, Weitz S, Horoupian DS. Cerebral granular cell tumor: immunohistochemical and electron microscopic study. J Neuropathol Exp Neurol 1986;45:304–14.

163. Harris CP, Townsend JJ, Brockmeyer DL, Heilbrun MP. Cerebral granular cell tumor occurring with glioblastoma multiforme: case report. Surg Neurol 1991;36:202–6.

164. Kornfeld M. Granular cell glioblastoma: a malignant granular cell neoplasm of astrocytic origin. J Neuropathol Exp Neurol 1986;45:447–62.

165. Markesbery WR, Duffy PE, Cowen D. Granular cell tumors of the central nervous system. J Neuropathol Exp Neurol 1973;32:92–109.

166. Nakamura T, Hirato J, Hotchi M, Kyoshima K, Nakamura Y. Astrocytoma with granular cell tumor-like changes. Report of a case with histochemical and ultrastructural characterization of granular cells. Acta Pathol Jpn 1990;40:206–11.

167. Sakurama N, Matsukado Y, Marubayashi T, Kodama T. Granular cell tumour of the brain and its cellular identity. Acta Neurochir 1981;56:81–94.

Gliomatosis Cerebri

168. Artigas J, Cervos-Navarro J, Iglesias JR, Ebhardt G. Gliomatosis cerebri: clinical and histological findings. Clin Neuropathol 1985;4:135–48.
169. Balko MG, Blisard KS, Samaha FJ. Oligodendroglial gliomatosis cerebri. Hum Pathol 1992;23:706–7.
170. Couch JR, Weiss SA. Gliomatosis cerebri: report of four cases and review of the literature. Neurology 1974;24:504–11.
171. Dunn J Jr, Kernohan JW. Gliomatosis cerebri. Arch Pathol 1957;64:82–91.
172. Kandler RH, Smith CM, Broome JC, Davies-Jones GA. Gliomatosis cerebri: a clinical, radiological and patho-logical report of four cases. Br J Neurosurg 1991;5:187–93.
173. Kawano N, Miyasaka Y, Yada K, Atari H, Sasaki K. Diffuse cerebrospinal gliomatosis: case report. J Neurosurg 1978;49:303–7.
174. Nevin S. Gliomatosis cerebri. Brain 1938;61:170–91.
175. Ross IB, Robitaille Y, Villemure JG, Tampieri D. Diagnosis and management of gliomatosis cerebri: recent trends. Surg Neurol 1991;36:431–40.
176. Yanaka K, Kamezaki T, Kobayashi E, Matsueda K, Yoshii Y, Nose T. MR imaging of diffuse glioma. AJNR Am J Neuroradiol 1992;13:349–51.

Meningeal Gliomatosis

177. Bailey OT. Relation of glioma of the leptomeninges to neuroglia nests. Report of a case of astrocytoma of the leptomeninges. Arch Pathol 1936;21:584–600.
178. Cooper IS, Kernohan JW. Heterotopic glial nests in the subarachnoid space: histopathologic characteristics, mode of origin and relation to meningeal gliomas. J Neuropathol Exp Neurol 1951;10:16–29.
179. Heye N, Iglesias JR, Tönsen K, Graef G, Maier-Hauff K. Primary leptomeningeal gliomatosis with predominant involvement of the spinal cord. Acta Neurochir (Wein) 1990;102:145–8.
180. Kakita A, Wakabayashi K, Takahashi H, Ohama E, Ikurta F, Tokiguchi S. Primary leptomeningeal glioma: ultrastructural and laminin immunohisto-chemical studies. Acta Neuropathol (Berl) 1992;83:538–42.
181. Kalyan-Raman UP, Cancilla PA, Case MJ. Solitary, primary malignant astrocytoma of the spinal leptomeninges. J Neuropathol Exp Neurol 1983;42:517–21.
182. Kitahara M, Katakura R, Wada T, Namiki T, Suzuki J. Diffuse form of primary leptomeningeal gliomatosis: case report. J Neurosurg 1985;63:283–7.
183. Korein J, Feigin I, Shapiro MF. Oligodendrogliomatosis with intracranial hypertension. Neurology 1957;7:589–94.
184. Polmeteer FE, Kernohan JW. Meningeal gliomatosis: a study of forty-two cases. Arch Neurol Psychiatry 1947;57:593–616.
185. Ramsay DA, Goshko V, Nag S. Primary spinal lepto-meningeal astrocytoma. Acta Neuropathol (Berl) 1990;80:338–41.
186. Sceats DJ Jr, Quisling R, Rhoton AL Jr, Ballinger WE, Ryan P. Primary leptomeningeal glioma mimicking an acoustic neuroma: case report with review of the literature. Neurosurgery 1986;19:649–54.
187. Sumi SM, Leffman H. Primary intracranial leptomeningeal glioma with persistent hypoglycorrhachia. J Neurol Neurosurg Psychiatry 1968;31:190–4.
188. Whelan HT, Sung JH, Mastri AR. Diffuse leptomeningeal gliomatosis: report of three cases. Clin Neuropathol 1987;6:164–8.
189. Yung WK, Horten BC, Shapiro WR. Meningeal gliomatosis: a review of 12 cases. Ann Neurol 1980;8:605–8.

Pilocytic Astrocytoma

190. Albright AL, Guthkelch AN, Packer RJ, Price RA, Rourke LB. Prognostic factors in pediatric brain-stem gliomas. J Neurosurg 1986;65:751–5.
191. Alvord EC Jr, Lofton S. Gliomas of the optic nerve or chiasm. J Neurosurg 1988;68:85–98.
192. Bernell WR, Kepes JJ, Seitz EP. Late malignant recurrence of childhood cerebellar astrocytoma. J Neurosurg 1972;37:470–4.
193. Civitello LA, Packer RJ, Rorke LB, Siegel K, Sutton LN, Schut L. Leptomeningeal dissemination of low-grade gliomas in childhood. Neurology 1988;38:562–6.
194. Clark GB, Henry JM, McKeever PE. Cerebral pilocytic astrocytoma. Cancer 1985;56:1128–33.
195. Daumas-Duport C, Scheithauer BW, O'Fallon J, Kelly P. Grading of astrocytomas: a simple and reproducible method. Cancer 1988;62:2152–65.
195a. Dirks PB, Jay V, Becker LE, et al. Development of anaplastic changes in low-grade astrocytomas of childhood. Neurosurgery 1994;34:68–78.
196. Forsyth PA, Shaw EG, Scheithauer BW, O'Fallon JR, Layton DD, Katzmann JA. 51 cases of supratentorial pilocytic astrocytomas: a clinicopathologic, prognostic, and flow cytometric study. Cancer. 1993;72:1335–42.
197. Geissinger JD, Bucy PC. Astrocytomas of the cerebellum in children: long-term study. Arch Neurol 1971;24:125–35.
198. Gjerris F, Klinken L. Long-term prognosis in children with benign cerebellar astrocytoma. J Neurosurg 1978;49:179–84.
199. Hayostek C, Shaw EG, Scheithauer BW, et al. Astrocytomas of the cerebellum. A comparative clinicopathologic study of pilocytic and diffuse astrocytomas. Cancer 1993;72:856–69.
200. Hoffman HJ, Becker L, Craven MA. A clinically and pathologically distinct group of benign brain stem gliomas. Neurosurgery 1980;7:243–8.
201. Ito S, Hoshino T, Shibuya M, Prados MD, Edwards MS, Davis RL. Proliferative characteristics of juvenile pilocytic astrocytomas determined by bromode-oxyuridine labeling. Neurosurgery 1992;31:413–9.
202. Katsetos CD, Friedberg E, Reidy J, et al. Localization of serine protease inhibitors α-1-antichymotrypsin and α-1-antitrypsin in eosinophilic granular bodies of pilocytic astrocytomas. J Neuropathol Exp Neurol 1991;50:293.
203. Khatib Z, Heidemann R, Kovnar E, et al. Pilocytic dorsally exophytic brainstem gliomas: a distinct clinicopathological entity. Ann Neurol 1992;32:458–9.
204. Kleinman GM, Schoene WC, Walshe TM III, Richardson EP Jr. Malignant transformation in benign cerebellar astrocytoma. Case report. J Neurosurg 1978;49:111–8.

205. Kocks W, Kalff R, Reinhardt V, Grote W, Hilke J. Spinal metastasis of pilocytic astrocytoma of the chiasma opticum. Childs Nerv Syst 1989;5:118–20.

206. Lach B, Sikorska M, Rippstein P, Gregor A, Staines W, Davie TR. Immunoelectron microscopy of Rosenthal fibers. Acta Neuropathol (Berl) 1991;81:503–9.

207. Lombardi D, Scheithauer BW, Piepgras D, Meyer FB, Forbes GS. "Angioglioma" and the arteriovenous malformation-glioma association. J Neurosurg 1991;75:589–96.

208. Longee DC, Friedman HS, Phillips PC, et al. Osteoblastic metastases from astrocytomas: a report of two cases. Med Pediatr Oncol 1991;19:318–24.

209. McGirr SJ, Kelly PJ, Scheithauer BW. Stereotactic resection of juvenile pilocytic astrocytoma of the thalamus and basal ganglia. Neurosurgery 1987;20:447–52.

209a. Minehan K, Scheithauer B, Shaw E, Onofrio B. Astrocytic tumors of the spinal cord [Abstract]. J Neuropathol Exp Neurol 1993;52:289.

210. Murayama S, Bouldin TW, Suzuki K. Immunocytochemical and ultrastructural studies of eosinophilic granular bodies in astrocytic tumors. Acta Neuropathol (Berl) 1992;83:408–14.

211. Nishio S, Takeshita I, Fukui M, Yamashita M, Tateishi J. Anaplastic evolution of childhood optico-hypothalamic pilocytic astrocytoma: report of an autopsy case. Clin Neuropathol 1988;7:254–8.

212. Obana WG, Cogen PH, Davis RL, Edwards MS. Metastatic juvenile pilocytic astrocytoma. Case report. J Neurosurg 1991;75:972–5.

213. Packer RJ, Sutton LN, Bilaniuk LT, et al. Treatment of chiasmatic/hypothalamic gliomas of childhood with chemotherapy: an update. Ann Neurol 1988;23:79–85.

214. Pagni CA, Giordana MT, Canavero S. Benign recurrence of a pilocytic cerebellar astrocytoma 36 years after radical removal: case report. Neurosurgery 1991;28:606–9.

215. Palma L, Guidetti B. Cystic pilocytic astrocytomas of the cerebral hemispheres. Surgical experience with 51 cases and long-term results. J Neurosurg 1985;62:811–5.

216. _____, Russo A, Celli P. Prognosis of the so-called "diffuse" cerebellar astrocytoma. Neurosurgery 1984;15:315–7.

216a. Pollack IF, Hoffman HJ, Humphreys RP, Becker L. The long-term outcome after surgical treatment of dorsally exophytic brain-stem gliomas. J Neurosurg 1993;78:859–63.

217. Rauhut F, Reinhardt V, Budach V, Wiedemayer H, Nau HE. Intramedullary pilocytic astrocytomas—a clinical and morphological study after combined surgical and photon or neutron therapy. Neurosurg Rev 1989;12:309–13.

218. Ringhertz N, Nordenstam H. Cerebellar astrocytoma. J Neuropathol Exp Neurol 1951;10:343–67.

219. Rodriguez LA, Edwards MS, Levin VA. Management of hypothalamic gliomas in children: an analysis of 33 cases. Neurosurgery 1990;26:242–7.

220. Rossitch E Jr, Zeidman SM, Burger PC, et al. Clinical and pathological analysis of spinal cord astrocytomas in children. Neurosurgery 1990;27:193–6.

221. Rush JA, Younge BR, Campbell RJ, MacCarty CS. Optic glioma. Long-term follow-up of 85 histopathologically verified cases. Ophthalmology 1982;89:1213–9.

222. Russell DS, Rubinstein LJ. Pathology of tumours of the nervous system. 5th ed. Baltimore: Williams & Wilkins, 1989:100–1.

223. Schneider JH Jr, Raffel C, McComb JG. Benign cerebellar astrocytomas of childhood. Neurosurgery 1992;30:58–63.

224. Schwartz AM, Ghatak NR. Malignant transformation of benign cerebellar astrocytoma. Cancer 1990;65:333–6.

225. Shaw EG, Daumas-Duport C, Scheithauer BW, et al. Radiation therapy in the management of low-grade supratentorial astrocytomas. J Neurosurg 1989;70:853–61.

226. Soffer D, Sahar A. Cystic glioma of the brain stem with prolonged survival. Neurosurgery 1982;10:499–502.

226a. Stern J, Jakobiec FA, Housepian EM. The architecture of optic nerve gliomas with and without neurofibromatosis. Arch Ophthalmol 1980;98:505–11.

227. Tomlinson FH, Scheithauer BW, Hayostek CH, Parisi JE, Meyer FB, Shaw EG. Atypia and malignancy in pilocytic astrocytoma of the cerebellum: a clinicopathologic and flow cytometric study. J Neuropathol Exp Neurol 1992;51:331.

228. Wilson WB, Feinsod M, Hoyt WF Nielsen SL. Malignant evolution of childhood chiasmal pilocytic astrocytoma. Neurology 1976;26:322–5.

Pleomorphic Xanthoastrocytoma

229. Allegranza A, Ferraresi S, Bruzzone M, Giombini S. Cerebromeningeal pleomorphic xanthoastrocytoma. Report on four cases: clinical, radiologic and pathological features. (Including a case with malignant evolution.) Neurosurg Rev 1991;14:43–9.

230. Furuta A, Takahashi H, Ikuta F, Onda K, Takeda N, Tanaka R. Temporal lobe tumor demonstrating ganglioglioma and pleomorphic xanthoastrocytoma components. Case report. J Neurosurg 1992;77:143–7.

231. Grant JW, Gallagher PJ. Pleomorphic xanthoastrocytoma: immunohistochemical methods for differentiation from fibrous histiocytomas with similar morphology. Am J Surg Pathol 1986;10:336–41.

232. Iwaki T, Fukui M, Kondo A, Matsushima T, Takeshita I. Epithelial properties of pleomorphic xanthoastrocytomas determined in ultrastructural and immunohistochemical studies. Acta Neuropathol (Berl) 1987;74:142–50.

232a. Kepes JJ. Pleomorphic xanthoastrocytoma: the birth of a diagnosis and a concept. Brain Pathol 1993;3:269–74.

233. Kepes JJ, Rubinstein LJ, Ansbacher L, Schreiber DJ. Histopathological features of recurrent pleomorphic xanthoastrocytomas: further corroboration of the glial nature of this neoplasm. A study of 3 cases. Acta Neuropathol (Berl) 1989;78:585–93.

234. _____, Rubinstein LJ, Eng LF. Pleomorphic xanthoastrocytoma: a distinctive meningocerebral glioma of young subjects with relatively favorable prognosis. A study of 12 cases. Cancer 1979;44:1839–52.

235. Kros JM, Vecht CJ, Stefanko SZ. The pleomorphic xanthoastrocytoma and its differential diagnosis: a study of five cases. Hum Pathol 1991;22:1128–35.

236. Lindboe CF, Cappelen J, Kepes JJ. Pleomorphic xanthoastrocytoma as a component of a cerebellar ganglioglioma: case report. Neurosurgery 1992;31:353–5.

236a. Lipper MH, Eberhard DA, Phillips CD, Vezina LG, Cail WS. Pleomorphic xanthoastrocytoma, a distinctive astroglial tumor: neuroradiologic and pathologic features. Am J Neuroradiol 1993;14:1397–404.

237. MacCaulay RJ, Becker LE, Jay V. Transformation of pleomorphic xanthoastrocytoma to glioblastoma: a case documented with immunogold electron microscopy [Abstract]. J Neuropathol Exp Neurol 1992;51:365.

237a. _____, Jay V, Hoffman HJ, Becker LE. Increased mitotic activity as a negative prognositc indicator in pleomorphic xanthrocytoma: case report. J Neurosurg 1993;79:761–8.

238. Paulus W, Peiffer J. Does the pleomorphic xanthoastrocytoma exist? Problems in the application of immunological techniques to the classification of brain tumors. Acta Neuropathol (Berl) 1988;76:245–52.

239. Sugita Y, Kepes JJ, Shigemori M, et al. Pleomorphic xanthoastrocytoma with desmoplastic reaction: angiomatous variant. Report of two cases. Clin Neuropathol 1990;9:271–8.

240. Weldon-Linne CM, Victor TA, Groothuis DR, Vick NA. Pleomorphic xanthoastrocytoma: ultrastructural and immunohistochemical study of a case with a rapidly fatal outcome following surgery. Cancer 1983;52:2055–63.

241. Whittle IR, Gordon A, Misra BK, Shaw JF, Steers AJ. Pleomorphic xanthoastrocytoma: report of four cases. J Neurosurg 1989;70:463–8.

242. Yoshino MT, Lucio R. Pleomorphic xanthoastrocytoma. AJNR Am J Neuroradiol 1992;13:1330–2.

Subependymal Giant Cell Astrocytoma (Tuberous Sclerosis)

243. Bender BL, Yunis EJ. Central nervous system pathology of tuberous sclerosis in children. Ultrastruct Pathol 1980;1:287–99.

244. Boesel CP, Paulson GW, Kosnik EJ, Earle KM. Brain hamartomas and tumors associated with tuberous sclerosis. Neurosurgery 1979;4:410–7.

245. Bonnin JM, Rubinstein LJ, Papasozomenos SC, Marangos PJ. Subependymal giant cell astrocytoma: significance and possible cytogenetic implications of an immunohistochemical study. Acta Neuropathol (Berl) 1984;62:185–93.

246. Chow CW, Klug GL, Lewis EA. Subependymal giant-cell astrocytoma in children: an unusual discrepancy between histological and clinical features. J Neurosurg 1988;68:880–3.

247. Iwaki T, Wisniewski T, Iwaki A, Corbin E, Tomokane N, Tateishi J, Goldman JE. Accumulation of alpha-β-crystallin in central nervous system glia and neurons in pathologic conditions. Am J Pathol 1992;140:345–56.

248. McMurdo SK Jr, Moore SG, Brant-Zawadzki M, et al. MR imaging of intracranial tuberous sclerosis. Am J Neuroradiol 1987;8:77–82.

249. Morimoto K, Mogami H. Sequential CT study of subependymal giant-cell astrocytoma associated with tuberous sclerosis: case report. J Neurosurg 1986; 65:874–7.

250. Nakamura Y, Becker LE. Subependymal giant-cell tumor: astrocytic or neuronal? Acta Neuropathol (Berl) 1983;60:271–7.

251. Padmalatha C, Harruff RC, Ganick D, Hafez GB. Glioblastoma multiforme with tuberous sclerosis: report of a case. Arch Pathol Lab Med 1980;104:649–50.

252. Shepherd CW, Scheithauer BW, Gomez MR, Altermatt HJ, Katzmann JA. Subependymal giant cell astrocytoma: a clinical, pathological and flow cytometric study. Neurosurgery 1991;28:864–8.

253. Trombley IK, Mirra SS. Ultrastructure of tuberous sclerosis: cortical tuber and subependymal tumor. Ann Neurol 1981;9:174–81.

Infantile Desmoplastic Astrocytoma

254. Aydin F, Ghatak NR, Salvant J, Muizelaar P. Desmoplastic cerebral astrocytoma of infancy. A case report with immunohistochemical, ultrastructural and proliferation studies. Acta Neuropathol 1993;86:666–70.

254a. de Chadarévian JP, Pattisapu JV, Faerber EN. Desmoplastic cerebral astrocytoma of infancy. Light microscopy, immunocytochemistry, and ultrastructure. Cancer 1990;66:173–9.

255. Taratuto AL, Monges J, Lylyk P, Leiguarda R. Superficial cerebral astrocytoma attached to dura. Report of six cases in infants. Cancer 1984;54:2505–12.

Gliofibroma

256. Budka H, Sunder-Plassmann M. Benign mixed glial-mesenchymal tumour ("glio-fibroma") of the spinal cord. Acta Neurochir (Wein) 1980;55:141–5.

257. Cerda-Nicolas M, Kepes JJ. Gliofibromas (including malignant forms), and gliofibromas: a comparative study and review of the literature. Acta Neuropathol 1993;85:349-61.

258. Friede RL. Gliofibroma: a peculiar neoplasia of collagen forming glia-like cells. J Neuropathol Exp Neurol 1978;37:300–13.

259. Iglesias JR, Richardson EP Jr, Collia F, Santos A, Garcia MC, Redondo C. Prenatal intramedullary gliofibroma: a light and electron microscope study. Acta Neuropathol (Berl) 1984;62:230–4.

260. Schober R, Bayindir C, Canbolat A, Urich H, Wechsler W. Gliofibroma: immunohistochemical analysis. Acta Neuropathol (Berl) 1992;83:207–10.

261. Snipes GJ, Steinberg GK, Lane B, Horoupian DS. Gliofibroma: case report. J Neurosurg 1991;75:642–6.

262. Vazquez M, Miller DC, Epstein F, Allen JC, Budzilovich GN. Glioneurofibroma: renaming the pediatric "gliofibroma": a neoplasm composed of Schwann cells and astrocytes. Mod Pathol 1991;4:519–23.

Oligodendroglioma and Anaplastic Oligodendroglioma

263. Burger PC, Rawlings CE, Cox EB, McLendon RE, Schold SC Jr, Bullard DE. Clinicopathologic correlations in the oligodendroglioma. Cancer 1987;59:1345–52.

264. Cairncross JG, Macdonald DR. Successful chemotherapy for recurrent malignant oligodendroglioma. Ann Neurol 1988;23:360–4.

265. _____, Macdonald DR, Ramsay DA. Aggressive oligodendroglioma: a chemosensitive tumor. Neurosurgery 1992;81:78–82.

266. de la Monte SM. Uniform lineage of oligodendrogliomas. Am J Pathol 1989;135:529–40.

267. Glass J, Hochberg FH, Gruber ML, Louis DN, Smith D, Rattner B. The treatment of oligodendrogliomas and mixed oligodendroglioma-astrocytomas with PCV chemotherapy. J Neurosurg 1992;76:741–5.

268. Herpers MJ, Budka H. Glial fibrillary acidic protein (GFAP) in oligodendroglial tumors: gliofibrillary oligodendroglioma and transitional oligoastrocytoma as subtypes of oligodendroglioma. Acta Neuropathol (Berl) 1984;64:265–72.

269. James TG, Pagel W. Oligodendroglioma with extracranial metastases. Br J Surg 1951;39:56–65.

270. Jellinger K, Minauf M, Salzer-Kuntschik M. Oligodendroglioma with extraneural metastases. J Neurol Neurosurg Psychiatry 1969;32:249–53.

271. Kros JM, de Jong AA, van der Kwast TH. Ultrastructural characterization of transitional cells in oligodendrogliomas. J Neuropathol Exp Neurol 1992;51:186–93.

272. _____, Stefanko SZ, de Jong AA, van Vroonhoven CC, van der Heul RO, van der Kwast TH. Ultrastructural and immunohistochemical segregation of gemistocytic subsets. Hum Pathol 1991;22:33–40.

273. _____, Troost D, van Eden CG, van der Werf AJ, Uylings HB. Oligodendroglioma: a comparison of two grading systems. Cancer 1988;61:2251–9.

274. _____, van Eden CG, Stefanko SZ, Waayer-Van Batenburg M, van der Kwast TH. Prognostic implications of glial fibrillary acidic protein containing cell types in oligodendrogliomas. Cancer 1990;66:1204–12.

275. _____, van Eden CG, Vissers CJ, Mulder AH, van der Kwast TH. Prognostic relevance of DNA flow cytometry in oligodendroglioma. Cancer 1992;69:1791–8.

276. Lindegaard KF, Mørk SJ, Eide GE, et al. Statistical analysis of clinicopathological features, radiotherapy, and survival in 170 cases of oligodendroglioma. J Neurosurg 1987;67:224–30.

277. Lombardi D, Scheithauer BW, Piepgras D, Meyer FB, Forbes GS. "Angioglioma" and the arteriovenous malformation-glioma association. J Neurosurg 1991;75:589–96.

278. Ludwig CL, Smith MT, Godfrey AD, Armbrustmacher VW. A clinicopathological study of 323 patients with oligodendrogliomas. Ann Neurol 1986;19:15–21.

279. Mørk SJ, Halvorsen TB, Lindegaard KF, Eide GE. Oligodendroglioma. Histologic evaluation and prognosis. J Neuropathol Exp Neurol 1986;45:65–78.

280. _____, Lindegaard KF, Halvorsen TB, et al. Oligodendroglioma: incidence and biological behavior in a defined population. J Neurosurg 1985;63:881–9.

281. Nakagawa Y, Perentes E, Rubinstein LJ. Immunohistochemical characterization of oligodendrogliomas: an analysis of multiple markers. Acta Neuropathol (Berl) 1986;72:15–22.

282. Nazek M, Mandybur TI, Kashiwagi S. Oligodendroglial proliferative abnormality associated with arteriovenous malformation: report of three cases with review of the literature. Neurosurgery 1988;23:781–5.

283. Packer RJ, Sutton LN, Rorke LB, et al. Oligodendroglioma of the posterior fossa in childhood. Cancer 1985;56:195–9.

284. Robertson DM, Vogel FS. Concentric lamination of glial processes in oligodendrogliomas. J Cell Biol 1962; 15:313–34.

285. Sarkar C, Roy S, Tandon PN. Oligodendroglial tumors: an immunohistochemical and electron microscopic study. Cancer 1988;61:1862–6.

286. Shaw EG, Scheithauer BW, O'Fallon JR, Tazelaar HD, Davis DH. Oligodendrogliomas: the Mayo Clinic experience. J Neurosurg 1992;76:428–34.

287. Smith MT, Ludwig CL, Godfrey AD, Armbrustmacher VW. Grading of oligodendrogliomas. Cancer 1983;52:2107–14.

287a. Tice H, Barnes PD, Goumneroval L, Scott RM, Tarbell NJ. Pediatric and adolescent oligodendrogliomas. Am J Neuroradiol 1993;14:1293–300.

288. Wallner KE, Gonzales M, Sheline GE. Treatment of oligodendrogliomas with or without postoperative irradiation. J Neurosurg 1988;68:684–8.

289. Whitton AC, Bloom HJ. Low grade glioma of the cerebral hemispheres in adults: a retrospective analysis of 88 cases. Int J Radiat Oncol Biol Phys 1990;18:783–6.

Ependymoma and Anaplastic Ependymoma

290. Áfra D, Müller W, Slowik F, Wilcke O, Budka H, Túróczy L. Supratentorial lobar ependymomas: reports on the grading and survival periods in 80 cases, including 46 recurrences. Acta Neurochir (Wein) 1983;69:243–51.

291. Ang, LC, Taylor AR, Bergin D, Kaufmann JC. An immunohistochemical study of papillary tumors in the central nervous system. Cancer 1990;65:2712–9.

292. Cruz-Sanchez FF, Rossi ML, Esiri MM, Reading M. Epithelial membrane antigen expression in ependymomas. Neuropathol Appl Neurobiol 1988;14:197–205.

293. _____, Rossi ML, Hughes JT, Cervos-Navarro J. An immunohistological study of 66 ependymomas. Histopathology 1988;13:443–54.

294. Davis C, Barnard RO. Malignant behavior of myxopapillary ependymoma: report of three cases. J Neurosurg 1985;62:925–9.

295. Ernestus RI, Wilcke O, Schröder R. Supratentorial ependymomas in childhood: clinicopathological findings and prognosis. Acta Neurochir (Wien) 1991;111:96–102.

296. Figarella-Branger D, Gambarelli D, Dollo C, et al. Infratentorial ependymomas of childhood. Correlation between histological features, immunohistological phenotype, silver nucleolar organizer region staining values and post-operative survival in 16 cases. Acta Neuropathol (Berl) 1991;82:208–16.

297. Friede RL, Pollak A. The cytogenetic basis for classifying ependymomas. J Neuropathol Exp Neurol 1978;37:103–18.

298. Goldwein JW, Glauser TA, Packer RJ, et al. Recurrent intracranial ependymomas in children. Survival, patterns of failure, and prognostic factors. Cancer 1990;66:557–63.

299. Ho KL. Microtubular aggregates within rough endoplasmic reticulum in myxopapillary ependymoma of the filum terminale. Arch Pathol Lab Med 1990;114:956–60.

300. Ilgren EB, Stiller CA, Hughes JT, Silberman D, Steckel N, Kaye A. Ependymomas: a clinical and pathologic study. Part II. Survival features. Clin Neuropathol 1984;3:122–7.

301. Kaneko Y, Takeshita I, Matsushima T, Iwaki T, Tashima T, Fukui M. Immunohistochemical study of ependymal neoplasms: histological subtypes and glial and epithelial characteristics. Virchows Arch [A] 1990;417:97–103.

302. Kawano N, Yada K, Yagishita S. Clear cell ependymoma: a histological variant with diagnostic implications. Virchows Arch [A] 1989;415:467–72.

303. Kramer GW, Rutten E, Sloof J. Subcutaneous sacro-coccygeal ependymoma with inguinal lymph node metastasis: case report. J Neurosurg 1988;68:474–7.

304. Lyons MK, Kelly PJ. Posterior fossa ependymomas: report of 30 cases and review of the literature. Neurosurgery 1991;28:659–65.

305. Mannoji H, Becker LE. Ependymal and choroid plexus tumors: cytokeratin and GFAP expression. Cancer 1988;61:1377–85.

306. Maruyama R, Koga K, Nakahara T, Kishida K, Nabeshima K. Cerebral myxopapillary ependymoma. Hum Pathol 1992;23:960–2.

307. Mathews T, Moossy J. Gliomas containing bone and cartilage. J Neuropathol Exp Neurol 1974;33:456–71.

308. Miralbell R, Louis DN, O'Keeffe D, Rosenberg AE, Suit HD. Metastatic ependymoma of the sacrum. Cancer 1990;65:2353–5.

309. Mørk SJ, Løken AC. Ependymoma: a follow-up study of 101 cases. Cancer 1977;40:907–15.

310. Nagashima T, Hoshino T, Cho KG, Edwards MS, Hudgins RJ, Davis RL. The proliferative potential of human ependymomas measured by in situ bromodeoxyuridine labeling. Cancer 1988;61:2433–8.

311. Nazar GB, Hoffman HJ, Becker LE, Jenkin D, Humphreys RP, Hendrick EB. Infratentorial ependymomas in childhood: prognostic factors and treatment. J Neurosurg 1990;72:408–17.

312. Nobles E, Lee R, Kircher T. Mediastinal ependymoma. Hum Pathol 1991;22:94–6.

313. Pulitzer DR, Martin PC, Collins PC, Ralph DR. Subcutaneous sacrococcygeal ("myxopapillary") ependymal rests. Am J Surg Pathol 1988;12:672–7.

314. Rawlings CE III, Giangaspero F, Burger PC, Bullard DE. Ependymomas: a clinicopathologic study. Surg Neurol 1988;29:271–81.

315. Rawlinson DG, Herman MM, Rubinstein LJ. The fine structure of a myxopapillary ependymoma of the filum terminale. Acta Neuropathol (Berl) 1973;25:1–13.

316. Rosenblum MK, Erlandson RA, Aleksic SN, Budzilovich GN. Melanotic ependymoma and subependymoma. Am J Surg Pathol 1990;14:729–36.

317. Schiffer D, Chiò A, Cravioto H, et al. Ependymoma: internal correlations among pathological signs: the anaplastic variant. Neurosurgery 1991;29:206–10.

318. Schweitzer JS, Batzdorf U. Ependymoma of the cauda equina region: diagnosis, treatment, and outcome in 15 patients. Neurosurgery 1992;30:202–7.

319. Shaw EG, Evans RG, Scheithauer BW, Ilstrup DM, Earle JD. Radiotherapeutic management of adult intraspinal ependymomas. Int J Radiat Oncol Biol Phys 1986;12:323–7.

320. Sonneland PR, Scheithauer BW, Onofrio BM. Myxopapillary ependymoma: a clinicopathologic and immunocytochemical study of 77 cases. Cancer 1985;56:883–93.

321. Specht CS, Smith TW, DeGirolami U, Price JM. Myxopapillary ependymoma of the filum terminale: a light and electron microscopic study. Cancer 1986;58:310–7.

322. Spoto GP, Press GA, Hesselink JR, Solomon M. Intracranial ependymoma and subependymoma: MR manifestations. AJNR Am J Neuroradiol 1990;11:83–91.

323. Uematsu Y, Rojas-Corona RR, Llena JF, Hirano A. Distribution of epithelial membrane antigen in normal and neoplastic human ependyma. Acta Neuropathol (Berl) 1989;78:325–8.

324. Wen BC, Hussey DH, Hitchon PW, et al. The role of radiation therapy in the management of ependymomas of the spinal cord. Int J Radiat Oncol Biol Phys 1991;20:781–6.

325. Wolff M, Santiago H, Duby MM. Delayed distant metastasis from a subcutaneous sacrococcygeal ependymoma: case report, with tissue culture, ultrastructural observations, and review of the literature. Cancer 1972;30:1046–67.

Subependymoma

326. Azzarelli B, Rekate HL, Roessmann U. Subependymoma: a case report with ultrastructural study. Acta Neuropathol (Berl) 1977;40:279–82.

327. Boykin FC, Cowen D, Iannucci CA, Wolf A. Subependymal glomerate astrocytomas. J Neuropathol Exp Neurol 1954;13:30–49.

328. Changaris DG, Powers JM, Perot PL Jr, Hungerford GD, Neal GB. Subependymoma presenting as subarachnoid hemorrhage: case report. J Neurosurg 1981;55:643–5.

329. French JD, Bucy PC. Tumors of the septum pellucidum. J Neurosurg 1948;5:433–49.

330. Fu YS, Chen AT, Kay S, Young HF. Is subependymoma (subependymal glomerate astrocytoma) an astrocytoma or ependymoma? A comparative ultrastructural and tissue culture study. Cancer 1974;34:1992–2008.

331. Gandolfi A, Brizzi RE, Tedeschi F, Paini P, Bassi P. Symptomatic subependymoma of the fourth ventricle: case report. J Neurosurg 1981;55:841–4.

332. Kondziolka D, Bilbao JM. Mixed ependymoma-astrocytoma (subependymoma?) of the cerebral cortex. Acta Neuropathol (Berl) 1988;76:633–7.

333. Lee KS, Angelo JN, McWhorter JM, Davis CH Jr. Symptomatic subependymoma of the cervical spinal cord: report of two cases. J Neurosurg 1987;67:128–31.

334. Lombardi D, Scheithauer BW, Meyer FB, et al. Symptomatic subependymoma: a clinicopathological and flow cytometric study. J Neurosurg 1991;75:583–8.

335. Louis DN, Hedley-Whyte ET, Martuza RL. Sarcomatous proliferation of the vasculature in a subependymoma. Acta Neuropathol (Berl) 1989;78:332–5.

336. Matsumura A, Hori A, Spoerri O. Spinal subependymoma presenting as an extramedullary tumor: case report. Neurosurgery 1988;23:115–7.

337. Pagni CA, Canavero S, Giordana MT, Mascalchi M, Arnetoli G. Spinal intramedullary subependymomas: case report and review of the literature. Neurosurgery 1992;30:115–7.

338. Rea GL, Akerson RD, Rockswold GL, Smith SA. Subependymoma in a 21 over 2-year-old boy: case report. J Neurosurg 1983;59:1088–91.

339. Salcman M, Mayer R. Intramedullary subependymoma of the cervical spinal cord: case report. Neurosurgery 1984;14:608–11.

340. Salvati M, Raco A, Artico M, Artizzu S, Ciappetta P. Subependymoma of the spinal cord. Case report and review of the literature. Neurosurg Rev 1992;15:65–9.

341. Scheinker IM. Subependymoma: a newly recognized tumor of subependymal derivation. J Neurosurg 1945;2:232–40.

342. Tomlinson FH, Scheithauer BW, Kelly PJ, Forbes GS. Subependymoma with rhabdomyosarcomatous differentiation: report of a case and literature review. Neurosurgery 1991;28:761–8.

343. Vaquero J, Martinez R, Vegazo I, Pontón P. Subependymoma of the cervical spinal cord. Neurosurgery 1989;24:625–7.

344. Yamasaki T, Kikuchi H, Higashi T, Yamabe H, Moritake K. Two surgically cured cases of subependymoma with emphasis on magnetic resonance imaging. Surg Neurol 1990;33:329–35.

Choroid Plexus Papilloma and Carcinoma

345. Albrecht S, Rouah E, Becker LE, Bruner J. Transthyretin immunoreactivity in choroid plexus neoplasms and brain metastases. Mod Pathol 1991;4:610–4.

346. Andreini L, Doglioni C, Giangaspero F. Tubular adenoma of choroid plexus: a case report. Clin Neuropathol 1991;10:137–40.

347. Ang LC, Taylor AR, Bergin D, Kaufmann JC. An immunohistochemical study of papillary tumors in the central nervous system. Cancer 1990;65:2712–9.

348. Bergsagel DJ, Finegold MJ, Butel JS, Kupsky WJ, Garcea RL. DNA sequences similar to those of simian virus 40 in ependymomas and choroid plexus tumors of childhood. N Engl J Med 1992;326:988–93.

349. Body G, Darnis E, Pourcelot D, Santini JJ, Gold F, Soutoul JH. Choroid plexus tumors: antenatal diagnosis and follow-up. JCU J Clin Ultrasound 1990;18:575–8.

350. Boesel CP, Suhan JP. A pigmented choroid plexus carcinoma: histochemical and ultrastructural studies. J Neuropathol Exp Neurol 1979;38:177–86.

351. Bonnin JM, Colon LE, Morawetz RB. Focal glial differentiation and oncocytic transformation in choroid plexus papilloma. Acta Neuropathol (Berl) 1987;72:277–80.

352. Cardozo J, Cepeda F, Quintero M, Mora E. Choroid plexus papilloma containing bone. Acta Neuropathol (Berl) 1985;68:83–5.

353. Coates TL, Hinshaw DB Jr, Peckman N, et al. Pediatric choroid plexus neoplasms: MR, CT, and pathologic correlation. Radiology 1989;173:81–8.

354. Coffin CM, Wick MR, Braun JT, Dehner LP. Choroid plexus neoplasms. Clinicopathologic and immunohistochemical studies. Am J Surg Pathol 1986;10:394–404.

355. Cruz-Sanchez FF, Garcia-Bachs M, Rossi ML, et al. Epithelial differentiation in gliomas, meningiomas, and choroid plexus papillomas. Virchows Arch [Cell Pathol] 1992;62:25–34.

356. _____, Rossi ML, Hughes JT, Coakham HB, Figols J, Eynaud PM. Choroid plexus papillomas: an immunohistological study of 16 cases. Histopathology 1989;15:61–9.

357. Davis RL, Fox GE. Acinar choroid plexus adenoma. Case report. J Neurosurg 1970;33:587–90.

358. Duckett S, Osterholm J, Schaefer D, Gonzales C, Schwartzman RJ. Ossified mucin-secreting choroid plexus adenoma: case report. Neurosurgery 1991;29:130–2.

359. Ellenbogen RG, Winston KR, Kupsky WJ. Tumors of the choroid plexus in children. Neurosurgery 1989;25:327–35.

360. Enomoto H, Mizuno M, Katsumata T, Doi T. Intracranial metastasis of a choroid plexus papilloma originating in the cerebellopontine angle region: a case report. Surg Neurol 1991;36:54–8.

361. Furness PN, Lowe J, Tarrant GS. Subepithelial basement membrane deposition and intermediate filament expression in choroid plexus neoplasms and ependymomas. Histopathology 1990;16:251–5.

361a. Gottschalk J, Jautzke G, Paulus W, Goebel S, Cervos-Navarro J. The use of immunomorphology to differentiate choroid plexus tumors from metastatic carcinomas. Cancer 1993;72:1343–9.

362. Gullotta F, de Melo AS. Das Karzinom des Plexus chorioideus. Klinische, lichtmikroskopische und elektronenoptische untersuchungen. Neurochirurgia (Stuttg) 1979;22:1–9.

363. Herbert J, Cavallaro T, Dwork AJ. A marker for primary choroid plexus neoplasms. Am J Pathol 1990;136:1317–25.

364. Ken JG, Sobel DF, Copeland B, Davis J, Kortman KE. Choroid plexus papillomas of the foramen of Luschka: MR appearance. AJNR Am J Neuroradiol 1991;12:1201–3.

365. Kepes JJ. Oncocytic transformation of choroid plexus epithelium. Acta Neuropathol (Berl) 1983;62:145–8.

365a. Lach B, Scheithauer BW, Gregor A, Wick MR. Colloid cyst of the third ventricle. A comparative immunohistochemical study of neuraxis cysts and choroid plexus epithelium. J Neurosurg 1993;78:101–11.

366. Lippa C, Abroms IF, Davidson R, DeGirolami U. Congenital choroid plexus papilloma of the fourth ventricle. J Child Neurol 1989;4:127–30.

367. Mannoji H, Becker LE. Ependymal and choroid plexus tumors. Cytokeratin and GFAP expression. Cancer 1988;61:1377–85.

368. Matsushima T. Choroid plexus papillomas and human choroid plexus: a light and electron microscopic study. J Neurosurg 1983;59:1054–62.

369. _____, Inoue T, Takeshita I, Fukui M, Iwaki T, Kitamoto T. Choroid plexus papillomas: an immunohistochemical study with particular reference to the coexpression of prealbumin. Neurosurgery 1988;23:384–9.

370. McComb RD, Burger PC. Choroid plexus carcinoma: report of a case with immunohistochemical and ultrastructural observations. Cancer 1983;51:470–5.

371. McGirr SJ, Ebersold MJ, Scheithauer BW, Quast LM, Shaw EG. Choroid plexus papillomas: long-term follow-up results in a surgically treated series. J Neurosurg 1988;69:843–9.

372. Miettinen M, Clark R, Virtanen I. Intermediate filament proteins in choroid plexus and ependyma and their tumors. Am J Pathol 1986;123:231–40.

373. Navas JJ, Battifora H. Choroid plexus papilloma: light and electron microscopic study of three cases. Acta Neuropathol (Berl) 1978;44:235–9.

374. Packer RJ, Perilongo G, Johnson D, et al. Choroid plexus carcinoma of childhood. Cancer 1992;69:580–5.

375. Paulus W, Jänisch W. Clinicopathologic correlations in epithelial choroid plexus neoplasms: a study of 52 cases. Acta Neuropathol (Berl) 1990;80:635–41.

376. Reimund EL, Sitton JE, Harkin JC. Pigmented choroid plexus papilloma. Arch Pathol Lab Med 1990;114:902–5.

377. Salazar J, Vaquero J, Aranda IF, Menèndez J, Jimenez MD, Bravo G. Choroid plexus papilloma with chondroma: case report. Neurosurgery 1986;18:781–3.

378. Stefanko SZ, Vuzevski VD. Oncocytic variant of choroid plexus papilloma. Acta Neuropathol (Berl) 1985;66:160–2.

379. Tomita T, Naidich TP. Successful resection of choroid plexus papillomas diagnosed at birth: report of two cases. Neurosurgery 1987;20:774–9.

380. Valladares JB, Perry RH, Kalbag RM. Malignant choroid plexus papilloma with extraneural metastasis. Case report. J Neurosurg 1980;52:251–5.

Mixed Gliomas

381. Bonnin JM, Colon LE, Morawetz RB. Focal glial differentiation and oncocytic transformation in choroid plexus papilloma. Acta Neuropathol (Berl) 1987;72:277–80.
382. de la Monte SM. Uniform lineage of oligodendrogliomas. Am J Pathol 1989;135:529–40.
383. Glass J, Hochberg FH, Gruber ML, Louis DN, Smith D, Rattner B. The treatment of oligodendrogliomas and mixed oligodendroglioma-astrocytomas with PCV chemotherapy. J Neurosurg 1992;76:741–5.
384. Hart MN, Petito CK, Earle KM. Mixed gliomas. Cancer 1974;33:134–40.
385. Kawano N, Yada K, Yagishita S. Clear cell ependymoma. A histological variant with diagnostic implications. Virchows Arch [A] 1989;415:467–72.
386. Kros JM, Van Eden CG, Stefanko SZ, Waayer-Van Batenburg M, van der Kwast TH. Prognostic implications of glial fibrillary acidic protein containing cell types in oligodendrogliomas. Cancer 1990;66:1204–12.
387. Scherer HJ. Cerebral astrocytomas and their derivatives. Am J Cancer 1940;40:159–198.
388. Shaw E, Scheithauer B, O'Fallon J. Astrocytomas (A), oligo-astrocytomas (OA), and oligodendrogliomas (O): a comparative survival study. Neurology 1992; 42(Suppl 3):342.

Astroblastoma

389. Bailey P, Bucy PC. Astroblastomas of the brain. Acta Psychiatr Neurol 1930;5:439–61.
390. Bonnin JM, Rubinstein LJ. Astroblastomas: a pathological study of 23 tumors, with a postoperative follow-up in 13 patients. Neurosurgery 1989;25:6–13.
391. Cabello A, Madero S, Castresana A, Diaz-Lobato R. Astroblastoma: electron microscopy and immunohisto-chemical findings: case report. Surg Neurol 1991; 35:116–21.
392. Rubinstein LJ, Herman MM. The astroblastoma and its possible cytogenic relationship to the tanycyte. An electron microscopic, immunohistochemical, tissue- and organ-culture study. Acta Neuropathol (Berl) 1989;78:472–83.

Granular Cell Tumor of the Infundibulum

393. Becker DH, Wilson CB. Symptomatic parasellar granular cell tumors. Neurosurgery 1981;8:173–80.
394. Boecher-Schwarz HG, Fries G, Bornemann A, Ludwig B, Perneczky A. Suprasellar granular cell tumor. Neurosurgery 1992;31:751–4.
395. Jenevein EP. A neurohypophyseal tumor originating from pituicytes. Am J Clin Pathol 1964;41:522–6.
396. Liss L, Kahn EA. Pituicytoma. Tumor of the sella turcica. A clinicopathological study. J Neurosurg 1957;15:481–8.
397. Liwnicz BH, Liwnicz RG, Huff JS, McBride BH, Tew JM Jr. Giant granular cell tumor of the suprasellar area: immunocytochemical and electron microscopic studies. Neurosurgery 1984;15:246–51.
398. Luse SA, Kernohan JW. Granular-cell tumors of the stalk and posterior lobe of the pituitary gland. Cancer 1955;8:616–22.
399. Nishioka H, Ii K, Llena JF, Hirano A. Immunohistochemical study of granular cell tumors of the neurohypophysis. Virchows Arch [Cell Pathol] 1991;60:413–7.
400. Scheithauer BW, Horvath E, Kovacs K. Ultrastructure of the neurohypophysis. Microsc Res Tech 1992;20:177–86.
401. Shanklin WM. The origin, histology and senescence of tumorettes in the human neurohypophysis. Acta Anatomica 1953;18:1–19.
402. Takei Y, Seyama S, Pearl GS, Tindall GT. Ultrastructural study of the human neurohypophysis. II. Cellular elements of neural parenchyma, the pituicytes. Cell Tissue Res 1980;205:273–87.
403. Vinores SA. Demonstration of glial fibrillary acidic (GFA) protein by electron immunocytochemistry in the granular cells of a choristoma of the neurohypophysis. Histochemistry 1991;96:265–9.

4

NEURONAL AND GLIO-NEURONAL TUMORS

Gangliocytoma and Ganglioglioma

Definition. Neoplasms consisting entirely or in part of large mature neurons.

General Comments. Ganglion cell tumors are sufficiently diverse in their microscopic appearance that they overlap with a number of primary tumors of the brain and spinal cord. Since surgery alone is generally curative, it is extremely important that they not be confused with other tumors that require radiotherapy or chemotherapy (see Appendices B, C). Unnecessarily aggressive treatment may result when this neoplasm is misdiagnosed, particularly if considered an infiltrating glioma.

The designation ganglioglioma is applied to tumors with a neoplastic glial component while the term gangliocytoma is reserved for the less common situation in which only abnormal neurons are present. Since these two entities are not always distinct, the umbrella term *ganglion cell tumor* is a useful compromise for lesions in which the neoplastic nature of the glial component remains in doubt.

Clinical and Radiographic Features. Ganglion cell tumors arise throughout the neuraxis including the spinal cord (1,13,17) (see Appendix G), but most are supratentorial: the temporal lobe is a favorite site. Patients of all ages are affected, but the majority of tumors present in the first two decades of life. Seizures or the consequences of increased intracranial pressure are most often observed.

Radiographically, ganglion cell tumors assume a variety of appearances (2,20,21). Some lesions are cystic (see Appendix D) with much of the mass effect due to the cyst rather than the solid component (fig. 4-1). A mural nodule may be seen. Calcification is common (see Appendix E). The cyst margins can enhance, mimicking the ring enhancement of malignant glioma. This same misrepresentation as a malignant tumor is created when a ganglion cell tumor extends into the subarachnoid space (4,21). The cyst-mural nodule configuration is shared with pilocytic astrocytoma as well as pleomorphic xantho-

astrocytoma, both of which also are seizure-associated tumors of the young.

Macroscopic Findings. In some ganglion cell tumors, a mural nodule projects into a cyst filled with clear fluid. Even solid examples are usually well circumscribed. Any type may be gritty if extensively calcified.

Microscopic Findings. The microscopic appearance of ganglion cell tumors varies from paucicellular lesions containing only clustered abnormal neurons to complex cellular masses consisting of mature ganglion cells, smaller neurons, lymphocytes, and fibrous stroma. Extension into the subarachnoid space with entrapment of large blood vessels is frequent (4).

Although histologic diversity precludes a single concise description of ganglion cell tumors, they fall into several somewhat overlapping categories. The most elementary and benign form is an essentially hamartomatous process consisting of abnormal neurons in a fibrillar background of low cellularity (fig. 4-2). Some of these tumors are rather diffuse and the ganglion cells difficult to identify without immunohistochemistry

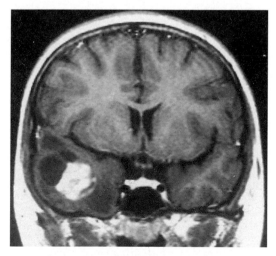

Figure 4-1
GANGLION CELL TUMOR
Some ganglion cell tumors are an enhancing nodule in the wall of a cyst. In contrast to rapidly evolving malignant neoplasms, there is little mass effect or peritumoral edema.

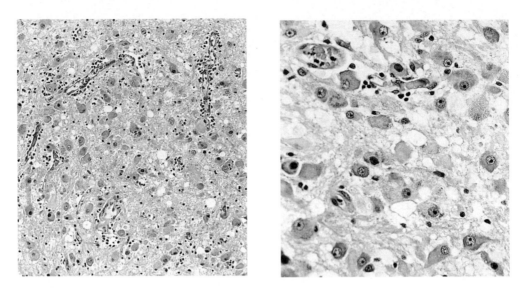

Figure 4-2
GANGLIOCYTOMA

Left: Well-formed ganglion cells are dispersed within a paucicellular neuropil. The sprinkling of perivascular lymphocytes is common.

Right: The neoplastic nature of the ganglion cells is evident at higher magnification due to their increased cell density, lack of orientation, and abnormal cytologic features.

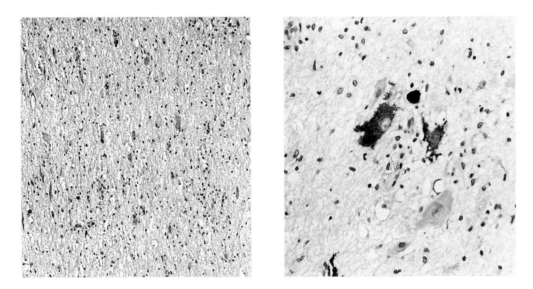

Figure 4-3
GANGLIOCYTOMA

Left: Some gangliocytomas are diffuse lesions in which ganglion cells are inapparent at low or even high magnification in H&E stained sections.

Right: In this case, some cells are highlighted by immunoreactivity for chromogranin.

(fig. 4-3). The ganglion cells can closely resemble normal large neurons, but are abnormally clustered and lack the orderly distribution and polarity of their normal cortical counterparts. Most have large nuclei with prominent nucleoli as well as the basophilic Nissl substance which lies at the periphery of the cytoplasm. Although in some instances smaller neurons are admixed, mitotically active neuroblasts are not seen. Scattered binucleated neurons are often present. A sprinkling of perivascular lymphocytes or calcospherites may be seen.

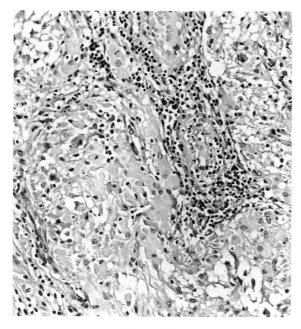

Figure 4-4
GANGLION CELL TUMOR

Lobules of neoplastic cells set in a collagen and lymphocyte-rich stroma are a common feature of ganglion cell tumors. The glassy, fibrillated cytoplasm of many cells creates a glioma-like appearance.

Another histologic pattern of ganglion cell tumor features a lobular architecture and reticulin-rich stroma entrapping nests of neoplastic cells (fig. 4-4). Other similar lesions are less lobular and resemble glioma if studied only by low magnification (fig. 4-5). In any ganglion cell tumor some neoplastic elements are obviously ganglionic, with vesicular nuclei, large nucleoli, and prominent Nissl substance. Other cells are less readily identified as neuronal since their nucleoli are smaller, the cytoplasm more glassy, and the Nissl substance more difficult to find (fig. 4-5, right). In such lesions, more typically neuronal cells are usually situated at the center of the lobules. Although, at first glance, large cells with appropriate nuclear features may appear neuronal, many are seen on close scrutiny to project multipolar cytoplasmic processes suggesting astrocytic rather than neuronal differentiation. The cellular pleomorphism so typical of ganglioglioma understandably results in the diagnostic confusion discussed below under Differential Diagnosis.

A third histologic pattern is one of highly desmoplastic tumor in which ganglion cells are

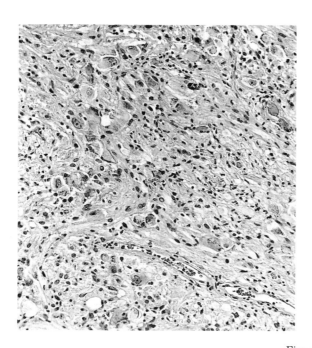

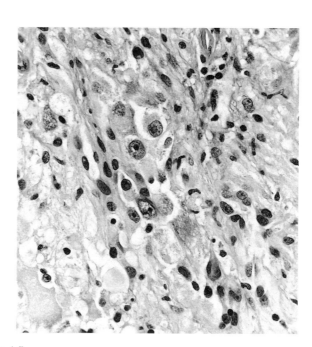

Figure 4-5
GANGLION CELL TUMOR

Left: A common variant of ganglion cell tumor includes both large neurons and a dense, often spindle cell, astrocytic stroma.
Right: At higher magnification, some of the cells are obviously ganglionic, but others with glassy cytoplasm and process formation appear astrocytic.

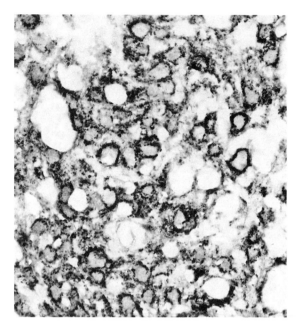

Figure 4-14
GANGLION CELL TUMOR
Constituent neurons show granular surface immunoreactivity for synaptophysin, a feature not seen on normal neurons.

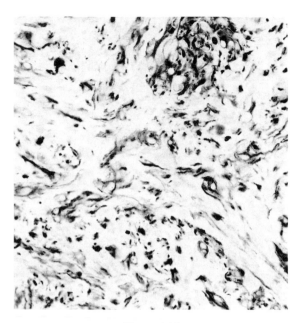

Figure 4-15
GANGLIOGLIOMA
Gangliogliomas typically contain numerous astrocytes positive for GFAP.

immunoreactivity for neuronal markers is proportional to nucleolar size. Obviously, neuronal cells with large nucleoli are generally positive, whereas those with small nucleoli may not be. In some cells, cytoplasmic whorls may be labeled by immunohistochemistry for neurofilament protein but, in most cases, the perikaryon of the ganglion cells is immunonegative and reactivity is confined to cell processes. These often cannot be distinguished from normal axons trapped within the lesion. Synaptophysin may show focal paranuclear staining but exhibits granular cell surface reactivity on large ganglion cells, but not on normal large neurons (fig. 4-14) (3,12). Immunopositivity for neuron-specific enolase (NSE), although least specific, is nonetheless helpful in many cases.

Ganglion cells may stain for neuropeptides such as vasoactive intestinal peptide (VIP), metenkephalin, leuenkephalin, dopamine, tyrosine hydroxylase, serotonin, somatostatin, substance P, and beta hydrolyase (3,5,7,19). More than one may be found in a single tumor (19). In contrast to the weak staining of normal neurons (7), some neoplastic ganglion cells are positive for chromogranin

A (see fig. 4-3, right) (3,7). Such staining presumably reflects the presence of dense core granules in many ganglion cell tumors, a finding discussed below under Ultrastructural Findings.

Astrocytes in ganglion cell tumors are reactive for GFAP (fig. 4-15), but it may be difficult to decide whether such immunopositive cells are reactive or neoplastic. In tumors with a lobular architecture, GFAP-positive tumor cells are usually easy to identify and are more numerous at the periphery of the lobules. The monomorphism or pleomorphism of these cells and their lack of long, radially symmetric processes are indicators that they are participants in the tumor rather than mere reactive bystanders.

Ultrastructural Findings. Electron microscopy plays a role in the diagnosis of ganglion cell tumors by revealing the dense core granules which are a distinctive feature of neoplastic ganglion cells (fig. 4-16) (3,5,15,19). Such granules are lacking or inconspicuous in most normal central nervous system neurons. Also seen are long axonal processes containing microtubules. Clear secretory vesicles and even synapses may be seen in cell terminations.

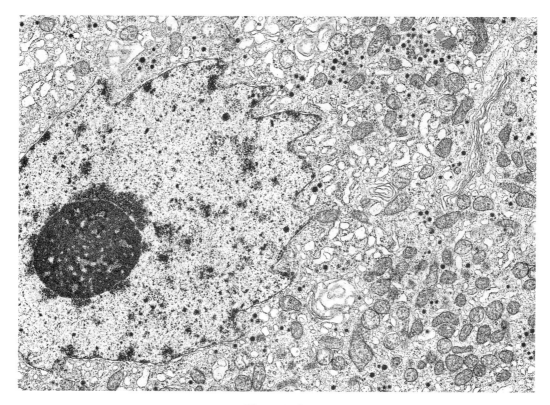

Figure 4-16
GANGLION CELL TUMOR
The presence of dense core neurosecretory granules is a classic ultrastructural feature of ganglion cell tumors, but not generally of normal cortical neurons.

Differential Diagnosis. Given the great heterogeneity of ganglion cell tumors, as well as the difficulty in distinguishing trapped neoplastic neurons in some gliomas, ganglion cell tumors can be both over- and underdiagnosed (see Appendix B).

Overdiagnosis can occur when infiltrating gliomas entrap large cortical or subcortical neurons which are then misinterpreted as part of the neoplasm. Given the propensity of oligodendrogliomas to undergo cortical extension, it is this tumor that is most often interpreted as ganglioglioma (figs. 3-118, 4-17). The mistake can be avoided if it is recognized that the lesion in question is an infiltrating neoplasm rather than a compact mass, as is typical of ganglion cell tumors. In addition, trapped normal neurons are uniform, fully differentiated, and, in favorable sections, polar in their orientation. The presence of satellitosis about the ganglion cells is a distinctive feature of infiltrating gliomas such as oligodendrogliomas, but not of ganglion cell tumors.

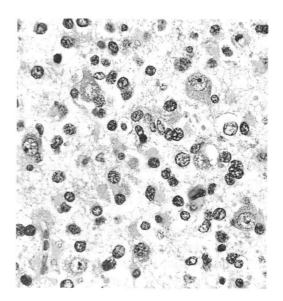

Figure 4-17
OLIGODENDROGLIOMA SIMULATING
GANGLION CELL TUMOR
Preexisting neurons trapped in an infiltrating oligodendroglioma should not be interpreted as evidence of a ganglion cell neoplasm.

171

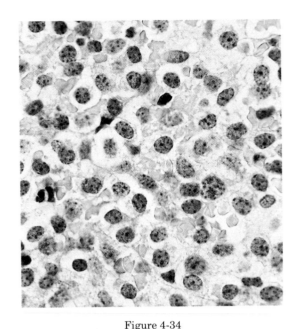

Figure 4-34
CENTRAL NEUROCYTOMA
A "salt and pepper" chromatin pattern is typical of neurocytic and neuroendocrine neoplasms.

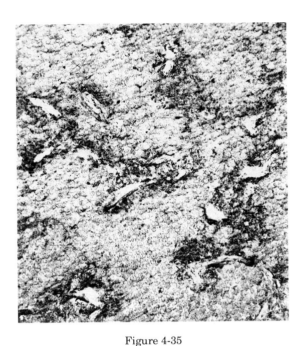

Figure 4-35
CENTRAL NEUROCYTOMA
Synaptophysin immunoreactivity in the fibrillar zones is an important diagnostic feature.

Structures resembling Homer Wright rosettes are uncommon in neurocytomas. Large ganglion cells are rare (39), although maturation through ganglioid cells to mature neurons is occasionally achieved (46). The cells of most neurocytomas, therefore, appear to be arrested at the neurocyte stage, neither regressing to neuroblasts nor advancing to mature neurons.

The strikingly uniform nuclei of neurocytomas exhibit finely speckled chromatin and small nucleoli (fig. 4-34). They lack the vesicular chromatin and prominent nucleoli of ganglion cells, but differ from the smudgy or coarse chromatin-containing nuclei of neuroblastomas or of other embryonal or primitive tumors. Multinucleation and pleomorphism are generally absent and mitoses are rare or absent. The low Ki-67 cell proliferation index is not surprising in light of the benign histologic and cytologic features of typical tumors (38). A minority of neurocytomas show an accelerated mitotic rate, with or without necrosis. The necrosis is often microscopic in extent but may be accompanied by pseudopalisading of nuclei. According to some, atypical tumors may be associated with invasive growth and recurrence (49). The clinical behavior of these tumors remains to be characterized.

Immunohistochemical Findings. Fibrillar zones are immunoreactive for both synaptophysin and NSE (fig. 4-35) (39,41a,42). A high incidence of reactivity for other neuronal epitopes (class III beta-tubulin and neurofilament protein) has been noted in some studies as well (42). Immunoreactivity for GFAP is usually confined to scattered reactive astrocytes, most of which are perivascular in location, but focal abundant reactivity may be seen (fig. 4-36). One investigation utilizing double labeling suggested that in some neurocytomas individual neoplastic cells express both glial (GFAP) and neuronal markers (48). In contrast, GFAP-positive tumor cells have not been found in other studies (39,42). Neurocytomas are typically immunonegative for chromogranin.

Ultrastructural Findings. The neuropil produced by neurocytoma cells consists of a dense feltwork of cytoplasmic processes containing microtubules (fig. 4-37) (39). A few neurosecretory granules are often seen, either within the processes or the perinuclear cytoplasm. In some cases they may be sparse. Clear vesicles, synapses, and synapse-like membrane thickenings are infrequent (39,41,41a).

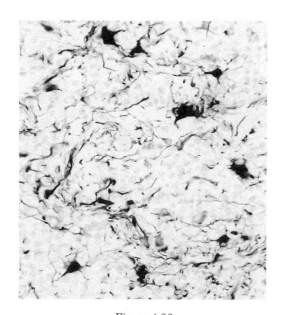

Figure 4-36
CENTRAL NEUROCYTOMA
Scattered reactive astrocytes immunopositive for GFAP are commonly found.

Frozen Section and Cytology. Awareness of neurocytoma and its stereotypical appearance is essential to its intraoperative identification. At low magnification, the neoplasm is markedly cellular and resembles oligodendroglioma, ependymoma, or neuroblastoma, as discussed above. High cellularity and the fibrillar zones that may mimic necrosis even bring malignant tumors such as glioblastoma into the differential diagnosis (fig. 4-38). Cytologic preparations are highly recommended since they capture the neurocytoma's remarkable nuclear uniformity, delicate chromatin pattern, and virtual lack of mitoses (pl. VIA, p. 183).

Neurocytomas lose much of their neurocytic character in paraffin-embedded tissues that have been utilized for a frozen section. Such tissue may resemble a generic small cell neoplasm. If, however, the location of the tumor is considered, as well as its cellular uniformity and lack of mitotic activity, the correct diagnosis usually comes to mind.

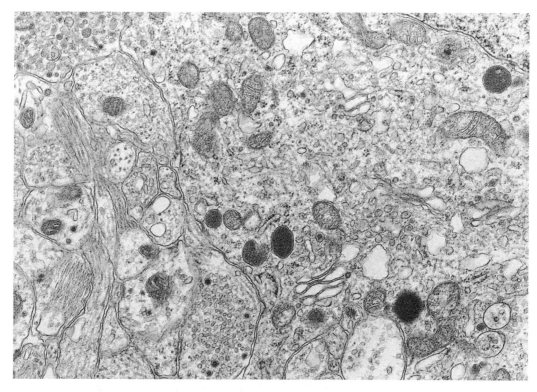

Figure 4-37
CENTRAL NEUROCYTOMA
Dense core granules are often seen within cell processes and, to a lesser extent, within perinuclear cytoplasm. Despite the frequent presence of clear synaptic vesicles, as are seen at the bottom of the illustration, synapses are rare. Note the microtubule-rich processes characteristic of neuronal neoplasms.

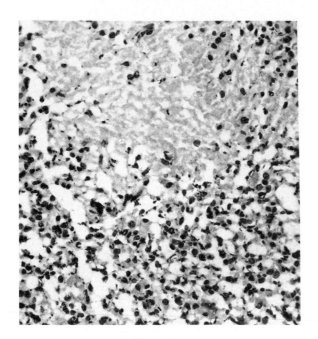

Figure 4-38
CENTRAL NEUROCYTOMA: FROZEN SECTION
In frozen sections, neurocytomas may be mistaken for malignant gliomas in view of the high cellularity and fibrillar zones which resemble necrosis.

Differential Diagnosis. Oligodendroglioma, cellular ependymoma, and neuroblastoma are the main diagnostic contenders.

In light of the cellular monotony, perinuclear halos, and frequent calcification of neurocytomas, oligodendroglioma becomes the principal entity in the differential diagnosis (fig. 4-33). The residual white matter in infiltrative oligodendrogliomas may closely resemble the fibrillar background of the neurocytoma, but consists of aligned regimented axons as seen with special stains. If present, stellate perivascular fibrillar zones and cellular streaming are diagnostic features of neurocytoma; however, some neurocytomas lack these diagnostic features and oligodendrogliomas and neurocytomas are then virtually indistinguishable at the H&E level. Most tumors previously reported as intraventricular oligodendrogliomas are in fact neurocytomas.

Immunostaining for synaptophysin is the simplest way to distinguish neurocytoma from oligodendroglioma since the latter is nonreactive. While reactivity for NSE is less specific and can be seen in some oligodendrogliomas, strong staining is, nevertheless, evidence in support of neurocytoma.

Ultrastructurally, both intercellular accumulations of diminutive cell processes containing microtubules as well as small lysosomes mimicking secretory granules may be seen in oligodendrogliomas. The extent of process formation, their larger size, and the presence of uniform neurosecretory granules or vesicles favor a diagnosis of neurocytoma.

The ependymoma enters into the differential diagnosis from both a clinical and radiographic perspective, given its paraventricular or intraventricular location and frequent calcification. Of all ependymomas, the clear cell variant most closely shares an oligodendroglioma-like appearance with neurocytomas. Most ependymoma, however, intrude unilaterally into a ventricle and also involve paraventricular tissue, whereas neurocytomas lie in the midline involving the septum pellucidum and are exclusively intraventricular. The ependymoma nevertheless remains in the differential since the perivascular fibrillar zones of neurocytomas closely resemble the perivascular pseudorosettes of ependymoma (fig. 4-31). In contrast to the roundness of ependymal pseudorosettes, the perivascular fibrillar zones of neurocytomas are often stellate in configuration and associated with cell streaming. Most important is the immunoreactivity of neurocytomas for synaptophysin and the lack of GFAP staining. Ependymal pseudorosettes usually contain at least some strongly GFAP-positive processes.

The cerebral neuroblastoma, a largely pediatric tumor, is intraparenchymal rather than intraventricular in location. It is also highly cellular, cytologically atypical, and often shows brisk mitotic activity. Desmoplasia, an occasional feature of neuroblastoma, is alien to neurocytoma. Necrosis, parenchymal invasion, and a tendency to cerebrospinal seeding further contrast neuroblastoma with the histologically well-differentiated appearance and macroscopic discreteness of most neurocytomas. The immunohistochemical and electron microscopic features of these two tumors are sufficiently similar to be of little differential diagnostic utility.

Treatment and Prognosis. When central neurocytomas lend themselves to gross total resection, cure results. Given the location of the lesion, residual neoplasm often remains. Regrowth is therefore a possibility. Nevertheless, clinical recurrence comes about only slowly

PLATE VI

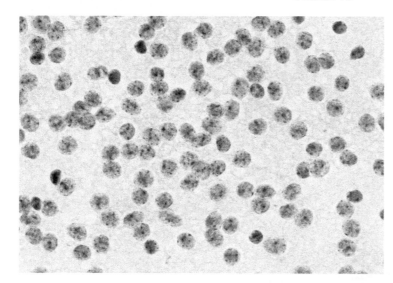

A. CENTRAL NEUROCYTOMA
Remarkably uniform round nuclei with a "salt and pepper" chromatin pattern are typical of this lesion. Cytoplasm and processes are inapparent.

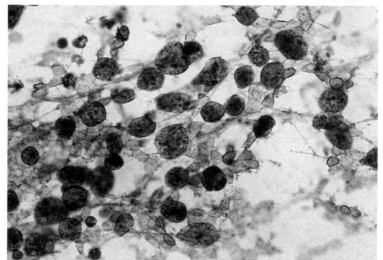

B. CEREBRAL NEUROBLASTOMA
In contrast to the neurocytoma, this embryonal neoplasm is composed of cytologically malignant cells.

C. MEDULLOBLASTOMA
Dense, coarse, and moderately pleomorphic nuclei are common.

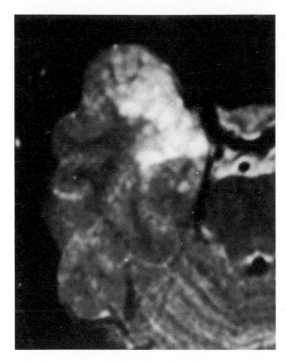

Figure 4-39
DYSEMBRYOPLASTIC NEUROEPITHELIAL TUMOR
Magnetic resonance imaging in the T2 mode visualizes the characteristic intracortical nodules.

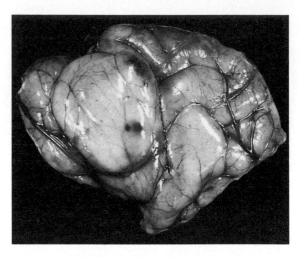

Figure 4-40
DYSEMBRYOPLASTIC
NEUROEPITHELIAL TUMOR
Gyral expansion and, on occasion, blister-like elevations are typical gross features. The latter reflect the presence of superficial cortical nodules.

(43,49). As noted above, the significance of examples with increased mitotic activity remains to be established (41a,49). Although the intraventricular location of neurocytoma should favor cerebrospinal fluid spread, this is rare. The prognosis of patients with neurocytoma is thus excellent. The role of radiation therapy remains to be defined but is often administered to subtotally resected tumors (39,45a).

Dysembryoplastic Neuroepithelial Tumor

Definition. A quasi-hamartomatous, multinodular intracortical mass composed mainly of glia and, to a lesser extent, neurons.

Clinical and Radiographic Features. Although this uncommon lesion typically becomes symptomatic during the first two decades of life, an additional decade or two may pass before surgery is undertaken. Seizures of the partial complex type are the almost exclusive symptom (50,50a, 52). All reported dysembryoplastic neuroepithelial tumors (DNTs) have been supratentorial, with the temporal lobe being the most common site.

The MRI spectrum remains to be defined, but in favorable planes the superficial intracortical location of these lesions is readily evident (fig. 4-39) (51). Especially fortuitous views resolve its multiple constituent nodules (52). In accord with the growth characteristics of DNT, the lesion lacks the peritumoral edema seen around most infiltrative or malignant gliomas. Deformation of the overlying skull further attests to the chronicity of some examples. Occasional lesions are calcified or in part cystic.

Macroscopic Findings. There is considerable variation in the macroscopic appearance of DNTs. They vary in size from only millimeters in greatest dimension to those that are nearly lobar in extent, although most measure several centimeters at best. Some degree of gyral expansion is generally seen. Close inspection of the cortical surface shows blister-like nodules in some fully developed examples (fig. 4-40). Many are ill-defined and only vaguely nodular or cystic. Calcification, if present, is a focal microscopic feature.

Microscopic Findings. Despite considerable morphologic variation, all DNTs exhibit one common characteristic: multiple intracortical nodules (fig. 4-41). These range from larger profiles spanning, if not expanding, the entire cortical ribbon to small subtle foci with only a mild hypercellularity and faintly basophilic background (fig. 4-42, left).

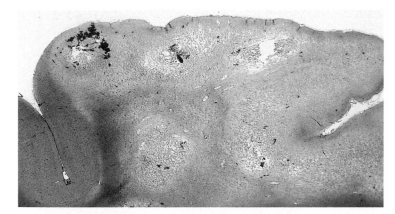

Figure 4-41
DYSEMBRYOPLASTIC
NEUROEPITHELIAL TUMOR
This whole mount histologic section reveals
the intracortical location of this lesion, including its constituent nodules. The darkly staining
foci are artifactual consequences of excision.

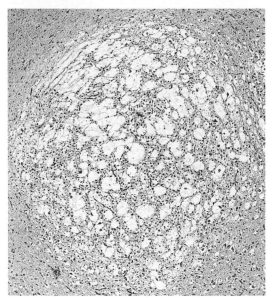 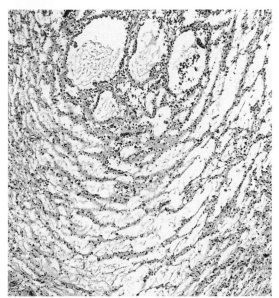

Figure 4-42
DYSEMBRYOPLASTIC NEUROEPITHELIAL TUMOR
Dysembryoplastic neuroepithelial tumors show considerable variation in the architecture of the cortical nodules. Some are uniform
masses interrupted by microcysts (left), whereas others have a highly patterned, and sometimes targetoid, appearance (right).

Regardless of their size, the nodules are rich in acid mucopolysaccharide and accordingly stand out after Alcian blue staining. For the most part, cells of these nodules closely resemble those of well-differentiated oligodendroglioma, sometimes with cell clustering or a ribbon-like architecture producing a targetoid pattern (fig. 4-42, right). Indeed, taken out of context and at high magnification, both the nodules and internodular tissue can be readily mistaken for this glioma which is many times more common than DNT. The intranodular cells are often arranged in clusters or intricate patterns, unlike the cells of oligodendroglioma. Perineuronal satellitosis is not conspicuous.

Instead, neurons within nodules lie randomly and unaccompanied, floating in clear spaces (figs. 4-43, 4-44). The neurons of DNT are also very well differentiated. In addition to the usual predominant oligodendroglial cells, an astrocytic component may be seen as well (fig. 4-45).

An additional feature of DNT, one furthering the similarity to oligodendroglioma, is an extranodular cortical alteration characterized by diffuse oligodendroglial hypercellularity and mucin accumulation (fig. 4-46). The cells permeate the cortex, resulting in isolation of neurons within mucous pools ("floating neurons") rather than engaging in satellitosis.

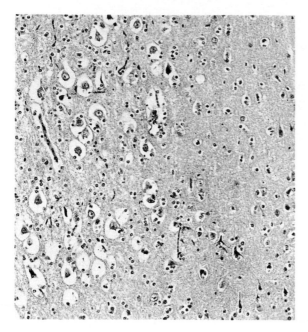

Figure 4-43
DYSEMBRYOPLASTIC NEUROEPITHELIAL TUMOR
A cluster of large neurons and oligodendroglia-like cells abuts normal cortex.

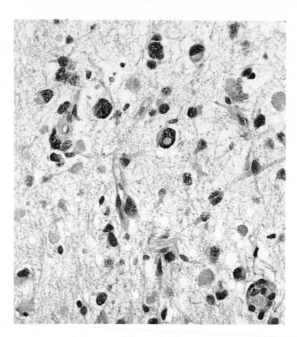

Figure 4-45
DYSEMBRYOPLASTIC NEUROEPITHELIAL TUMOR
Although most of the cells within the nodules resemble oligodendrocytes, astrocytes are not uncommon.

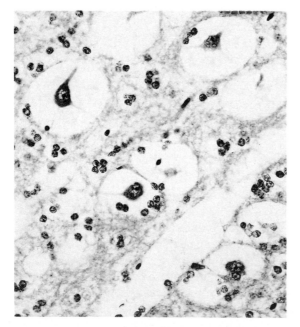

Figure 4-44
DYSEMBRYOPLASTIC NEUROEPITHELIAL TUMOR
The uniformity of the component cells is often noted on high magnification examination of the nodules. Note the large disordered neurons as well as the lack of perineuronal satellitosis.

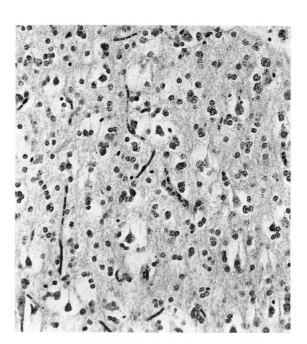

FIGURE 4-46
DYSEMBRYOPLASTIC NEUROEPITHELIAL TUMOR
The paranodular and internodular cortices typically show an oligodendroglioma-like hypercellularity, but not the perineuronal satellitosis characteristic of oligodendrogliomas. The neurons appear to "float" in mucin-rich spaces.

186

DNTs also exhibit other architectural patterns. These variations involve primarily the nodules. Although aggregates or ribbons of oligodendrocytes predominate, compact masses of elongated bipolar astrocytes resembling pilocytic astrocytoma may also be seen. Also common is the loose microcystic pattern so frequently noted in pilocytic astrocytoma. A finding in some nodules is glomeruloid capillary proliferation.

These obvious changes are often, but not invariably, associated with cortical dysplasia which takes the form of disturbed lamination and architectural disarray in surrounding cerebral cortex, and abnormal neurons. The latter may be present in nodules, where cells can be difficult to distinguish from trapped neurons. Abnormal neurons are more readily recognized between and around nodules where their polymorphism, lack of polarity, and occasional binucleation are more evident.

Immunohistochemical Findings. The identification of neurons is simplified by their reactivity for synaptophysin, neurofilament protein, and NSE. For the most part, the usually minor astrocytic component reacts for GFAP.

Differential Diagnosis. The principal differential diagnosis of dysembryoplastic neuroepithelial tumor is oligodendroglioma; in occasional cases in which abnormal neurons are prominent, ganglion cell tumor is considered (see Appendix B). Since the diagnosis of DNT is based in large part upon recognition of architectural changes, particularly patterned nodules, its distinction from oligodendroglioma may not be possible in small biopsies. It should be suspected, however, even in the presence of a single, round, intracortical mucin-rich nodule of oligodendrocytes. Technically, the nodules of DNT are composed of cells more uniform in size and chromasia than those of oligodendroglioma. They are also less likely to exhibit prominent perineuronal satellitosis. In practice, these are subtle rather than diagnostic distinctions. A definitive diagnosis of DNT, therefore, rests more upon low magnification features, particularly the finding of cortical multinodularity. Multiplicity of nodules, when associated with extranodular floating neurons and cortical dysplasia, provides the basis for a sound diagnosis. Unlike the nodules occasionally seen in oligodendroglioma, nodules of DNT are more discrete and patterned. Some do, however, tend to merge with the oligodendroglial hypercellularity so often seen in extranodular cortex.

In contrast to ganglion cell tumor, which usually features a large astrocytic component, DNT exhibits oligodendroglia and lacks a reticulin-rich collagenous stroma, inflammatory cells, and the neuronal pleomorphism so typical of ganglioglioma.

Treatment and Prognosis. DNTs are extremely slow-growing masses, as evidenced by their ability to deform the overlying skull. They appear also to be largely noninfiltrative. Even subtotal resection has reportedly been curative, but a full understanding of the nature of this lesion awaits further clinical experience (50,50a).

Other Glio-Neuronal Lesions

There is a wide variety of generally small, often epileptogenic lesions containing neurons, glia, or cells with intermediate neuronal-glial phenotypes. These may be encountered at autopsy or in surgical specimens, usually of the temporal lobes, removed for seizure control (53, 55–60). Some are relatively well-characterized abnormalities as occur in syndromes such as neurofibromatosis 2 and tuberous sclerosis. Others are minute foci which are not well understood, particularly with regard to their proliferative potential. Some lesions present as radiographically detectable foci but many come to light only when lobectomy specimens are systematically studied. The former are particularly relevant to this volume (61–63). One such lesion is noted for abrupt transition from normal cortical architecture to prominent neuronal giantism. Such an abnormality may be focal but often involves much of one cerebral hemisphere (figs. 4-47, 4-48). These large neurons are generally well oriented with their apical dendrites pointing to the cortical surface, but are irregularly laminated horizontally and create considerable disarray in the cortical architecture (fig. 4-49). Such giant neurons, which possess prominent Nissl substance, are several times larger than their normal counterparts in unaffected cortex and may be accompanied by aggregates of large atypical astrocytic elements with glassy pink cytoplasm (fig. 4-49). These elements are found throughout the cortex but are especially prominent in the superficial molecular layer. The same elements may be even more conspicuous in underlying white matter where they are accompanied by extensive gliosis

26. Ng TH, Fung CF, Ma LT. The pathological spectrum of desmoplastic infantile gangliogliomas. Histopathology 1990;16:235–41.

27. Parisi JE, Scheithauer BW, Priest JR, Okazaki H, Komori T. Desmoplastic infantile ganglioglioma (DIG): a form of ganglioglioma. J Neuropathol Exp Neurol 1992;51:365.

28. Taratuto AL, Monges J, Lylyk P, Leiguarda R. Superficial cerebral astrocytoma attached to dura. Report of six cases in infants. Cancer 1984;54:2505–12.

29. VandenBerg SR. Desmoplastic infantile ganglioglioma and desoplastic cerebral astrocytoma of infnacy. Brain Pathol 1993;275–81.

29a. VandenBerg SR, May EE, Rubinstein LJ, et al. Desmoplastic supratentorial neuroepithelial tumors of infancy with divergent differentiation potential ("desmoplastic infantile gangliogliomas"). Report on 11 cases of a distinctive embryonal tumor with favorable prognosis. J Neurosurg 1987;66:58–71.

Dysplastic Cerebellar Gangliocytoma (Lhermitte-Duclos Disease)

30. Ambler M, Pogacar S, Sidman R. Lhermitte-Duclos disease (granule cell hypertrophy of the cerebellum). Pathological analysis of the first familial cases. J Neuropathol Exp Neurol 1969;28:622–47.

31. Milbouw G, Born JD, Martin D, et al. Clinical and radiological aspects of dysplastic gangliocytoma (Lhermitte-Duclos disease): a report of two cases with review of the literature. Neurosurgery 1988;22:124–8.

32. Pritchett PS, King TI. Dysplastic gangliocytoma of the cerebellum—an ultrastructural study. Acta Neuropathol (Berl) 1978;42:1–5.

33. Reeder RF, Saunders RL, Roberts DW, Fratkin JD, Cromwell LD. Magnetic resonance imaging in the diagnosis and treatment of Lhermitte-Duclos disease (dysplastic gangliocytoma of the cerebellum). Neurosurgery 1988;23:240–5.

34. Shiurba RA, Gessaga EC, Eng LF, Sternberger LA, Sternberger NH, Urich H. Lhermitte-Duclos disease.

An immunohistochemical study of the cerebellar cortex. Acta Neuropathol (Berl) 1988;75:474–80.

35. Stapleton SR, Wilkins PR, Bell BA. Recurrent dysplastic cerebellar gangliocytoma (Lhermitte-Duclos disease) presenting with subarachnoid haemorrhage. Br J Neurosurg 1992;6:153–6.

36. Williams DW III, Elster AD, Ginsberg LE, Stanton C. Recurrent Lhermitte-Duclos disease: report of two cases and association with Cowden's disease. AJNR Am J Neuroradiol 1992;13:287–90.

37. Yachnis AT, Trojanowski JQ, Memmo M, Schlaepfer WW. Expression of neurofilament proteins in the hypertrophic granule cells of Lhermitte-Duclos disease: an explanation for the mass effect and the myelination of parallel fibers in the disease state. J Neuropathol Exp Neurol 1988;47:206–16.

Central Neurocytoma

38. Barbosa MD, Balsitis M, Jaspan T, Lowe J. Intraventricular neurocytoma: a clinical and pathological study of three cases and review of the literature. Neurosurgery 1990;26:1045–54.

39. Figarella-Branger D, Pellissier JF, Daumas-Duport C, et al. Central neurocytomas. Critical evaluation of a small-cell neuronal tumor. Am J Surg Pathol 1992;16:97–109.

40. Goergen SK, Gonzales MF, McLean CA. Intraventricular neurocytoma: radiologic features and review of the literature. Radiology 1992;182:787–92.

41. Hassoun J, Gambarelli D, Grisoli F, et al. Central neurocytoma. An electron-microscopic study of two cases. Acta Neuropathol (Berl) 1982;56:151–6.

41a. Hassoun J, Söylemezoglu F, Gambarelli D, Figarella-Branger D, von Ammon K, Kleihues P. Central neurocytoma: a synopsis of clinical and histological features. Brain Pathol 1993;3:297–306.

42. Hessler RB, Lopes MB, Frankfurter A, Reidy J, VandenBerg SR. Cytoskeletal immunohistochemistry of central neurocytomas. Am J Surg Pathol 1992;16:1031–8.

43. Kim DG, Chi JG, Park SH, et al. Intraventricular neurocytoma: clinicopathological analysis of seven cases. J Neurosurg 1992;76:759–65.

44. Louis DN, Swearingen B, Linggood RM, et al. Central nervous system neurocytoma and neuroblastoma in adults—report of eight cases. J Neurooncol 1990; 9:231–8.

45. Miller DC, Kim R, Zagzag D. Neurocytomas: non-classical sites and mixed elements. J Neuropathol Exp Neurol 1992;51:364.

45a. Nakagawa K, Aoki Y, Sakata K, Sasaki Y, Matsutani M, Akanuma A. Radiation therapy of well-differentiated neuroblastoma and central neurocytoma. Cancer 1993;72:1350–5.

46. Nishio S, Takeshita I, Fukui M. Primary cerebral ganglioneurocytoma in an adult. Cancer 1990;66:358–62.

47. Smoker WR, Townsend JJ, Reichman MV. Neurocytoma accompanied by intraventricular hemorrhage: case report and literature review. AJNR Am J Neuroradiol 1991;12:765–70.

48. von Deimling A, Kleihues P, Saremaslani P, et al. Histogenesis and differentiation potential of central neurocytomas. Lab Invest 1991;64:585–91.

49. Yasargil MG, von Ammon K, von Deimling A, Valavanis A, Wichmann W, Wiestler OD. Central neurocytoma: histopathological variants and therapeutic approaches. J Neurosurg 1992;76:32–7.

Dysembryoplastic Neuroepithelial Tumor

50. Daumas-Duport C. Dysembryoplastic neuroepithelial tumors. Brain Pathol 1993;3:283–95.

50a. _____, Scheithauer BW, Chodkiewicz JP, Laws ER Jr, Vedrenne C. Dysembryoplastic neuroepithelial tumor: a surgically curable tumor of young patients with intractable partial seizures. Report of thirty-nine cases. Neurosurgery 1988;23:545–56.

51. Koeller KK, Dillon WP. Dysembryoplastic neuroepithelial tumors: MR appearance. AJNR Am J Neuroradiol 1992;13:1319–25.

52. Prayson RA, Estes ML. Dysembryoplastic neuroepithelial tumor. Am J Clin Pathol 1992;97:398–401.

Other Glio-Neuronal Lesions

53. Armstrong DD, Bruton CJ. Postscript: what terminology is appropriate for tissue pathology? How does it predict outcome? In: Engel J Jr, ed. Surgical treatment of the epilepsies. New York: Raven Press, 1987:541–52.

54. Caccamo D, Herman MM, Urich H, Rubinstein LJ. Focal neuronal gigantism and cerebral cortical thickening after therapeutic irradiation of the central nervous system. Arch Pathol Lab Med 1989;113:880–5.

55. Daumas-Duport C, Scheithauer BW, Chodkiewicz JP, Laws ER Jr, Vedrenne C. Dysembryoplastic neuroepithelial tumor: a surgically curable tumor of young patients with intractable partial seizures. Report of thirty-nine cases. Neurosurgery 1988;23:545–56.

56. Farrell MA, DeRosa MJ, Curran JG, et al. Neuropathologic findings in cortical resections (including hemispherectomies) performed for the treatment of intractable childhood epilepsy. Acta Neuropathol (Berl) 1992;83:246–59.

57. Hardiman O, Burke T, Phillips J, et al. Microdysgenesis in resected temporal neocortex: incidence and clinical significance in focal epilepsy. Neurology 1988;38:1041–7.

58. Kaufmann WE, Galaburda AM. Cerebrocortical microdysgenesis in neurologically normal subjects: a histopathologic study. Neurology 1989;39(2 Pt 1):238–44.

59. Lévesque MF, Nakasato N, Vinters H, Babb TL. Surgical treatment of limbic epilepsy associated with extrahippocampal lesions: the problem of dual pathology. J Neurosurg 1991;75:364–70.

60. Meencke HJ. Pathology of childhood epilepsies Cleve Clin J Med 1989;56(Suppl):S111–23.

61. Robain O, Floquet C, Heldt N, Rozenberg F. Hemimegalencephaly: a clinicopathological study of four cases. Neuropathol Appl Neurobiol 1988;14:125–35.

62. Taylor DC, Falconer MA, Bruton CJ, Corsellis JA. Focal dysplasia of the cerebral cortex in epilepsy. J Neurol Neurosurg Psychiatry 1971;34:369–87.

63. Townsend JJ, Nielsen SL, Malamud N. Unilateral megalencephaly: hamartoma or neoplasm? Neurology 1975;25:448–53.

5

EMBRYONAL TUMORS

The term embryonal tumor is used in this Fascicle for the small or blue cell tumors commonly identified by the suffix *blastoma*. Some are undifferentiated, whereas others exhibit specific architectural or immunohistochemical features which direct the entity into one of the several categories described below. Thus, a neoplasm becomes a medulloepithelioma if medullary-type epithelium is prominent; a neuroblastoma if clearly defined neuroblastic features, usually Homer Wright rosettes and a fine fibrillar background, are identified; an ependymoblastoma if ependymoblastic rosettes prevail, etc. Although medulloblastomas are recognized in part by location, many have a distinctive nodular pattern of growth rarely seen in supratentorial neoplasms of embryonal type. Given the considerable intertumoral and intratumoral heterogeneity of embryonal neoplasms arising in an organ in which diverse cell types are derived from common progenitors, it is no surprise that mixed and hybrid lesions are common.

We consider this classification system a useful framework based upon histologic, immunohistochemical, or electron microscopy criteria, modalities generally available to diagnostic pathologists. While comparison of the features of these neoplasms to the embryonic stages of development formed the original basis for this classification, and remains an issue germane to their histogenesis, we are not committed to the hypothesis that embryonal neoplasms faithfully recreate stages of embryogenesis or that all the cells in, for example, a cerebral neuroblastoma represent neuroblasts. When, in time, the cell lineages in normal and neoplastic differentiation become defined, the information will no doubt facilitate more accurate tumor classification. Until that time, we are wary of classification schemes based upon unproven or general theories as to how embryonal neoplasms arise. For instance, we are reluctant to accept the system in which the majority of embryonal tumors are considered primitive neuroectodermal tumors.

There is no denying that neither the system used here, nor any other scheme, short of the vague concept by which all embryonal tumors become primitive neuroectodermal tumors, can provide a niche for the spectrum of embryonal neoplasms with its considerable variability. For this reason, we use "other" embryonal tumors as a repository for unclassifiable lesions. Given these uncertainties, an entity may be described or discussed in more than one location.

Primitive Neuroectodermal Tumor

The term primitive neuroectodermal tumor (PNET) was first applied to a cellular form of embryonal central nervous system (CNS) tumor showing divergent differentiation along neuronal, glial, and often mesenchymal lines (2). More recently, the term was reintroduced under the assumption that most densely cellular embryonal tumors of the CNS have a common origin from primitive undifferentiated cells, and that they differ only in their location and in the type and degree of differentiation attained (1,5).

Reservations regarding this approach appeared quickly, expressing the view that embryonal tumors can arise from cells already committed to pathways of differentiation, not just from undifferentiated cells, and that the PNET system represented an oversimplification (4,6,7). It was also predicted that the term PNET would become, as it has, a wastebasket diagnosis for almost any small blue cell CNS tumor in children. There was also concern that clinicians would assume PNETs shared biologic properties, being basically similar lesions differing only in "minor" details such as the extent and types of differentiation.

In recent years the term PNET has become uncoupled from its original histogenetic underpinnings and is often used as a synonym for cellular embryonal tumors of the CNS. Thus, the term can be used without implying that the histogenesis of a tumor is understood. Applied in this sense it is a harmless, but unnecessary, synonym for embryonal tumor. It must be remembered that PNETs are not all the same tumor and that their histogenesis remains unsettled.

In the present World Health Organization (WHO) classification, many of the lesions originally

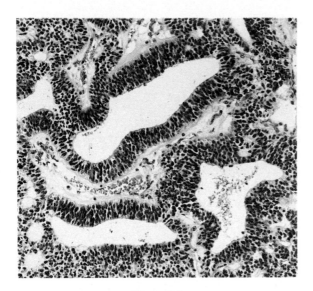

Figure 5-1
MEDULLOEPITHELIOMA
Well-defined gland-like structures with defined epithe-
lial surfaces are an essential diagnostic feature.

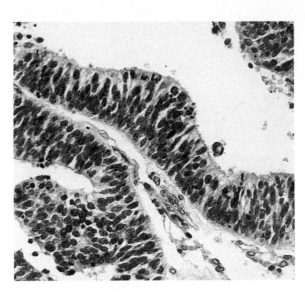

Figure 5-2
MEDULLOEPITHELIOMA
The tall columnar cells of medulloepithelioma rest upon
an external basement membrane. The inner or luminal
surface features a thin, often PAS-positive amorphous layer
as well as small projections. Mitotic figures, sometimes
numerous, lie near the apical surface of the cells. (Courtesy
of Professor D. Schiffer, Turin, Italy.)

included under the PNET umbrella, for instance
neuroblastoma, are given a separate niche (3).
The term PNET is found in the WHO classification but is applied in a limited fashion to small
cell lesions exhibiting divergent differentiation.
Examples include medulloblastomas and morphologically similar tumors in the supratentorial compartment. Whether this placement for
the term is justified is a matter of debate. In any
case, the designation PNET is used either as a
generic equivalent to small cell embryonal tumor
or in a restricted sense for a subset of embryonal
tumors with divergent differentiation much as
originally suggested (2). In this Fascicle, we consider PNET a concept, somewhat akin to the
APUD (amine precursor uptake and decarboxyl-
ation) system, rather than the basis for a
morphologic classification.

Medulloepithelioma

Definition. A neoplasm composed largely or
in part of epithelium resembling that of embryonic neural tube.

Clinical and Radiographic Features. Not
only do most medulloepitheliomas occur during
the first 5 years of life, but many present before
1 year of age. Even congenital examples have
been reported (18). The majority are large masses

which elevate intracranial pressure or produce
neurologic abnormalities reflecting their location. Most medulloepitheliomas arise supra-
tentorially (13–15,17), but examples have been
reported in the posterior fossa (8,9,18). Supratentorial lesions are often deep-seated and lie
close to the ventricular system.

Radiographically, medulloepitheliomas appear as circumscribed, contrast-enhancing lesions. Cysts and calcification may be noted.

Macroscopic Findings. Medulloepitheliomas
are generally discrete, solid, gray-tan tumors
which, although basically soft, may be modified
by cystic change, hemorrhage, calcification, fibrosis, or on rare occasion, bone formation.

Microscopic Findings. The hallmark of
medulloepitheliomas is a pseudostratified, primitive-appearing epithelium disposed in glands,
tubules, or canals (figs. 5-1, 5-2). Papillary patterns are less frequent. The extent to which medullary epithelium is represented varies considerably, being prominent in some cases but only focal
in others. It is mitotically active and delineated
by a well-defined periodic acid–Schiff (PAS)- or
collagen IV-positive basement membrane on its

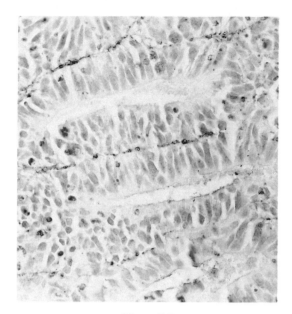

Figure 5-3
MEDULLOEPITHELIOMA
Immunostaining for type IV collagen highlights the basement membrane that underlies the neoplastic epithelium.

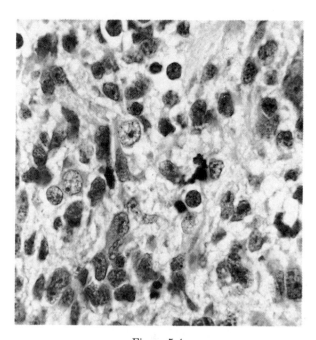

Figure 5-4
MEDULLOEPITHELIOMA
Neuronal differentiation, ranging from neuroblasts to ganglion cells, is seen in some medulloepitheliomas.

outer surface and an ill-defined amorphous pseudomembrane on its internal or luminal face (fig. 5-3). Mitotic figures are frequent and often lie adjacent to the lumen, a distribution similar to that observed in the epithelium of a developing neural tube. Small cytoplasmic blebs protrude from luminal cell surfaces in some lesions.

In addition to its eye-catching epithelium, medulloepitheliomas may exhibit not only the full spectrum of glial and neuronal, but also mesenchymal, differentiation. Markedly cellular regions of undifferentiated-appearing neoplasm, without specific architectural or immunohistochemical features, may be seen.

Neuronal components vary considerably in extent and maturation. In some instances they consist largely of neuroblasts, whose identification requires immunohistochemical studies when Homer Wright rosettes are not in evidence. Immature or well-formed ganglion cells are seen in other tumors (fig. 5-4).

Astrocytic components, if present, may also exhibit a spectrum of maturation. In poorly differentiated areas even immunostains for glial fibrillary acidic protein (GFAP) may show only scant reactivity about nuclei and within processes (fig. 5-5). In other areas, overtly astrocytic

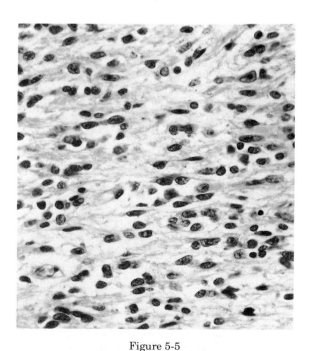

Figure 5-5
MEDULLOEPITHELIOMA
Glial differentiation is often apparent as diffuse areas of spindle cells in a fibrillar background, but may take the form of oligodendroglioma or ependymoma.

cells with radiating processes may abound. Care must be taken not to interpret incorporated reactive astrocytes as neoplastic cells. The inference that finely fibrillar areas on hematoxylin and eosin (H&E) stained sections are glial without support from immunohistochemistry is ill-advised, since the processes of immature neurons form a similar background. Patently astrocytic components vary from better differentiated areas resembling astrocytoma to cellular tumor with vascular proliferation, necrosis, and sometimes pseudopalisading, features typical of glioblastoma.

As in the case of astrocytic differentiation, ependymal components vary considerably in appearance from ependymoblastoma to more mature-appearing typical ependymoma. The former is more common and may cause diagnostic confusion with the neoplastic medullary epithelium of medulloepithelioma (12) (see Differential Diagnosis). The distinction is not always easy, since both forms of epithelium may be intimately associated.

Areas with the cell density, nuclear uniformity, and perinuclear halos of oligodendroglioma may also be observed. These may be interpreted as evidence of oligodendroglial differentiation but they may be neuronal or neuroblastic.

Mesenchymal components including bone, cartilage, muscle, and adipose tissue have also been described (8).

Immunohistochemical Findings. The epithelium of medulloepithelioma is generally immunonegative for S-100 protein, GFAP, and synaptophysin, whereas the neoplasm's differentiated components, e.g., neurons, are appropriately reactive for synaptophysin, tubulin, microtubule-associated protein, and neuron-specific enolase (NSE). GFAP reactivity is limited to glial elements (10,11,19).

Ultrastructural Findings. Given the rarity of medulloepithelioma, information is limited regarding its ultrastructural features. As expected, the primitive columnar epithelium rests upon a basal lamina and its component cells are joined by intermediate junctions (16,19).

Differential Diagnosis. In light of the largely undifferentiated nature of many embryonal neoplasms and of the practical difficulties inherent in distinguishing between the epithelium of medulloepithelioma and that of ependymoblastoma, it may be hard to identify these

tumors in small specimens. The rosettes of ependymoblastoma possess a clear-cut lumen, but lack an outer and inner membrane as well as a relationship between mitoses and the luminal surface. Apical cytoplasmic blebs are also not seen. A conspicuous, undifferentiated small cell element, so much a feature of ependymoblastoma, is less often seen in medulloepithelioma.

The differential diagnosis of medulloepithelioma also includes choroid plexus carcinoma. The distinction is not difficult since choroid plexus carcinoma is often overtly papillary, at least in part, and lacks the divergent differentiation so often seen in medulloepitheliomas. Choroid plexus tumors are also immunoreactive for vimentin, S-100 protein, and cytokeratin.

Since medullary epithelium is a common feature of immature teratomas, this common germ cell tumor is included in the differential diagnosis. The resemblance is augmented if other neuroectodermal elements are included in the teratoma. Distinguishing features of immature teratoma include fetal-appearing tissues of other germ layers, the concurrence of embryonal carcinoma or endodermal sinus tumor elements, and immunoreactivity for placental alkaline phosphatase and other markers such as alpha-fetoprotein and carcinoembryonic antigen (CEA).

Treatment and Prognosis. Most patients die within a year of diagnosis (8,15–17,19). Appropriate therapies remain to be determined. Cerebrospinal dissemination is not uncommon, but systemic metastases to bone, lymph nodes, or other viscera are rare.

Neuroblastoma and Ganglioneuroblastoma

Definition. Small cell neoplasms with neuroblastic differentiation.

General Comments. The neuroblastoma described here is to be distinguished from cerebellar neuroblastoma and central neurocytoma. Justification for the distinction from cerebellar neuroblastoma is found in the numerical predominance of the latter as well as the occurrence of transitional tumors bridging the common desmoplastic medulloblastoma and cerebellar neuroblastoma. Neurocytomas are set apart from neuroblastomas by their stereotypic intraventricular location, largely benign histologic features, and favorable prognosis.

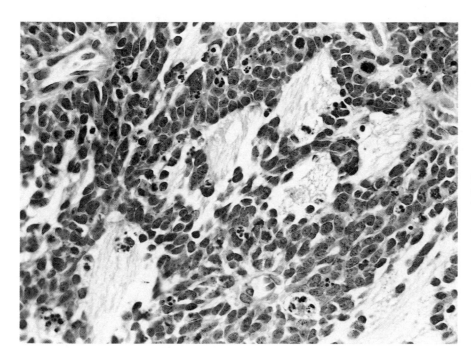

Figure 5-6
CEREBRAL
NEUROBLASTOMA
Distinctive anuclear zones of high fibrillarity permit recognition of many neuroblastomas without recourse to special stains.

Clinical and Radiographic Features. Although neuroblastomas occasionally occur in young adults, most patients present in the first decade of life, usually before the age of five. As a rule, neuroblastomas lie deep within the cerebral hemispheres (22,23,26).

Radiographically, neuroblastomas are large, discrete, and contrast enhancing. Cysts and calcification are common. The tumors can be hyperdense on noncontrast computerized tomographic (CT) images.

Macroscopic Findings. The tumors are circumscribed, gray, fleshy, variably desmoplastic, and cystic. Hemorrhage and necrosis may be seen.

Microscopic Findings. Cerebral neuroblastomas vary in their histologic appearance, but in many a fine fibrillarity interrupts otherwise dense sheets of tumor cells. Such fibrillar areas represent neuronal cell processes or neurites, and vary in extent as well as configuration. They include the cores of Homer Wright rosettes, perivascular anuclear zones, and larger unpatterned regions (fig. 5-6). Classic Homer Wright rosettes, relatively infrequent in cerebral neuroblastoma, consist of small round zones of fibrillarity surrounded by a somewhat palisaded row of tumor nuclei. Caution is in order when interpreting perivascular, nuclei-free fibrillar zones since they resemble the perivascular pseudorosettes of

ependymoma. Larger areas of fibrillarity, when circumscribed, can be viewed either as extensions of the perivascular pattern or as markedly exaggerated Homer Wright rosettes.

Cells within densely cellular regions often exhibit variation in nuclear shape, chromatin content, texture, and mitotic activity. As a rule, in the absence of neuronal differentiation, nucleoli are inconspicuous. Some tumors show little nuclear pleomorphism and mitotic activity, whereas others are overly malignant, both in histologic and cytologic terms. Virtually all are small cell neoplasms with arrangements of cells varying from patternless sheets to rosettes, ribbons, palisades, or fascicles (fig. 5-7). In one variant, nuclear palisading closely resembles that seen in primitive polar spongioblastoma (fig. 5-7C) (24,27).

The connective tissue content of neuroblastoma and ganglioneuroblastoma varies from scant to abundant, and is the basis of the classification of these tumors into classic, transitional, and desmoplastic forms (26). Collagen and reticulin in the intermediate or transitional variant produces a lobular pattern, but not with the precision and extent seen in the cerebellar neuroblastoma. As in medulloblastomas, the connective tissue component of cerebral neuroblastomas is most conspicuous when tumor reaches the leptomeninges.

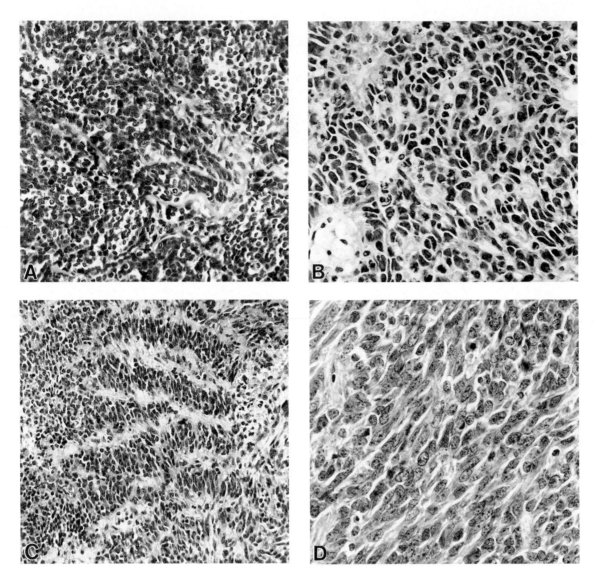

Figure 5-7
CEREBRAL NEUROBLASTOMA: VARIATIONS IN HISTOLOGIC APPEARANCE
Neuroblastomas present a variety of histologic patterns in addition to the classic lesion illustrated in figure 5-6. One variant is a densely cellular neoplasm with ill-defined lucent areas wherein the cells have a somewhat oligodendroglial character (A). Another is a cellular, pleomorphic neoplasm without specific architectural features (B). A compact palisading pattern (C) may be seen in some instances. A fascicular architecture is present in other cases (D).

Focal or partial differentiation to neurons is not rare in neuroblastomas, but occurs much less often than in neuroblastomas arising in peripheral autonomic ganglia. Although maturation in the central tumors may approach ganglion cell formation, in most instances it proceeds only to the intermediate ganglioid stage. Such cells are particularly prominent in lesions exhibiting large areas of fibrillarity. They must be distinguished from trapped normal small neurons.

Neuroblastic tumors known as *ganglioneuroblastoma* or *differentiating neuroblastomas* are less common than are classic neuroblastomas (20,30). In contrast to neuroblastoma in which ganglioid or mature ganglion cells are a focal feature, the designation ganglioneuroblastoma is reserved for rare lesions with widespread neuronal differentiation, in which cells transitional between neuroblasts and mature ganglion cells abound (fig. 5-8).

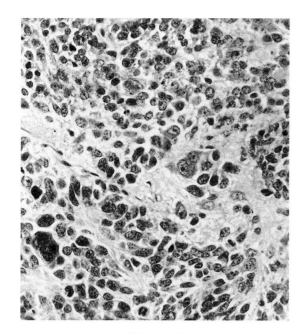

Figure 5-8
GANGLIONEUROBLASTOMA
Neuroblastic neoplasms with extensive maturation to ganglion cells are termed ganglioneuroblastomas.

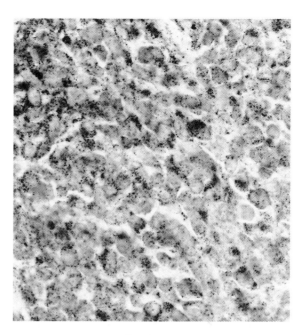

Figure 5-9
NEUROBLASTOMA
Immunohistochemistry may be required to identify neuroblastomas. Granular surface reactivity for synaptophysin is noted in the undifferentiated neoplasm shown in figure 5-7D.

In addition to large areas of high fibrillarity with streaming of cells and scattered plump ganglion-like cells, some cerebral neuroblastomas exhibit rosettes with clearly defined lumina resembling Flexner-Wintersteiner, or even ependymoblastic, rosettes. Such rosettes may lie within paucicellular or densely cellular portions of the tumor.

Cytology. The smear preparations of the neuritic processes, in aggregate, form a limited fibrillar background (pl. VIB, p. 183). The round to somewhat elongated nuclei are small and dark.

Immunohistochemical Findings. Highly fibrillar areas, including the cores of Homer Wright rosettes and the cytoplasm of ganglioid cells and neurons, are immunoreactive for NSE and synaptophysin (fig. 5-9). Of the two, staining for NSE is usually more intense but less specific. As a result, reactivity must be interpreted in light of routine histochemical and other immunostains, particularly when apparent staining is widespread, faint, or accentuated around areas of evolving necrosis. Impressive cytoplasmic NSE staining may be noted in perinecrotic regions of a wide variety of tumors. Synaptophysin, on the

other hand, is considered a neuron-specific marker. Unlike NSE reactivity, cytoplasmic staining is minor when compared to the staining of fibrillar zones rich in neuroblastic processes. Immunopositivity for neurofilament protein, heavily dependent upon optimal fixation and advanced differentiation, may be lacking or restricted to rare neuronal cell bodies or processes.

Some degree of immunoreactivity for GFAP is noted in virtually all cases and is usually attributable to scattered reactive astrocytes whose long processes concentrate about vessels. Such cells are especially prominent at the periphery of the lesion where the processes may be segmented linearly between streams of infiltrating tumor cells. In other neuroblastomas, the presence of neoplastic astrocytes is incontrovertible since GFAP positivity appears in the small neoplastic cells with an eccentric skirt of pink cytoplasm. Such tumors fall into the category of embryonal tumors with mixed neuronal and glial differentiation. In some cases, even within the center of the lesion, the neoplastic versus reactive nature of the glial component may be difficult to determine, particularly when only a feltwork of GFAP-positive processes is seen. It is not clear whether the presence of a glial component is of prognostic significance.

Ultrastructural Findings. Neoplastic neuroblasts are noted for their high nuclear-cytoplasmic ratios and microtubule-containing bipolar processes. Neurosecretory granules or vesicles are present, although usually sparse (21,24,28,31). Synapse formation is generally lacking.

Differential Diagnosis. The differential diagnosis of cerebral neuroblastoma proceeds by first identifying the tumor as one with neuroblastic elements; neoplastic glia or histologic features of other embryonal tumors are then excluded.

The identification of the lesion as neuroblastic is easiest in the presence of Homer Wright rosettes. Immunohistochemistry is not necessary in this setting. More often, the appearance of the tumor in H&E stained sections is less specific, although fibrillar rosette-like clearings suggest the diagnosis. Reactivity for synaptophysin then becomes essential, particularly in the absence of ganglioid cells or mature neurons. Caution is advised against over-interpreting small zones of fibrillarity as Homer Wright rosettes, especially when circumferential palisading of nuclei is vague or when immunohistochemical confirmation is lacking. In most instances, reactivity for synaptophysin or NSE is widespread, both in fibrillated areas and within the cytoplasm and minute processes of small cells.

A densely cellular neoplasm is occasionally encountered in young patients which, because of its cellularity, resembles neuroblastoma but in which no specific neuroblastic features can be identified by either light microscopy or immunohistochemistry. In such cases, ultrastructural studies may be diagnostic. Undifferentiated small cell tumors form a heterogeneous group for which a simple, descriptive diagnosis of undifferentiated embryonal tumor is appropriate.

A rare neoplasm occurring in the first 2 years of life, the desmoplastic infantile ganglioglioma (DIG), may exhibit a minor small cell component. This distinctive tumor is easily distinguished by its superficial location, accompanying cyst, predominant desmoplastic component containing enmeshed astrocytes, minor component of ganglioid cells, and immunoreactivity for both GFAP and neuronal markers.

The central neurocytoma, a neuronal neoplasm related to neuroblastoma, is briefly mentioned above and is discussed in detail later. The term differentiating cerebral neuroblastoma had once been applied to this now well-known low-grade intraventricular lesion. Like neuroblastoma, the neurocytoma is cellular, but does not appear particularly "primitive" since it exhibits remarkable cytologic uniformity with precise, round, mitotically inactive nuclei with delicate "salt and pepper" chromatin and inconspicuous micronucleoli. Neurocytomas typically arise near the septum pellucidum of young adults.

Treatment and Prognosis. Neuroblastomas appear to be somewhat less aggressive than other small cell tumors, particularly undifferentiated embryonal tumors. Given the paucity of published reports, there is little available information regarding prognostic factors, either clinical or histological. In one study the only significant factor was patient age, with recurrences more likely in younger patients (22). Although radiation has generally been administered to the tumor bed, the role of neuraxis radiation remains a subject of debate (22,23). Full maturation of a neuroblastoma to a ganglion cell tumor, as occasionally occurs in peripheral neuroblastoma, is rare (30). Extracranial metastasis has been reported (25,29).

Olfactory Neuroblastoma (Esthesioneuroblastoma)

Definition. A tumor composed primarily of neuroblasts, which arises in the vault of the nose overlying the cribriform plate.

Clinical and Radiographic Features. Olfactory neuroblastomas occur throughout life but exhibit a bimodal age distribution with a small peak in adolescence and a larger one in later adulthood. The tumors form polypoid masses that present as epistaxis or nasal obstruction, often longstanding (35,37,38). Involvement of the cribriform plate is so typical that in its absence a diagnosis of olfactory neuroblastoma should be questioned. Subfrontal intracranial extension may produce a midline intradural mass that elevates the frontal lobes. In such cases, neuroimaging discloses an enhancing dumbbell-shaped mass, centered upon the cribriform plate, extending at one pole as a polyp into the nose and

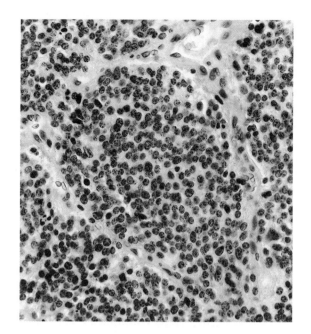

Figure 5-10
OLFACTORY NEUROBLASTOMA
Monotonous round cells in smooth contoured lobules comprise the classic lesion.

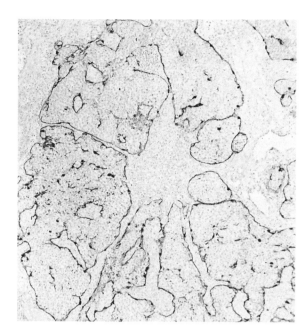

Figure 5-11
OLFACTORY NEUROBLASTOMA
The lobules are typically surrounded by, and may contain, cells that are immunoreactive for S-100 protein. Such cells are similar to the sustentacular cells of paraganglioma.

at the other as an intracranial subfrontal mass. Secondary involvement of the ethmoid or frontal sinuses may also be seen.

Macroscopic Findings. When partially resected by snare, the lesion consists of a smooth-surfaced polyp overlain by respiratory mucosa. In most cases, however, the tumor is fragmented and consists of gray-red vascular tissue. When portions of the cribriform plate are submitted, decalcification often reveals bone invasion.

Microscopic Findings. Although olfactory neuroblastomas are thought to originate from specialized neurosecretory cells of the olfactory mucosa, no in situ or intraepithelial precursor lesion is seen. Indeed, tumor usually occupies the submucosa and stroma. At low magnification, two principal growth patterns are seen: smooth contoured cellular nests within a vascular stroma (fig. 5-10) and, less often, diffuse sheet-like growth supported only by delicate capillaries (37,38). At higher magnification, cellular monomorphism is conspicuous. Although a suggestion of rosetting is often evident, well-formed Homer Wright rosettes are present in only a minority of lesions. Flexner-Wintersteiner–like

rosettes, also termed olfactory rosettes, are rare. As in other neuroblastic tumors, olfactory neuroblastomas usually exhibit a delicate fibrillary background composed of neuroblastic processes: in essence, a neoplastic neuropil. Ganglion cell differentiation is infrequent. As a rule, the cells are small with round nuclei and delicate, stippled or salt and pepper chromatin; inconspicuous nucleoli and necrosis is uncommon. Nuclear pleomorphism is minimal.

Immunohistochemical Findings. Key among the immunoreactivities of olfactory neuroblastoma is the high frequency of positivity of the nested cells for neuronal markers and reactivity of the cells at the edge of the lobules for S-100 protein (fig. 5-11) (32). Scattered S-100 protein–positive cells are also present internally within lobules. The neuronal markers include NSE, synaptophysin, neurofilament protein, microtubule-associated protein, and class III beta-tubulin (34). The nature of the S-100–positive cells is unsettled, but a parallel has been drawn with Schwann cells as well as with the sustentacular cells of paraganglioma. Although classic olfactory neuroblastomas are not cytokeratin positive, some are reportedly reactive (34). When the definition of olfactory neuroblastoma becomes sufficiently broad as to include other tumors, for instance neuroendocrine carcinoma, keratin reactivity can be expected. We do not include such tumors in the spectrum of olfactory neuroblastoma.

Ultrastructural Findings. As with neuroblastomas at other sites, the cell processes contain microtubules and scant intermediate filaments, the basis of tubulin and neurofilament immunoreactivity, respectively. Dense core or neurosecretory granules are most evident within cell processes. Clear vesicles, and particularly synapses, are infrequent (32). The S-100–positive cells defining the edge of the lobules are covered on their outer aspect by a basal lamina (32).

Differential Diagnosis. Other cellular lesions, both neoplastic and reactive, occur high in the nasal cavity (37,38). Among these are undifferentiated carcinomas of various types, sarcomas, malignant melanoma, and, on rare occasion, anterior extension of a pituitary adenoma.

The two principal lesions in the differential diagnosis of olfactory neuroblastoma are sinonasal undifferentiated carcinoma (SNUC) and neuroendocrine carcinoma (37,38). SNUC, although no doubt a heterogeneous entity, is a light microscopically undifferentiated carcinoma (33). It is highly malignant and aggressive and involves the ethmoid sinus, maxillary sinus, or both at presentation. The cribriform plate may also be affected. Unlike olfactory neuroblastoma, symptoms are of short duration. With sufficient tissue sampling, an in situ mucosal component is apparent. Histologically, sinonasal undifferentiated carcinoma exhibits a variety of growth patterns including lobules, sheets, and trabeculation. The cells have large, oval to irregular nuclei with prominent nucleoli and moderate quantities of eosinophilic cytoplasm. Mitoses are numerous. A tendency to invade mucosal vessels and lymphatics is seen.

Neuroendocrine carcinoma of the nose, like olfactory neuroblastoma SNUC, may affect the nasal vault and cribriform region. The histologic patterns include lobules, trabeculae, ribbons, and gland-like spaces. Cytologically, the tumor varies from a well-differentiated carcinoid-like lesion to an overtly malignant tumor with both a high nuclear grade and mitotic index. Keratin, chromogranin, and NSE reactivities are regular

features. Epithelial membrane antigen staining may also be seen. When present, neurofilament positivity is usually paranuclear in distribution. As in similar tumors of the respiratory tract, synaptophysin reactivity may also occur. Ultrastructural features include secretory granules and well-formed junctions but microtubule-containing processes are absent. Paranuclear whorls of intermediate filaments underlie the neurofilament protein immunoreaction. The behavior of neuroendocrine carcinomas varies according to the degree of differentiation. Distinction between high-grade neuroendocrine carcinoma and SNUC is not sharp, since they exhibit a degree of overlap in their immunohistochemical (see Appendix H) and ultrastructural features.

Melanomas arising high in the nasal cavity are amelanotic and composed of cells that are small and round rather than spindled or epithelioid. Melanomas are strongly S-100 protein immunopositive, but lack neuronal marker reactivity. Pituitary adenomas originate in the sella turcica, a site unaffected by olfactory neuroblastomas.

Treatment and Prognosis. The prognosis of olfactory neuroblastoma is favorable, particularly when gross total excision is possible. In one study, only a few patients died of the disease (37,38). Not only can recurrent or residual tumor be locally destructive but dissemination to cervical lymph nodes and bone can occur (35). In most instances the disease is only slowly progressive (36–38). Given the infrequency of the lesion, its long-term prognosis is unclear.

Retinoblastoma

Retinoblastoma is a retinal neoplasm of neurosensory cells akin to neuroblasts.

Most retinoblastomas occur in children under the age of 3 years. Both hereditary and sporadic forms are recognized. Bilaterality and earlier onset characterize the former. A white reflex is commonly noted on ophthalmoscopic examination.

The tumors are gray-white, necrosis-prone, often calcified masses which extend into the vitreous or break through the retina to reach the subretinal space. Advanced tumors penetrate the optic nerve head, enter the surrounding subarachnoid space, extend into orbital soft tissue, or metastasize to distant sites.

Microscopically, the dense cellularity of retinoblastoma is interrupted only by foci of necrosis that are prone to dystrophic calcification, and the lumina of Flexner-Wintersteiner rosettes (48). The rosettes are an expression of photoreceptor differentiation. They consist of small lumina circumscribed by neoplastic cells joined at their apices to produce a form of internal limiting membrane. Nuclei are basally situated at the periphery of the rosettes. In less common, particularly well-differentiated neoplasms, referred to as *retinocytomas*, apical projections are prominent and contribute to the formation of so-called "fleurettes" (49,50). Similar luminal projections are occasionally seen in pineoblastomas.

The neuroblastic nature of retinoblastoma is evidenced by fleurette formation in some Homer Wright rosettes, as well as immunoreactivity for synaptophysin and retinal S-antigen. The Homer Wright rosettes also react for class III beta-tubulin and microtubule-associated protein (41,42,44).

The retinoblastoma is of interest since it is occasionally associated with an intracranial midline tumor of small cell type. In conjunction with the bilateral hereditary form of retinoblastoma, the often microscopically similar intracranial lesion affects either the pineal or suprasellar regions (39,43,45–47,51). This complex lesion is termed *trilateral retinoblastoma*. Variants include unilateral rather than bilateral retinoblastoma or instances of intracranial tumor antedating the retinal lesions (39,40,45). Intracranial retinoblastomas are densely cellular masses which resemble their ocular counterparts, replete with Homer Wright and Flexner-Wintersteiner rosettes as well as immunoreactivity for retinal S-antigen (42,46).

Melanotic Neuroectodermal Tumor of Infancy

The melanotic neuroectodermal tumor of infancy (MNTI) or *melanotic progonoma* is a rare neoplasm that generally arises in the maxilla (52–54). Involvement of bones of the cranial vault (53,55,58), or other extracranial bones (52), is rare.

Macroscopically, this gray-brown tumor expands surrounding bone. Compression and invasion of adjacent tissue may also occur. Microscopically, it contains both variably pigmented epithelium, as well as islands of neuroblastic cells, which may by

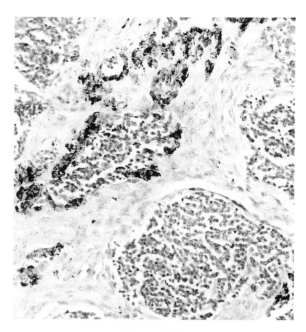

Figure 5-12
MELANOTIC NEUROECTODERMAL
TUMOR OF INFANCY
Lobules of monomorphous small cells and solid clusters, with associated gland-like or tubular arrangements of pigmented epithelium, comprise this highly distinctive lesion.

process formation create a fine fibrillar background (fig. 5-12). The pigmented cells form clusters, glands, or tubules which, in some cases, surround islands of neuroblasts. Maturation to ganglioid cells or neurons is infrequent.

On occasion, pigmented neoplasms similar to MNTI arise within the substance of the brain, but it is debatable whether these actually represent classic MNTI (55,56,58). We are reluctant to accept cerebellar tumors exhibiting pigmented epithelium as MNTI (57), since such biologically malignant lesions are more akin to medulloblastoma.

Classic MNTI is locally invasive, but usually amenable to resection and cure.

Ependymoblastoma

Definition. A small cell neoplasm with prominent ependymoblastic rosettes.

General Comments. The term ependymoblastoma denotes a small cell embryonal neoplasm with ependymoblastic rosettes, not a malignant or otherwise conventional ependymoma (64,65). Although it is easy to distinguish these lesions in most instances, in some cases it may

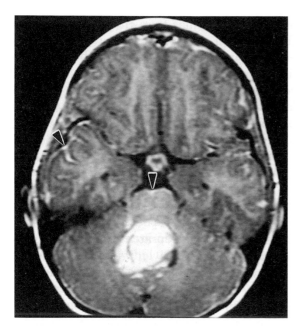

Figure 5-14
MEDULLOBLASTOMA
As seen in this MRI study of a vermian lesion, medulloblastomas are contrast-enhancing masses. Diffuse enhancement in the cerebral subarachnoid space (arrows) indicates leptomeningeal dissemination.

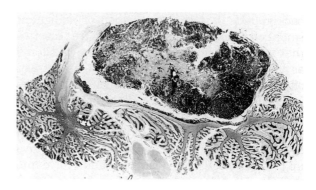

Figure 5-15
MEDULLOBLASTOMA
Medulloblastomas are densely cellular and usually rather discrete.

Classification. In the following discussion, medulloblastomas are classified as: 1) classic, i.e., light-microscopically undifferentiated; 2) those with neuroblastic or neuronal differentiation; 3) those with glial differentiation; and 4) those with mixed or glial-neuronal differentiation. The rare "medulloblastomas" with divergent differentiation toward melanotic or mesenchymal elements are discussed separately.

General Histologic and Cytologic Features. By definition, medulloblastomas are dense small cell tumors (fig. 5-15) (109). They can be homogeneously cellular, lacking apparent stroma or distinctive architectural features; nodular and reticulin rich; or desmoplastic but otherwise undifferentiated. In terms of histologic pattern, quantity and type of stroma, cytologic features, and mitotic activity, there is thus considerable heterogeneity, both intertumorally and intratumorally (fig. 5-16).

Although in large part a solid tumor, the medulloblastoma may be diffusely permeative at its periphery. Medulloblastomas frequently exit the cerebellum, invading the subarachnoid space to form an "icing"-like layer of neoplastic cells on the pial surface. In some cases, this superficial layer appears inordinately extensive relative to the underlying, more solid tumor and diffuse neoplastic transformation of the external granular cell layer is suggested (fig. 5-16C) (90). From the subarachnoid space, tumor often reenters the cerebellum by way of perivascular (Virchow-Robin) spaces or intraparenchymatously, by moving down preexisting normal cellular processes of the molecular layer as do the granular cells during normal embryologic development. The result is a distinctive palisading, similar to the pattern noted when stacked Homer Wright rosettes are cut along their long axes (figs. 5-16D, 5-16E). A reactive meshwork of reticulin may be seen where tumor reaches the subarachnoid space. The distinctive reticulin deposition of desmoplastic medulloblastoma, although reactive, seems almost an intrinsic consequence of the tumor rather than simply a reflection of leptomeningeal invasion. Medulloblastomas seldom show extensive necrosis but are among the few tumors, other than high-grade gliomas, to exhibit perinecrotic pseudopalisading (fig. 5-16F).

As would be expected, given the heterogeneity of the lesion, the cytologic appearances are variable, but as a group the neoplasm is known for its small, hyperchromatic, condensed nuclei. Cytoplasm is inconspicuous (pl. VIC, p. 183).

Histologic Subtypes. Although the archetypical medulloblastoma is to many a monotonous undifferentiated neoplasm, routine histochemical stains show specific tissue patterns or evidence of differentiation in almost half of the

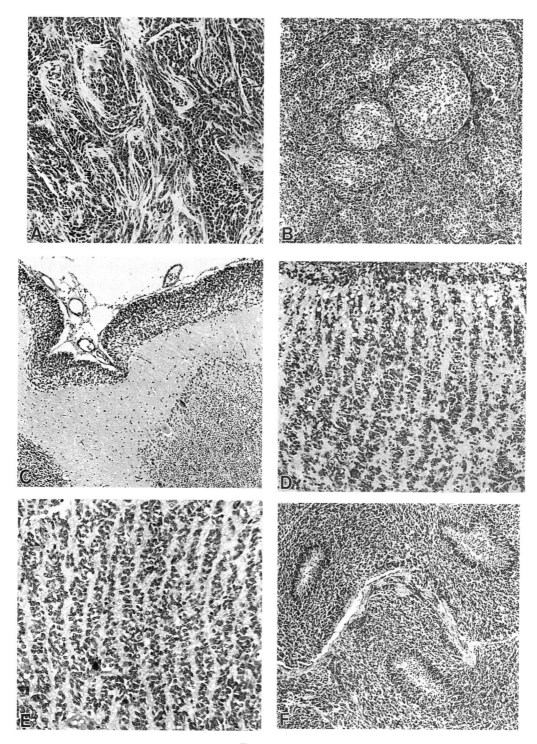

Figure 5-16
MEDULLOBLASTOMA

Medulloblastomas exhibit a broad range of histologic features. Some tumors are undifferentiated and often show considerable desmoplasia (A). Others have a nodular pattern (B). Medulloblastomas are prone to spread along the surface of the molecular layer and, in some cases, the pattern of infiltration is so extensive as to suggest the possibility of widespread neoplastic transformation of the external granular cell layer (C). Vertical, linear arrays of tumor cells are sometimes seen in the molecular layer (D) and deep cerebellar parenchyma (E). Medulloblastoma is one of the few neoplasms other than glioblastoma to exhibit necrosis with pseudopalisading (F).

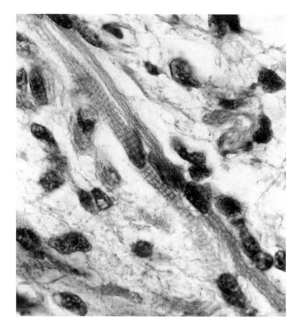

Figure 5-36
MEDULLOMYOBLASTOMA
Densely cellular neoplasms of the posterior fossa composed of primitive-appearing small cells as well as striated muscle cells are known as medullomyoblastomas. It is debatable whether such lesions represent variants of medulloblastoma or are distinct entities.

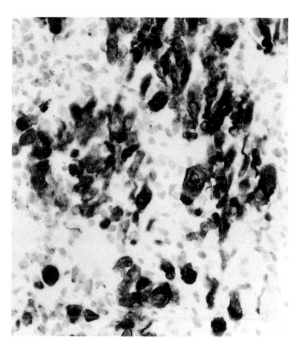

Figure 5-37
MEDULLOMYOBLASTOMA
Immunostains for muscle-related antigens such as desmin facilitate the identification of medullomyoblastoma since cross striations may be difficult to find.

Medullomyoblastoma and Melanotic Medulloblastoma

In light of their location and content of cellular small cell elements, these rare tumors are often considered variants of the medulloblastoma, but these "variants" often have a variety of tissue patterns foreign to most medulloblastomas. It thus remains to be established whether these two neoplasms are subtypes of medulloblastoma or are pathologic entities in their own right. Occasional cases appear to bridge the medullomyoblastoma and melanotic medulloblastoma categories by exhibiting both myoid and pigmented epithelial cells (115,118). Our hesitancy to accept melanotic medulloblastoma as a melanotic neuroectodermal tumor of infancy (MNTI or progonoma) is discussed below. The spectrum of medullomyoblastomas is limited and should not include primary CNS rhabdomyosarcoma or myogenic lesions also exhibiting teratomatous or malignant germ cell elements (116).

The medullomyoblastoma occurs most frequently in children, usually boys (114,117,122,

124). Adults are rarely affected (123). This unique tumor combines a small cell neuroectodermal element with foci of rhabdomyoblastic differentiation. Considerable variation is seen in the degree to which myoblasts or more mature myocytes are represented. Most often myoid differentiation is evidenced by round blast forms. Alternatively, in its consummate form, it results in the formation of cross-striated "strap cells" or even multinucleate myotubes which weave and crisscross through cellular and hypocellular regions (fig. 5-36). The latter are sometimes extensive. Desmin, myoglobin, and muscle-specific actin are diagnostically useful immunomarkers in that cross striations may be difficult to find (fig. 5-37).

The undifferentiated-appearing part of these tumors consists of small cells variably organized in terms of histologic pattern and cell density. A nodular pattern similar to that of desmoplastic medulloblastoma is occasionally seen. In addition to synaptophysin immunoreactivity, neuroblastic and ganglionic differentiation have both been noted (122,124), as have GFAP-positive cells indicative of glial differentiation (117).

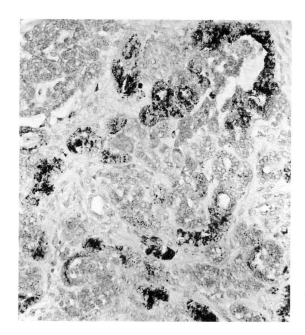

Figure 5-38
MELANOTIC MEDULLOBLASTOMA
Small tubules or clusters of epithelial-appearing cells
producing melanin are the basis for the designation melanotic medulloblastoma.

Densely cellular CNS neoplasms occurring
outside the cerebellum may also exhibit differentiation along myoid lines (112,120). Some are
considered neuroepithelial tumors with muscle
differentiation, whereas similar neoplasms are
classified by others as rhabdomyosarcomas, the
object of disagreement hinging upon the neuroectodermal versus the mesenchymal character
of the undifferentiated-appearing component.

Melanotic medulloblastoma is characterized
by the presence of small clusters or tubules of
pigmented epithelial cells containing finely
granular black pigment, identified ultrastructurally as true melanin (fig. 5-38) (114,121).
Scattered individual pigmented cells may also be
seen. As in more ordinary medulloblastomas, the
mitotic rate varies. Synaptophysin reactivity is
evident in small, more typical medulloblastoma
cells. Aggressive behavior is the rule and includes craniospinal dissemination (113,114,119,
125). These attributes distinguish the tumor
from melanotic neuroectodermal tumor of infancy (melanotic progonoma). With few exceptions, the latter is generally benign.

Other Embryonal Tumors

As mentioned in the introduction to this chapter, a number of small cell neoplasms cannot be
assigned readily to a histologic category. Some of
these misfits represent incompletely sampled
but otherwise classic entities, whereas others
are distinct neoplasms. The spectrum of these
lesions, as well as their clinical significance,
remain largely unexplored. Occasional tumors of
a mixed nature fall into more than one category.

Many of these embryonal tumors are undifferentiated small cell neoplasms without light microscopic evidence of differentiation. Such lesions
vary considerably in histologic pattern and in
nuclear characteristics. Some are composed of
closely packed, cytologically uniform cells,
whereas others are frankly malignant, exhibiting
coarse chromatin, frequent mitoses, and either
single cell or geographic necrosis. If these lesions
are immunoreactive for synaptophysin, a presumptive diagnosis of neuroblastoma is appropriate, effectively removing it from the undifferentiated category. It remains to be seen what impact
better tissue sampling, ultrastructural characterization, improved fixation, and newer staining
methods will have upon the ratio of "undifferentiated" and "differentiated" embryonal tumors. A
number of small cell cerebellar neoplasms, lacking routine light microscopic evidence of differentiation, fall into the undifferentiated category, but
are considered medulloblastomas.

Notably absent from most classifications of
embryonal tumors are astrocytic or oligodendroglial equivalents of ependymoblastoma or
neuroblastoma: embryonal neoplasms with differentiation only along glial lines. The primitive
polar spongioblastoma only partly fills this void,
although it is not a small round cell tumor. The
unqualified term spongioblastoma has been too
variably applied to now serve as a specific diagnosis. The designation glioblastoma, and perhaps astroblastoma, if one assumes that the
GFAP-positive cells in the latter tumor are astrocytes, would have been appropriate had not
these terms already been applied to other lesions. A largely undifferentiated embryonal
tumor with choroid plexus differentiation has
been reported (133).

Histologically, embryonal tumors with glial
differentiation vary in appearance but are in

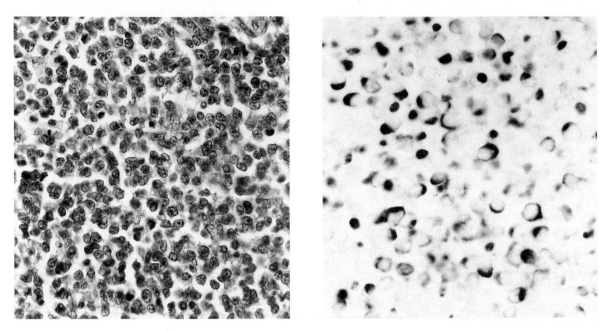

Figure 5-39
EMBRYONAL TUMOR WITH GLIAL DIFFERENTIATION
Left: This embryonal tumor with glial differentiation consists of small undifferentiated-appearing cells.
Right: The glial nature is apparent only on immunostains for GFAP.

large part diffusely cellular, monomorphous, and round cell in composition. They lack the marked cellular elongation and generally low to medium cellularity of primitive polar spongioblastoma. Most are highly cellular and exhibit cytoplasm so scanty that the possibility of glial differentiation may not come to mind (fig. 5-39, left). Reactivity for GFAP, usually confined to the immediate perinuclear region, may nevertheless be impressive (fig. 5-39, right). Immunopositive fields may alternate with expanses of nonreactivity. Largely undifferentiated neoplasms occasionally possess foci with a distinctly "rhabdoid" appearance, with large vesicular nuclei and prominent glassy or faintly fibrillar GFAP- and vimentin-positive cytoplasm (see fig. 7-13). The relationship of such lesions to GFAP-negative rhabdoid tumors and atypical teratoid tumors (127,134) is unclear but an apparently consistent cytogenetic abnormality may unify these tumors.

Embryonal tumors with glial differentiation must be distinguished from embryonal tumors of neuroblastic type and from anaplastic gliomas. The first issue is readily resolved by immunostaining for synaptophysin. The distinction from anaplastic gliomas, on the other hand,

may be more of a problem, particularly in small biopsies in which a morphologic overlap exists between embryonal tumors and highly anaplastic gliomas. The latter are not usually as monomorphous as embryonal tumors, more often contain better differentiated areas, and are far more likely to occur in adults. Malignant gliomas also tend to exhibit nuclear pleomorphism and vascular ("endothelial") proliferation or necrosis, features uncommon in most embryonal tumors.

The prototypic embryonal tumor with mixed neuronal/neuroblastic and glial differentiation is the medulloepithelioma when it expresses its potential for divergent differentiation (fig. 5-30). Neuroblastic tumors that contain ependymoblastic rosettes are also mixed. Neuronal medulloblastomas, usually nodular neoplasms with glial differentiation, fit into the mixed neuronal/glial category but are considered separately.

On rare occasion, other mixed neuronal/glial embryonal tumors arise in the supratentorial compartment. Analogous to medulloblastoma, these tumors are densely cellular, often contain Homer Wright rosettes, synaptophysin-positive perivascular zones of fibrillarity, and some GFAP-reactive cells (135). In yet other extracerebellar embryonal tumors, both the neuronal and glial components are better differentiated (130).

An additional neoplasm with divergent differentiation is the infantile desmoplastic ganglioglioma. Although this tumor is curable in most instances, it can in a broad sense be considered an embryonal tumor with divergent differentiation. The same can be said for certain rare "unconventional" gangliogliomas which are less well differentiated than classic ganglion cell tumors (see fig. 4-11), and neoplasms which contain both densely cellular regions and gangliocytomatous foci (see fig. 4-12). If divergent differentiation is the sole criteria, even the classic ganglioglioma qualifies. If it is confirmed that some neurocytomas exhibit both neuronal and glial phenotypes, then such tumors could also be considered a form of embryonal tumor with divergent differentiation (136), albeit a better differentiated one than the classic cerebral neuroblastoma.

In addition to the above "other" embryonal tumors with neuronal, glial, or mixed differentiation is a mixed group of miscellaneous embryonal tumors. One such lesion is an embryonal tumor that follows prophylactic irradiation of the nervous system. These are densely cellular, mitotically active lesions which may exhibit neuroblastic neuronal features, glial differentiation, or both (128).

Some densely cellular tumors, most of which occur in infants, contain numerous GFAP-positive rhabdoid cells (see fig. 7-13). A similar and possibly related tumor with rhabdoid, neuroepithelial, epithelial, and mesenchymal features has been designated atypical teratoid tumor (127,134), and is discussed in chapter 7. An additional interesting lesion contains glial and neuronal differentiation with a desmin-positive mesenchymal component (137).

A desmoplastic response is common in many embryonal tumors, such as neuroblastoma, medulloblastoma, and the primitive neuroectodermal tumors as defined by Hart and Earle (131). A neoplastic mesenchymal component is occasionally present in embryonal tumors and has generally been expressed as differentiation toward muscle (126,132,137). Fat has been observed as well (129). There is not always a clear distinction between an embryonal tumor with rhabdomyoblasts and a largely undifferentiated rhabdomyosarcoma.

REFERENCES

Primitive Neuroectodermal Tumor

1. Becker LE, Hinton D. Primitive neuroectodermal tumors of the central nervous system. Hum Pathol 1983;14:538–50.
2. Hart MN, Earle KM. Primitive neuroectodermal tumors of the brain in children. Cancer 1973;32:890–7.
3. Kleihues P, Burger PC, Scheithauer BW. Histologic typing of tumours of the central nervous system. World Health Organization. Berlin: Springer-Verlag, 1993.
4. McLendon, RE, Burger PC. The primitive neuroectodermal tumor: a cautionary view. J Pediatr Neurosci 1987;3:1–8.
5. Rorke LB. The cerebellar medulloblastoma and its relationship to primitive neuroectodermal tumors. J Neuropathol Exp Neurol 1983;42:1–15.
6. Rubinstein LJ. Embryonal central neuroepithelial tumors and their differentiating potential. A cytogenetic view of a complex neuro-oncological problem. J Neurosurg 1985;62:795–805.
7. Russell DS, Rubinstein LJ. Pathology of tumours of the nervous system. 5th ed. Baltimore: Williams & Wilkins, 1989:247–89.

Medulloepithelioma

8. Auer RN, Becker LE. Cerebral medulloepithelioma with bone, cartilage, and striated muscle. J Neuropathol Exp Neurol 1983;42:256–67.
9. Best PV. Posterior fossa medulloepithelioma. Report of a case. J Neurol Sci 1974;22:511–8.
10. Caccamo DV, Herman MM, Rubinstein LJ. An immunohistochemical study of the primitive and maturing elements of human cerebral medulloepitheliomas. Acta Neuropathol (Berl) 1989;79:248–54.
11. Cruz-Sanchez FF, Rossi ML, Hughes JT, Moss TH. Differentiation in embryonal neuroepithelial tumors of the central nervous system. Cancer 1991;67:965–76.
12. Deck JH. Cerebral medulloepithelioma with maturation into ependymal cells and ganglion cells. J Neuropathol Exp Neurol 1969;28:442–54.
13. Greenfield JG. Two cases of medulloepithelioma (Bailey and Cushing) with special reference to the relative malignancy of this type of tumour. J Pathol Bacteriol 1934;38:11–6.

14. Jellinger K. Cerebral medulloepithelioma. Acta Neuropathol (Berl) 1972;22:95–101.
15. Karch SB, Urich H. Medulloepithelioma: definition of an entity. J Neuropathol Exp Neurol 1972;31:27–53.
16. Pollak A, Friede RL. Fine structure of medulloepithelioma. J Neuropathol Exp Neurol 1977;36:712–25.
17. Scheithauer BW, Rubinstein LJ. Cerebral medulloepithelioma. Report of a case with multiple divergent neuroepithelial differentiation. Childs Brain 1979;5:62–71.
18. Treip CS. A congenital medulloepithelioma of the midbrain. J Pathol Bacteriol 1957;74:357–63.
19. Troost D, Jansen GH, Dingemans KP. Cerebral medulloepithelioma—electron microscopy and immunohistochemistry. Acta Neuropathol 1990;80:103–7.

Neuroblastoma and Ganglioneuroblastoma

20. Ahdevaara P, Kalimo H, Törmä T, Haltia M. Differentiating intracerebral neuroblastoma. Report of a case and review of the literature. Cancer 1977;40:784–8.
21. Azzarelli B, Richards DE, Anton AH, Roessmann U. Central neuroblastoma. Electron microscopic observations and catecholamine determinations. J Neuropathol Exp Neurol 1977;36:384–97.
22. Bennett JP Jr, Rubinstein LJ. The biological behavior of primary cerebral neuroblastoma: a reappraisal of the clinical course in a series of 70 cases. Ann Neurol 1984;16:21–7.
23. Berger MS, Edwards MS, Wara WM, Levin VA, Wilson CB. Primary cerebral neuroblastoma. Long-term follow-up review and therapeutic guidelines. J Neurosurg 1983;59:418–23.
24. Dehner LP, Abenoza P, Sibley RK. Primary cerebral neuroectodermal tumors: neuroblastoma, differentiated neuroblastoma, and composite neuroectodermal tumor. Ultrastruct Pathol 1988;12:479–94.
25. Henriquez AS, Robertson DM, Marshall WJ. Primary neuroblastoma of the central nervous system with spontaneous extracranial metastases. Case report. J Neurosurg 1973;38:226–31.
26. Horten BC, Rubinstein LJ. Primary cerebral neuroblastoma. A clinicopathological study of 35 cases. Brain 1976;99:735–56.
27. Ojeda VJ, Spagnolo DV, Vaughan RJ. Palisades in primary neuroblastoma simulating so-called polar spongioblastoma. A light and electron microscopical study of an adult case. Am J Surg Pathol 1987;11:316–22.
28. Rhodes RH, Davis RL, Kassel SH, Clague BH. Primary cerebral neuroblastoma: a light and electron microscopic study. Acta Neuropathol (Berl) 1978;41:119–24.
29. Sakaki S, Mori Y, Motozaki T, Nakagawa K, Matsuoka K. A cerebral neuroblastoma with extracranial metastases. Surg Neurol 1981;16:53–60.
30. Torres LF, Grant N, Harding BN, Scaravilli F. Intracerebral neuroblastoma. Report of a case with neuronal maturation and long survival. Acta Neuropathol (Berl) 1985;68:110–14.
31. Yagishita S, Itoh Y, Chiba Y, Yuda K. Cerebral neuroblastoma. Virchows Arch [A] 1978;381:1–11.

Olfactory Neuroblastoma (Esthesioneuroblastoma)

32. Choi HS, Anderson PJ. Olfactory neuroblastoma: an immuno-electron microscopic study of S-100 protein-positive cells. J Neuropathol Exp Neurol 1986;45:576–87.
33. Frierson HF Jr, Mills SE, Fechner RE, Taxy JB, Levine PA. Sinonasal undifferentiated carcinoma. An aggressive neoplasm derived from scheiderian epithelium and distinct from olfactory neuroblastoma. Am J Surg Pathol 1986;10:771–9.
34. _____, Ross GW, Mills SE, Frankfurter A. Olfactory neuroblastoma. Additional immunohistochemical characterization. Am J Clin Pathol 1990;94:547–53.
35. Mack EE, Prados MD, Wilson CB. Late manifestations of esthesioneuroblastomas in the central nervous system: report of two cases. Neurosurgery 1992;30:93–7.
36. Meneses MS, Thurel C, Mikol J, et al. Esthesioneuroblastoma with intracranial extension. Neurosurgery 1990;27:813–20.
37. Mills SE, Fechner RE. "Undifferentiated" neoplasms of the sinonasal region: differential diagnosis based on clinical, light microscopic, immunohistochemical, and ultrastructural features. Semin Diagn Pathol 1989;6:316–28.
38. _____, Frierson HF Jr. Olfactory neuroblastoma. A clinicopathologic study of 21 cases. Am J Surg Pathol 1985;9:317–27.

Retinoblastoma

39. Bader JL, Meadows AT, Zimmerman LE, et al. Bilateral retinoblastoma with ectopic intracranial retinoblastoma: trilateral retinoblastoma. Cancer Genet Cytogenet 1982;5:203–13.
40. Bullitt E, Crain BJ. Retinoblastoma as a possible primary intracranial tumor. Neurosurgery 1981;9:706–9.
41. Donoso LA, Folberg R, Arbizo V. Retinal S antigen and retinoblastoma. A monoclonal antibody histopathologic study. Arch Ophthalmol 1985;103:855–7.
42. _____, Rorke LB, Shields JA, Augsburger JJ, Brownstein S, Lahoud S. S-antigen immunoreactivity in trilateral retinoblastoma. Am J Ophthalmol 1987;103:57–62.
43. Johnson DL, Chandra R, Fisher WS, Hammock MK, McKeown CA. Trilateral retinoblastoma: ocular and pineal retinoblastomas. J Neurosurg 1985;63:367–70.
44. Katsetos CD, Herman MM, Frankfurter A, Uffer S, Perentes E, Rubinstein LJ. Neuron-associated class III beta-tubulin isotype, microtubule-associated protein 2, and synaptophysin in human retinoblastomas in situ. Further immunohistochemical observations on the Flexner-Wintersteiner rosettes. Lab Invest 1991;64:45–54.
45. Kingston JE, Plowman PN, Hungerford JL. Ectopic intracranial retinoblastoma in childhood. Br J Ophthalmol 1985;69:742–8.
46. Schwartz AM, Ghatak NR, Laine FJ. Intrasellar primitive neuroectodermal tumor (PNET) in familial retinoblastoma: a variant of "trilateral retinoblastoma." Clin Neuropathol 1990;9:55–9.
47. Stannard C, Knight BK, Sealy R. Pineal malignant neoplasm in association with hereditary retinoblastoma. Br J Ophthalmol 1985;69:749–53.
48. Ts'o MO, Fine BS, Zimmerman LE. The Flexner-Wintersteiner rosettes in retinoblastoma. Arch Pathol 1969;88:664–71.

49. _____, Fine BS, Zimmerman LE. The nature of retinoblastoma. II. Photoreceptor differentiation: an electron microscopic study. Am J Ophthalmol 1970;69:350–9.
50. _____, Zimmerman LE, Fine BS. The nature of retinoblastoma. I. Photoreceptor differentiation: a clinical and histopathologic study. Am J Ophthalmol 1970;69:339–49.

Melanotic Neuroectodermal Tumor of Infancy

52. Johnson RE, Scheithauer BW, Dahlin DC. Melanotic neuroectodermal tumor of infancy. A review of seven cases. Cancer 1983;52:661–6.
53. Mirich DR, Blaser SI, Harwood-Nash DC, Armstrong DC, Becker LE, Posnick JC. Melanotic neuroectodermal tumor of infancy: clinical, radiologic, and pathologic findings in five cases. AJNR Am J Neuroradiol 1991;12:689–97.
54. Nožicka Z, Špacek J. Melanotic neuroectodermal tumor of infancy with highly differentiated neuronal component. Light and electron microscopic study. Acta Neuropathol (Berl) 1978;44:229–33.
55. Parizek J, Nemecek S, Cernoch Z, Heger L, Nožicka Z, Špacek J. Melanotic neuroectodermal neurocranial

tumor of infancy of extra- intra- and subdural right temporal location: CT examination, surgical treatment, literature review. Neuropediatrics 1986;17:115–23.
56. Stowens D, Lin TH. Melanotic progonoma of the brain. Hum Pathol 1974;5:105–13.
57. Sung JH, Mastri AR, Segal EL. Melanotic medulloblastoma of the cerebellum. J Neuropathol Exp Neurol 1973;32:437–45.
58. Yu JS, Moore MR, Kupsky WJ, Scott RM. Intracranial melanotic neuroectodermal tumor of infancy: two case reports. Surg Neurol 1992;37:123–9.

Ependymoblastoma

59. Cruz-Sanchez FF, Rossi ML, Hughes JT, Moss TH. Differentiation in embryonal neuroepithelial tumors of the central nervous system. Cancer 1991;67:965–76.
60. Deck JH. Cerebral medulloepithelioma with maturation into ependymal cells and ganglion cells. J Neuropathol Exp Neurol 1969;28:442–54.
61. Kleinert R. Immunohistochemical characterization of primitive neuroectodermal tumors and their possible relationship to the stepwise ontogenetic development of the central nervous system. 2. Tumor studies. Acta Neuropathol (Berl) 1991;82:508–15.
62. Langford LA. The ultrastructure of the ependymoblastoma. Acta Neuropathol 1986;71:136–41.
63. Lorentzen M, Hägerstrand I. Congenital ependymoblastoma. Acta Neuropathol (Berl) 1980;49:71–4.
64. Mørk SJ, Rubinstein LJ. Ependymoblastoma. A reappraisal of a rare embryonal tumor. Cancer 1985;55:1536–42.
65. Rubinstein LJ. The definition of the ependymoblastoma. Arch Pathol 1970;90:35–45.

Medulloblastoma

66. Anwer UE, Smith TW, DeGirolami U, Wilkinson HA. Medulloblastoma with cartilaginous differentiation. Arch Pathol Lab Med 1989;113:84–8.
67. Badiali M, Pession A, Basso G, et al. N-myc and c-myc oncogenes amplification in medulloblastomas. Evidence of particularly aggressive behavior of a tumor with c-myc amplification. Tumori 1991;77:118–21.
68. Belza MG, Donaldson SS, Steinberg GK, Cox RS, Cogen PH. Medulloblastoma: freedom from relapse longer than 8 years—a therapeutic cure? J Neurosurg 1991;75:575–82.
69. Bonnin JM, Rubinstein LJ, Palmer NF, Beckwith JB. The association of embryonal tumors originating in the kidney and in the brain. Cancer 1984;54:2137–46.
70. Burger PC, Grahmann FC, Bliestle A, Kleihues P. Differentiation in the medulloblastoma. A histological and immunohistochemical study. Acta Neuropathol 1987;73:115–23.
71. Campbell AN, Chan HS, Becker LE, Daneman A, Park TS, Hoffman HJ. Extracranial metastases in childhood primary intracranial tumors. A report of 21 cases and review of the literature. Cancer 1984;53:974–81.
72. Caputy AJ, McCullough DC, Manz HJ, Patterson K, Hammock MK. A review of the factors influencing the prognosis of medulloblastoma. The importance of cell differentiation. J Neurosurg 1987;66:80–7.
73. Chatty EM, Earle KM. Medulloblastoma. A report of 201 cases with emphasis on the relationship of histologic variants to survival. Cancer 1971;28:977–83.
74. Chimelli L, Hahn MD, Budka H. Lipomatous differentiation in a medulloblastoma. Acta Neuropathol (Berl) 1991;81:471–3.
75. Coffin CM, Braun JT, Wick MR, Dehner LP. A clinicopathologic and immunohistochemical analysis of 53 cases of medulloblastoma with emphasis on synaptophysin expression. Mod Pathol 1990;3:164–70.
76. _____, Mukai K, Dehner LP. Glial differentiation in medulloblastomas. Histogenetic insight, glial reaction, or invasion of brain? Am J Surg Pathol 1983;7:555–65.
77. Czerwionka M, Korf HW, Hoffmann O, Busch H, Schachenmayr W. Differentiation in medulloblastomas: correlation between the immunocytochemical demonstration of photoreceptor markers (S-antigen, rodopsin) and the survival rate in 66 patients. Acta Neuropathol (Berl) 1989;78:629–36.
78. Evans DG, Farndon PA, Burnell LD, Gattamaneni HR, Birch JM. The incidence of Gorlin syndrome in 173 consecutive cases of medulloblastoma. Br J Cancer 1991;64:959–61.
79. Friedman HS, Oakes WJ, Bigner SH, Wikstrand CJ, Bigner DD. Medulloblastoma: tumor biological and clinical perspectives. J Neurooncol 1991;11:1–15.
80. Giangaspero F, Andreini L, Rigobello L, Asioli S, Galli G, Ceccarelli C. Vimentin immunoreactivity in medulloblastomas. J Neuropathol Exp Neurol 1990;49:274.
81. _____, Chieco P, Ceccarelli C, et al. "Desmoplastic" versus "classic" medulloblastoma: comparison of DNA content, histopathology and differentiation. Virchows Arch [A] 1991;418:207–14.

82. _____, Rigobello L, Badiali M, et al. Large cell medulloblastomas. A distinct variant with highly aggressive behavior. Am J Surg Pathol 1992;16:687–93.

83. Goldberg-Stern H, Gadoth N, Stern S, Cohen IJ, Zaizov R, Sandbank U. The prognostic significance of glial fibrillary acidic protein staining in medulloblastoma. Cancer 1991;68:568–73.

84. Gould VE, Jansson DS, Molenaar WM, et al. Primitive neuroectodermal tumors of the central nervous system. Patterns of expression of neuroendocrine markers, and all classes of intermediate filament proteins. Lab Invest 1990;62:498–509.

85. Hazuka MB, DeBiose DA, Henderson RH, Kinzie JJ. Survival results in adult patients treated for medulloblastoma. Cancer 1992;69:2143–8.

86. Herpers MJ, Budka H. Primitive neuroectodermal tumors including the medulloblastoma: glial differentiation signaled by immunoreactivity for GFAP is restricted to the pure desmoplastic medulloblastoma ("arachnoidal sarcoma of the cerebellum"). Clin Neuropathol 1985;4:12–8.

87. Hubbard JL, Scheithauer BW, Kispert DB, Carpenter SM, Wick MR, Laws ER Jr. Adult cerebellar medulloblastomas: the pathological, radiographic, and clinical disease spectrum. J Neurosurg 1989;70:536–44.

88. Hughes EN, Shillito J, Sallan SE, Loeffler JS, Cassady JR, Tarbell NJ. Medulloblastoma at the Joint Center for Radiation Therapy between 1968 and 1984. The influence of radiation dose on the patterns of failure and survival. Cancer 1988;61:1992–8.

89. Ito S, Hoshino T, Prados MD, Edwards MS. Cell kinetics of medulloblastomas. Cancer 1992;70:671–8.

90. Kadin ME, Rubinstein LJ, Nelson JS. Neonatal cerebellar medulloblastoma originating from the fetal external granular layer. J Neuropathol Exp Neurol 1970;29:583–600.

91. Katsetos CD, Frankfurter A, Christakos S, et al. Differential expression of neuronal class III β-tubulin isotype and calbindin D28k in the developing human cerebellar cortex and cerebellar neuroblastic tumors ("medulloblastomas"). J Neuropathol Exp Neurol 1991;50:293.

92. _____, Herman MM, Frankfurter A, et al. Cerebellar desmoplastic medulloblastomas. A further immunohistochemical characterization of the reticulin-free pale islands. Arch Pathol Lab Med 1989;113:1019–29.

93. Kleihues P, Burger PC, Scheithauer BW. Histologic typing of tumours of the central nervous system. World Health Organization. Berlin: Springer-Verlag, 1993.

94. Klériga E, Sher JH, Nallainathan SK, Stein SC, Sacher M. Development of cerebellar malignant astrocytoma at site of a medulloblastoma treated 11 years earlier. Case report. J Neurosurg 1978;49:445–9.

95. Kopelson G, Linggood RM, Kleinman GM. Medulloblastoma. The identification of prognostic subgroups and implications for multimodality management. Cancer 1983;51:312–9.

96. Krouwer HG, Vollmerhausen J, White J, Prados MD. Desmoplastic medulloblastoma metastatic to the pancreas: case report. Neurosurgery 1991;29:612–6.

97. Lefkowitz IB, Packer RJ, Ryan SG, et al. Late recurrence of primitive neuroectodermal tumor/medulloblastoma. Cancer 1988;62:826–30.

98. Mannoji H, Takeshita I, Fukui M, Ohta M, Kitamura K. Glial fibrillary acidic protein in medulloblastoma. Acta Neuropathol 1981;55:63–9.

99. Matakas F, Cervós-Navarro J, Gullotta F. The ultrastructure of medulloblastomas. Acta Neuropathol (Berl) 1970;16:271–84.

100. Molenaar WM, Jansson DS, Gould VE, et al. Molecular markers of primitive neuroectodermal tumors and other pediatric central nervous system tumors. Monoclonal antibodies to neuronal and glial antigens distinguish subsets of primitive neuroectodermal tumours. Lab Invest 1989;61:635–43.

101. Packer RJ, Sutton LN, Rorke LB, et al. Prognostic importance of cellular differentiation in medulloblastoma of childhood. J Neurosurg 1984;61:296–301.

102. Park TS, Hoffman HJ, Hendrick EB, Humphreys RP, Becker LE. Medulloblastoma: clinical presentation and management. Experience at the Hospital for Sick Children, Toronto, 1950–1980. J Neurosurg 1983;58:543–52.

103. Pearl GS, Mirra SS, Miles ML. Glioblastoma multiforme occurring 13 years after treatment of a medulloblastoma. Neurosurgery 1980;6:546–51.

104. _____, Takei Y. Cerebellar "neuroblastoma": nosology as it relates to medulloblastoma. Cancer 1981;47:772–9.

105. Rubinstein LJ. Embryonal central neuroepithelial tumors and their differentiating potential. A cytogenetic view of a complex neuro-oncological problem. J Neurosurg 1985;62:795–805.

106. Schofield DE, Yunis EJ, Geyer JR, Albright AL, Berger MS, Taylor SR. DNA content and other prognostic features in childhood medulloblastoma. Proposal of a scoring system. Cancer 1992;69:1307–14.

107. Tarbell NJ, Loeffler JS, Silver B, et al. The change in patterns of relapse in medulloblastoma. Cancer 1991;68:1600–4.

108. Tomlinson FH, Jenkins R, Scheithauer BW. Aggressive medulloblastoma with n-myc amplification. Mayo Clinic Proc. In press.

109. _____, Scheithauer BW, Jenkins RB. Medulloblastoma. II. A pathobiologic overview. J Child Neurol 1992;7:240–52.

110. _____, Scheithauer BW, Meyer FB, Smithason WA, Shaw EG, et al. Medulloblastoma. I. Clinical, diagnostic, and therapeutic overview. J Child Neurol 1992;7:142–55.

111. Yasue M, Tomita T, Engelhard H, Gonzalez-Crussi F, McLone DG, Bauer KD. Prognostic importance of DNA ploidy in medulloblastoma of childhood. J Neurosurg 1989;70:385–91.

Medulloblastoma and Melanotic Medulloblastoma

112. Abenoza P, Wick MR. Primitive cerebral neuroectodermal tumor with rhabdomyoblastic differentiation. Ultrastruct Pathol 1986;10:347–54.

113. Best PV. A medulloblastoma-like tumour with melanin formation. J Pathol 1973;110:109–11.

114. Boesel CP, Suhan JP, Sayers MP. Melanotic medulloblastoma. Report of a case with ultrastructural findings. J Neuropathol Exp Neurol 1978;37:531–43.

115. Bonnin JM, Wilson ER, Garcia JH. Medulloblastoma with neuronal, glial, striated muscle and pigment epithelium differentiation [Abstract]. Can J Neurol Sci 1989;16:227.

116. Chowdhury C, Roy S, Mahapatra AK, Bhatia R. Medullomyoblastoma. A teratoma. Cancer 1985;55:1495–500.

117. Dickson DW, Hart MN, Menezes A, Cancilla PA. Medulloblastoma with glial and rhabdomyoblastic differentiation. A myoglobin and glial fibrillary acidic protein immunohistochemical and ultrastructural study. J Neuropathol Exp Neurol 1983;42:639–47.

118. Duinkerke SJ, Slooff JL, Gabreëls FJ, Renier WO, Thijssen HO, Biesta JH. Melanotic rhabdomyomedulloblastoma or teratoid tumour of the cerebellar vermis. Clin Neurol Neurosurg 1981;83:29–33.

119. Fowler M, Simpson DA. A malignant melanin-forming tumour of the cerebellum. J Pathol Bacteriol 1984;62:307–11.

120. Hedley-Whyte ET. Primitive neuroectodermal tumor. Pediatr Pathol 1987;7:85–90.

121. Jimenez CL, Carpenter BF, Robb IA. Melanotic cerebellar tumor. Ultrastruct Pathol 1987;11:751–9.

122. Lata M, Mahapatra AK, Sarkar C, Roy S. Medullomyoblastoma. A case report. Indian J Can 1989;26:240–6.

123. Rao C, Friedlander ME, Klein E, Anzil AP, Sher JH. Medullomyoblastoma in an adult. Cancer 1990;65:157–63.

124. Smith TW, Davidson RI. Medullomyoblastoma. A histologic, immunohistochemical, and ultrastructural study. Cancer 1984;54:323–32.

125. Sung JH, Mastri AR, Segal EL. Melanotic medulloblastoma of the cerebellum. J Neuropathol Exp Neurol 1973:32:437–45.

Other Embryonal Tumors

126. Abenoza P, Wick MR. Primitive cerebral neuroectodermal tumor with rhabdomyoblastic differentiation. Ultrastruct Pathol 1986;10:347–54.

127. Biegel JA, Rorke LB, Packer RJ, Emanuel BS. Monosomy 22 in rhabdoid or atypical tumors of the brain. J Neurosurg 1990;73:710–4.

128. Brüstle O, Ohgaki H, Schmitt HP, Walter GF, Ostertag H, Kleihues P. Primitive neuroectodermal tumors after prophylactic central nervous system irradiation in children in association with an activated K-ras gene. Cancer 1992;69:2385–92.

129. Chimelli L, Hahn MD, Budka H. Lipomatous differentiation in a medulloblastoma. Acta Neuropathol (Berl) 1991;81:471–3.

130. Gambarelli D, Hassoun J, Choux M, Toga M. Complex cerebral tumor with evidence of neuronal, glial and Schwann cell differentiation. A histologic, immunocytochemical and ultrastructural study. Cancer 1982;49:1420–8.

131. Hart MN, Earle KM. Primitive neuroectodermal tumors of the brain in children. Cancer 1973;32:890–7.

132. Hedley-Whyte ET. Primitive neuroectodermal tumor. Pediatr Pathol 1987;7:85–90.

133. Janzer RC, Kleihues P. Primitive neuroectodermal tumor with choroid plexus differentiation. Clin Neuropathol 1985;4:93–8.

134. Lefkowitz IB, Rorke LB, Packer RJ, Sutton LN, Siegel KR, Katnick RJ. Atypical teratoid tumor of infancy: definition of an entity [Abstract]. Ann Neurol 1987;22:448–9.

135. Tang TT, Harb JM, Mork SJ, Sty JR. Composite cerebral neuroblastoma and astrocytoma. A mixed central neuroepithelial tumor. Cancer 1985;56:1404–12.

136. von Deimling A, Kleihues P, Saremaslani P, et al. Histogenesis and differentiation potential of central neurocytomas. Lab Invest 1991;64:585–91.

137. Yachnis AT, Rorke LB, Biegel JA, Perilongo G, Zimmerman RA, Sutton LN. Desmoplastic primitive neuroectodermal tumor with divergent differentiation. Broadening the spectrum of desmoplastic infantile neuroepithelial tumors. Am J Surg Pathol 1992;16:998–1006.

6
TUMORS OF THE PINEAL GLAND

Although both neurosensory and glial components of the pineal gland are potential sources of primary neoplasms, most parenchymatous tumors arise from pineocytes, the pineal parenchymal cells that represent specially modified neurons related to retinal photoreceptors (10a). The resulting spectrum of neoplasms ranges from the well-differentiated pineocytoma to the poorly differentiated pineoblastoma. Common differential diagnostic problems, germ cell neoplasms, are considered elsewhere in the text.

Criteria for the grading of pineal parenchymal tumors are unsettled, but most neoplasms are assigned to either the pineocytoma or the pineoblastoma category. The classification of the World Health Organization recognizes an additional lesion exhibiting features of both pineocytoma and pineoblastoma, the mixed pineocytoma/pineoblastoma (8). Additional tumors, which are intermediate rather than mixed in differentiation, represent a fourth division.

Morphologic criteria for the distinction of pineocytoma from pineoblastoma remain to be agreed upon, in large part due to the existence of intermediate lesions. According to the binary classification of Russell and Rubinstein (15), the pineocytoma group includes the well-recognized rosette-forming tumors and the more cellular mitotically active lesions, as long as they retain a lobular pattern. Other classifications restrict the designation pineocytoma to better differentiated lesions with pineocytomatous rosettes. Justification for this latter approach can be found in the shorter survival periods of patients with pineocytomas without such rosettes (2,20). It is our general practice, therefore, to include densely cellular pineal neoplasms within the pineoblastoma or intermediate category, especially if mitotic figures are noted. There is no clear line of distinction between these lesions and moderately cellular pineocytomas.

Pineocytoma

Clinical and Radiographic Features.
Pineocytomas occur primarily in mid to late adulthood, but children may be affected (2,20).

Radiographically, the tumors are discrete contrast-enhancing masses (fig. 6-1) in the posterior third ventricle (see Appendix F). Caution is required in the face of a cystic lesion since pineocytomas are usually solid and non-neoplastic pineal cysts are relatively common.

Macroscopic Findings. Pineocytomas displace rather than infiltrate surrounding brain parenchyma or leptomeninges. They are soft, homogeneous, and finely granular on cut surface.

Microscopic Findings. The classic and diagnostically inescapable pineocytoma is a moderately cellular neoplasm with fibrillar silver-positive zones representing pineocytomatous rosettes (figs. 6-2, 6-3). The size and number of the rosettes vary considerably. They are prominent in some lesions and sparse and incompletely formed in others. In contrast to the perivascular pseudorosettes of ependymoma, the rosettes of pineocytomas do not wheel about a vessel. Pineocytomatous rosettes are larger and more irregular than Homer Wright rosettes. In both types, however, the fibrillarity is produced by neoplastic cell processes emanating from the cells that palisade about the fibrillar core. In general, the cells of the

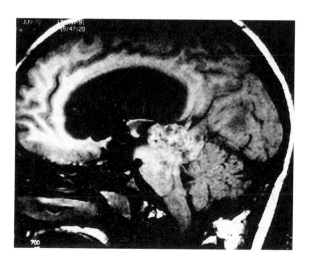

Figure 6-1
PINEOCYTOMA
In contrast to the pineoblastoma, pineocytomas are well-circumscribed masses showing neither a tendency to parenchymal invasion nor cerebrospinal dissemination.

7

TUMORS OF UNCERTAIN ORIGIN

Hemangioblastoma

Definition. A capillary-rich neoplasm containing variably lipidized interstitial or stromal cells.

Clinical and Radiographic Features. Hemangioblastomas arise either in the setting of von Hippel-Lindau disease or, more often, as solitary sporadic lesions without extracerebellar stigmata or family history (17). Von Hippel-Lindau syndrome includes intracranial or intraspinal hemangioblastoma, often multiple; retinal hemangioblastoma (see fig. 18-8); cystic lesions of the liver, kidney, pancreas, and epididymis; and benign and malignant renal cell tumors. This disease is discussed in chapter 18.

Hemangioblastomas are tumors of adulthood, generally occurring between the ages 30 and 65 years. A moderate male predominance is noted. While the cerebellum is by far the most frequent site, hemangioblastomas also arise in the medulla and spinal cord, particularly in syndrome-associated cases. Rare examples even appear in the supratentorial leptomeninges (9). Approximately 10 percent of patients present with polycythemia, a consequence of the tumoral production of erythropoietin (10,20).

Radiologically, hemangioblastomas are discrete, highly vascular, contrast-enhancing masses which, particularly in the cerebellum and spinal cord, are generally associated with a non-neoplastic cyst (fig. 7-1) (9) (see Appendix D). In the spinal cord the latter is referred to as a syrinx (see Appendix G).

Macroscopic Findings. In the cerebellum, most hemangioblastomas appear to the surgeon as highly vascular nodules. Although not always apparent intraoperatively, the tumors usually abut the leptomeninges. On cut section, they are generally dark red with a spongy texture and exude blood on compression. The degree to which hemangioblastomas appear yellow is proportionate to their content of lipid-laden stromal cells.

Spinal hemangioblastomas are intramedullary, discrete, and, as at other sites, abut the leptomeninges (see Appendix G). A prominent leptomeningeal blood supply may simulate a vascular malformation. In some cases, the associated syrinx dwarfs the tumor.

Rare hemangioblastomas occurring in the supratentorial leptomeninges produce discrete meningioma-like masses. Most are associated with von Hippel-Lindau disease.

Microscopic Findings. At low magnification, hemangioblastomas often vary considerably in their cell density: some regions are highly cellular while others consist of paucicellular tissue with a network of dilated vessels accompanying cyst-like spaces (fig. 7-2). Stromal or interstitial cells are distinctive at high magnification; they lie packed between abundant, often crisscrossing capillary channels (fig. 7-3). The cellularity and distribution of stromal cells varies considerably, as does their lipid content. In the *cellular variant*, such cells are more numerous than vascular elements and produce large cellular lobules, whereas in the *reticular variant* the vasculature is predominant enough to permit

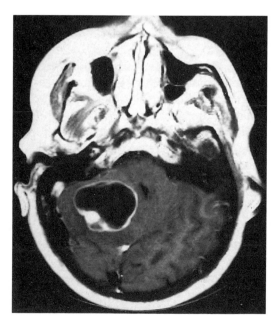

Figure 7-1
HEMANGIOBLASTOMA
The prototypic hemangioblastoma is a cystic cerebellar mass with a contrast-enhancing mural nodule.

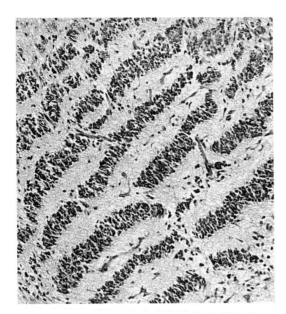 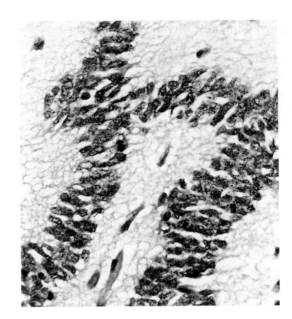

Figure 7-9
PRIMITIVE POLAR SPONGIOBLASTOMA
As seen at low (left) and high (right) magnification, the primitive polar spongioblastoma has striking columns of malignant cells. A blood vessel often lies equidistant from adjacent cords.

Macroscopic Findings. The primitive polar spongioblastoma is sufficiently rare that no specific gross characteristics have become evident. Circumscription has been noted in most reported cases. Leptomeningeal seeding may opacify the basal leptomeninges.

Microscopic Findings. This highly distinctive tumor is seen as regiments of palisaded cells assembling in long columns over several microscopic fields. The columns of nuclei are interrupted by highly fibrillar zones that are linear in longitudinal profile and circular when viewed on end (fig. 7-9, left). Thin and tapered, some cell processes extend from nuclei to nearby vessel walls (fig. 7-9, right). Accordingly, a delicate blood vessel is apparent in the center of many fibrillar areas. Nuclei are oval and chromatin rich, but are not particularly pleomorphic. Mitotic activity is generally scant but may be prominent in cases for which an entity status is most appropriate. Viewed in cross section, perinuclear clearing may mimic the appearance of oligodendroglioma.

Immunohistochemical Findings. Although in some cases the delicate processes are immunoreactive for S-100 protein, polar spongioblastomas have been largely negative for GFAP.

Ultrastructural Findings. Ultrastructural studies are too few in number to formulate diagnostic criteria, but several lesions had decidedly neuroblastic features, with the bipolar processes containing microtubules and neurosecretory granules (22,23).

Differential Diagnosis. In its most overt expression, the histologic pattern of polar spongioblastoma is so distinctive that it is immediately recognized. The issue of diagnosis thus gives way to more difficult problems of histogenesis and appropriate treatment. It is important to scan the nonpalisaded areas for evidence of more ordinary tumors in which the spongioblastoma pattern is known to occur. If an unequivocal pilocytic astrocytoma (fig. 7-10) or oligodendroglioma is found, the diagnosis should reflect their presence. We cautiously accept polar spongioblastoma as an entity only when palisading is overwhelmingly predominant, compact, and unaccompanied by other diagnostic tumor patterns. Frustratingly, in some tumors a rhythmic pattern arises in the background of a loose textured tissue not typical of any recognized neoplasm, and lacks the cellularity and mitotic activity of an embryonal tumor. The classification of such lesions is problematic and requires descriptive diagnoses.

244

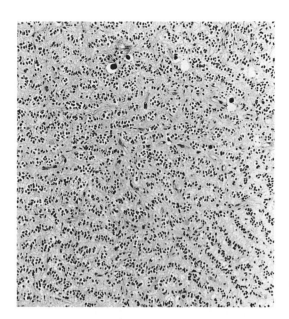 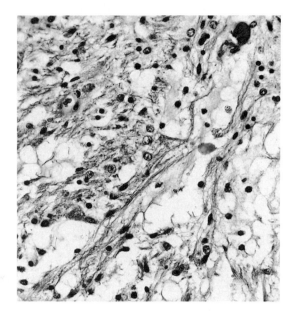

Figure 7-10
PILOCYTIC ASTROCYTOMA WITH
PALISADING RESEMBLING PRIMITIVE
POLAR SPONGIOBLASTOMA

Tissue with striking palisading (left) is associated with a typical pilocytic astrocytoma (right). Benign cytologic features distinguish the palisading tissue from the true primitive polar spongioblastoma. Note the calcification consistent with a longstanding and well-differentiated neoplasm.

Clinical Behavior and Treatment. The primitive polar spongioblastoma has been thought by some to behave so aggressively as to justify neuraxis radiation (28,29). Largely anecdotal experience suggests, however, that an aggressive course is not invariable, particularly if the spongioblastoma pattern is seen in an otherwise typical, well-differentiated tumor such as cerebellar astrocytoma or even in cases in which no other tissue pattern is observed (22,30,31). We recommend caution in considering aggressive radiotherapy and chemotherapy, particularly in the absence of mitotic activity. In the case of a "pure" lesion, it is appropriate to point out both the possibility of local recurrence and distant dissemination as well as to transmit present uncertainties regarding the classification and biologic behavior of this interesting tumor.

Atypical Teratoid/Rhabdoid Tumor

In the last several decades sporadic cases of intracranial "rhabdoid tumors" have been reported in both the supra- and infratentorial compartments (32–34,36–42,44). Histologically,

these neoplasms are high grade, with the classic plump cells with round or reniform nuclei and prominent nucleoli. Conspicuous eosinophilic hyaline or slightly fibrillar cytoplasmic masses displace nuclei. The tumors are biologically aggressive, with cerebrospinal fluid (CSF) dissemination a common terminal event.

It has become apparent recently that a similar, if not identical, tumor designated "atypical teratoid tumor" is a not uncommon neoplasm of infants and young children (46). While this tumor may have the prominent "rhabdoid" cytologic characteristics described above, it exhibits a broad range of other tissue patterns. The relationship of the atypical teratoid tumor to rhabdoid tumors thus remains to be defined. Nevertheless, there is unquestioned overlap in the histologic features of these two tumors; in one study both an atypical teratoid tumor and two central nervous system (CNS) lesions designated as pure rhabdoid tumors had a common cytogenetic abnormality: monosomy 22 (33). Similar cytogenetic changes were reported in two other cases classified as rhabdoid tumors (40), suggesting that the CNS rhabdoid tumor and the atypical teratoid tumor may be the same lesion. There is also some overlap of both cytogenetic (monosomy or translocation affecting chromosome 22) and immunohistochemical reactions between intracranial atypical teratoid/rhabdoid tumors and peripheral rhabdoid tumors (38, 45,47). It is not clear, however, to what extent the intracranial atypical teratoid/rhabdoid tumor relates to the renal tumor or to extrarenal rhabdoid tumors at non-CNS sites. Occasional renal rhabdoid tumors are associated with intracranial small cell embryonal neoplasms; in the cerebellum the latter are usually designated medulloblastomas as is discussed briefly on page 205 (35,43,48).

Patients with atypical teratoid/rhabdoid tumors are generally below the age of two; most, in our experience, are boys. The posterior fossa, sometimes the brain stem, is the common site (fig. 7-11).

Microscopically, the cellular sheets of neoplastic cells are interrupted by fibrovascular septa, which are often broad and edematous. Necrosis is common and mitoses are numerous. The Ki-67 staining index is high. Focal lateral alignment of cells to each other about septa or vessels can lend a vaguely epithelial appearance. Cytologically, most of the lesions are a jumble of medium-to-large cells with nuclei of moderate density. Nucleoli are prominent. Larger cells may appear as isolated forms, nests, or large lobules (fig. 7-12). Vacuolated cells are frequent, either as sheets or as individual forms giving a "starry sky" appearance. Cells with the prominent nuclear and cytoplasmic "rhabdoid" features may be evident, but tumors overall are not necessarily overtly rhabdoid. Some tumors have areas of smaller cells and are similar to the medulloblastoma in terms of high cell density and small nuclear size. Fascicular areas are common. Small nests and cords of cells can resemble the chordoma, resulting in the "trabecular pattern" of the renal rhabdoid tumor (49).

The histologic appearance can be distinctive or mundane, but in either case belies a remarkably complex immunophenotype (fig. 7-13). The tumors are consistently positive for vimentin, and reactivities for epithelial membrane antigen, glial fibrillary acidic protein, and cytokeratin are common. Reactivity for actin or desmin is sometimes seen, but the strap cells or rhabdo-

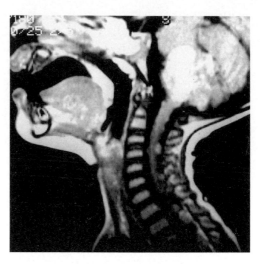

Figure 7-11
ATYPICAL TERATOID/RHABDOID TUMOR
As in this 19-month-old boy with a mass centered on the brain stem, most atypical teratoid/rhabdoid tumors arise in the posterior fossa. Note the multiple drop metastases on the medulla and cervical spinal cord present here at the time of initial presentation. (Courtesy of Dr. Gary S. Pearl, Orlando, FL.)

myoblasts of the medullomyoblastoma have not, in our experience, been present. Synaptophysin positivity is noted occasionally, but neuofilament staining is uncommon. Chromogranin-positive cells are occasionally seen. Masses of intermediate filaments are common ultrastrucural features (32,34,37,39,40,42,44). Neurosecretory granules are observed in some cases (39).

The differential diagnosis for lesions in the posterior fossa usually focuses on the medulloblastoma (see fig. 5-33). Distinguising the two neoplasms are the large paler cells of the atypical teratoid/rhabdoid tumor, although a small-cell component in some of the latter tumor can cause diagnostic confusion. Many atypical teratoid/rhabdoid tumors are lobular, but lack the distinctive nodules with neuritic differentiation common in the "desmoplastic" medulloblastoma with its "pale islands." The immunohistochemical repertoire of the atypical teratoid/rhabdoid tumor is clearly a decisive differential diagnostic feature, although staining may not be applied if the entity is not considered.

Reported cases of primary atypical teratoid/rhabdoid tumors are too few to include precise statements regarding their biologic behavior, but aggressive local recurrence and meningeal seeding are the rule. The latter is sometimes apparent at the time of presentation (fig. 7-11) (46).

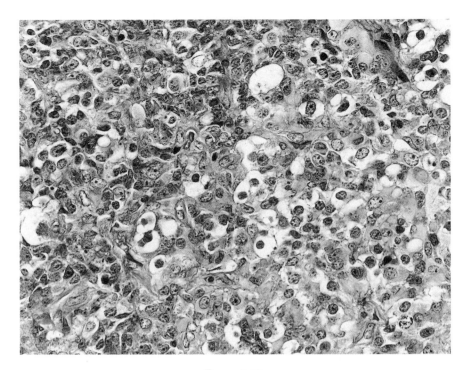

Figure 7-12
ATYPICAL TERATOID/RHABDOID TUMOR
The neoplasm is typically composed of large, pale cells in aggregates without specific architectural features.

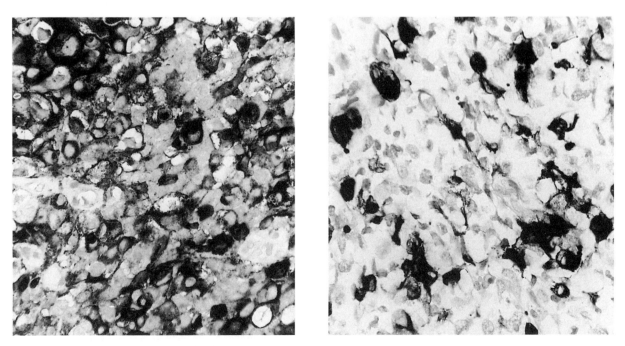

Figure 7-13
ATYPICAL TERATOID/RHABDOID TUMOR
An impressive display of immunoreactivity is common. The neoplasm illustrated in figures 7-11 and 7-12 is positive for epithelial membrane antigen (left) and glial fibrillary acidic protein (right). Other immunoreactivities in this case included those for vimentin, cytokeratin, actin, synaptophysin, neurofilament protein, chromogranin, and S-100 protein. Neurosecretory granules were seen ultrastructurally.

REFERENCES

Hemangioblastoma

1. Becker I, Paulus W, Roggendorf W. Histogenesis of stromal cells in cerebellar hemangioblastomas. An immunohistochemical study. Am J Pathol 1989;134:271–5.

2. Bonnin JM, Peña CE, Rubinstein LJ. Mixed capillary hemangioblastoma and glioma. A redefinition of the "angioglioma." J Neuropathol Exp Neurol 1983;42:504–16.

3. Chaudhry AP, Montes M, Cohn GA. Ultrastructure of cerebellar hemangioblastoma. Cancer 1978;42:1834–50.

4. de la Monte SM, Horowitz SA. Hemangioblastomas: clinical and histopathological factors correlated with recurrence. Neurosurgery 1989;25:695–8.

5. Deck JH, Rubinstein LJ. Glial fibrillary acidic protein in stromal cells of some capillary hemangioblastomas: significance and possible implications of an immunoperoxidase study. Acta Neuropathol (Berl) 1981;54:173–81.

6. Feldenzer JA, McKeever PE. Selective localization of gamma-enolase in stromal cells of cerebellar hemangioblastomas. Acta Neuropathol (Berl) 1987;72:281–5.

7. Frank TS, Trojanowski JQ, Roberts SA, Brooks JJ. A detailed immunohistochemical analysis of cerebellar hemangioblastoma: an undifferentiated mesenchymal tumor. Mod Pathol 1989;2:638–51.

8. Ho KL. Ultrastructure of cerebellar capillary hemangioblastoma. II. Mast cells and angiogenesis. Acta Neuropathol (Berl) 1984;64:308–18.

9. Ho VB, Smirniotopoulos JG, Murphy FM, Rushing EJ. Radiologic-pathologic correlation: hemangioblastoma. AJNR Am J Neuroradiol 1992;13:1343–52.

10. Horton JC, Harsh GR IV, Fisher JW, Hoyt WF. Von Hippel-Lindau disease and erythrocytosis: radioimmunoassay of erythropoietin in cyst fluid from a brainstem hemangioblastoma. Neurology 1991;41:753–4.

11. Hufnagel TJ, Kim JH, True LD, Manuelidis EE. Immunohistochemistry of capillary hemangioblastoma. Immunoperoxidase-labeled antibody staining resolves the differential diagnosis with metastatic renal cell carcinoma, but does not explain the histogenesis of the capillary hemangioblastoma. Am J Surg Pathol 1989;13:207–16.

12. Kepes JJ, Rengachary SS, Lee SH. Astrocytes in hemangioblastomas of the central nervous system and their relationship to stromal cells. Acta Neuropathol (Berl) 1979;47:99–104.

13. Lombardi D, Scheithauer BW, Piepgras D, Meyer FB, Forbes GS. "Angioglioma" and the arteriovenous malformation-glioma association. J Neurosurg 1991;75:589–96.

14. McComb RD, Jones TR, Pizzo SV, Bigner DD. Localization of factor VIII/von Willebrand factor and glial fibrillary acidic protein in the hemangioblastoma: implications for stromal cell histogenesis. Acta Neuropathol (Berl) 1982;56:207–13.

15. Mills SE, Ross GW, Perentes E, Nakagawa Y, Scheithauer BW. Cerebellar hemangioblastoma: immunohistochemical distinction from metastatic renal cell carcinoma. Surg Pathol 1990;3:121–32.

16. Nemes Z. Fibrohistiocytic differentiation in capillary hemangioblastoma. Hum Pathol 1992;23:805–10.

17. Neumann HP, Eggert HR, Weigel K, Friedburg H, Wiestler OD, Schollmeyer P. Hemangioblastomas of the central nervous system. A 10-year study with special reference to von Hippel-Lindau syndrome. J Neurosurg 1989;70:24–30.

18. Silverberg GD. Simple cysts of the cerebellum. J Neurosurg 1971;35:320–7.

19. Smalley SR, Schomberg PJ, Earle JD, Laws ER Jr, Scheithauer BW, O'Fallon JR. Radiotherapeutic considerations in the treatment of hemangioblastomas of the central nervous system. Int J Radiat Oncol Biol Phys 1990;18:1165–71.

20. Tachibana O, Yamashima T, Yamashita J. Immunohistochemical study of erythropoietin in cerebellar hemangioblastomas associated with secondary polycythemia. Neurosurgery 1991;28:24–6.

21. Zec N, Cera P, Towfighi J. Extramedullary hematopoiesis in cerebellar hemangioblastoma. Neurosurgery 1991;29:34–7.

Primitive Polar Spongioblastoma

22. de Chadarévian JP, Guyda HJ, Hollenberg RD. Hypothalamic polar spongioblastoma associated with the diencephalic syndrome: ultrastructural demonstration of a neuro-endocrine organization. Virchows Arch [A] 1984;402:465–74.

23. Jansen GH, Troost D, Dingemans KP. Polar spongioblastoma: an immunohistochemical and electron microscopical study. Acta Neuropathol (Berl) 1990;81:228–32.

24. Kleihues P, Burger PC, Scheithauer BW. Histological typing of tumours of the central nervous system. 2nd ed. New York: Springer-Verlag, 1993.

25. Langford LA, Camel MH. Palisading pattern in cerebral neuroblastoma mimicking the primitive polar spongioblastoma: an ultrastructural study. Acta Neuropathol (Berl) 1987;73:153–9.

26. Ojeda VJ, Spagnolo DV, Vaughan RJ. Palisades in primary cerebral neuroblastoma simulating so-called polar spongioblastoma: a light and electron microscop-ical study of an adult case. Am J Surg Pathol 1987;11:316–22.

27. Rubinstein LJ. Cytogenesis and differentiation of primitive central neuroepithelial tumors. J Neuropathol Exp Neurol 1972;31:7–26.

28. _____. Discussion on polar spongioblastomas. Acta Neurochir 1964;Suppl. X:126–32.

29. Russell DS, Rubinstein LJ. Pathology of tumours of the nervous system. Baltimore: Williams & Wilkins, 1989:169–72.

29a. Schiffer D, Cravioto H, Giordana MT, Migheli A, Pezzulo T, Vigliani MC. Is polar spongioblastoma a tumor entity? J Neurosurg 1993;78:587–91.

30. Schochet SS Jr, Violett TW, Nelson J, Pelofsky S, Barnes PA. Polar spongioblastoma of the cervical spinal cord: case report. Clin Neuropathol 1984;3:225–7.

31. Steinberg GK, Shuer LM, Conley FK, Hanbery JW. Evolution and outcome in malignant astroglial neoplasms of the cerebellum. J Neurosurg 1985;62:9–17.

Atypical Teratoid/Rhabdoid Tumor

32. Agranovich AL, Ang LC, Griebel RW, Kobrinsky NL, Lowry N, Tchang SP. Malignant rhabdoid tumor of the central nervous system with subarachnoid dissemination. Surg Neurol 1992;37:410–4.

33. Biegel JA, Rorke LB, Packer RJ, Emanuel BS. Monosomy 22 in rhabdoid or atypical tumors of the brain. J Neurosurg 1990;73:710–4.

34. Biggs PJ, Garen PD, Powers JM, Garvin AJ. Malignant rhabdoid tumor of the central nervous system. Hum Pathol 1987;18:332–7.

35. Bonnin JM, Rubinstein LJ, Palmer NF, Beckwith JB. The association of embryonal tumors originating in the kidney and in the brain. A report of seven cases. Cancer 1984;54:2137–46.

36. Briner J, Bannwart F, Kleihues P, et al. Malignant small cell tumor of the brain with intermediate filaments—a case of primary cerebral rhabdoid tumor [Abstract]. Pediatr Pathol 1985;3:117–8.

37. Chou SM, Anderson JS. Primary CNS malignant rhabdoid tumor (MRT): report of two cases and review of literature. Clin Neuropathol 1991;10:1–10.

38. Douglass EC, Valentine M, Rowe ST, et al. Malignant rhabdoid tumor: a highly malignant childhood tumor with minimal karyotypic changes. Genes Chromosom Cancer 1990;2:210–6.

39. Hanna SL, Langston JW, Parham DM, Douglass EC. Primary malignant rhabdoid tumor of the brain: clinical, imaging, and pathologic findings. AJNR Am J Neuroradiol 1993;14:107–15.

40. Hasserjian RP, Schofield D, Folkerth RF. Malignant rhabdoid tumor (MRT) of the central nervous system [Abstract]. J Neuropathol Exp Neurol 1992;51:367.

41. Ho PS, Lee WH, Chen CY, et al. Primary malignant rhabdoid tumor of the brain: CT characteristics. J Comput Assist Tomogr 1990;14:461–3.

42. Horn M, Schlote W, Lerch KD, Steudel WI, Harms D, Thomas E. Malignant rhabdoid tumor: primary intracranial manifestation in an adult. Acta Neuropathol (Berl) 1992;83:445–8.

43. Howat AJ, Gonzales MF, Waters KD, Campbell PE. Primitive neuroectodermal tumour of the central nervoussystem associated with malignant rhabdoid tumour of the kidney: report of a case. Histopathology 1986;10:643–50.

44. Jakate SM, Marsden HB, Ingram L. Primary rhabdoid tumour of the brain. Virchows Arch [A] 1988;412:393–7.

45. Karnes PS, Tran TN, Cui MY, Bogenmann E, Shimada H, Ying KL. Establishment of a rhabdoid tumor cell line with a specific chromosomal abnormality, 46,XY,t(11;22)(p15.5;q11.23). Cancer Genet Cytogenet 1991;56:31–8.

46. Lefkowitz IB, Rorke LB, Packer RJ, Sutton LN, Siegel KR, Katnick RJ. Atypical teratoid tumor of infancy: definition of an entity [Abstract]. Ann Neurol 1987;22:448–9.

47. Ota S, Crabbe DC, Tran TN, Triche TJ, Shimada H. Malignant rhabdoid tumor. A study with two established cell lines. Cancer 1993;71:2862–72.

48. Sotelo-Avila C, Gonzalez-Crussi F, deMello D, et al. Renal and extrarenal rhabdoid tumors in children: a clinicopathologic study of 14 patients. Semin Diagn Pathol 1986;3:151–63.

49. Weeks DA, Beckwith JB, Mierau GW. Rhabdoid tumor. An entity or a phenotype? Arch Pathol Lab Med 1989;113:113–4.

8

GERM CELL TUMORS

Definition. A histologically distinct group of variably differentiated germ cell neoplasms identical to those occurring in the gonads and at other extragonadal sites.

Clinical and Radiographic Features. Although most intracranial germ cell tumors arise in the midline, usually in the pineal or suprasellar regions (6,21,23,25), occasional examples are situated laterally in the basal ganglia or thalamus (7,26). Sometimes, simultaneous lesions appear at more than one locus (24). Teratomas, which may occur in utero or in the neonatal period, arise throughout the craniospinal axis. Some are so massive that they replace the brain or extend into adjacent cervical or cephalic soft tissues (10,17, 18,22). Rare teratomas appear in adults (8).

Germ cell tumors in the pineal gland and basal ganglia primarily affect males; no sex predilection is observed for lesions in the suprasellar region. Although intracranial germ cell neoplasms are uncommon, they appear to be more frequent in Japan.

Neuroradiologically, most lesions are well circumscribed and contrast enhancing (fig. 8-1). Understandably, teratomas are heterogeneous in their signal characteristics on magnetic resonance imaging.

Germ cell tumors have been associated with the production and secretion of alpha-fetoprotein, beta-human chorionic gonadotrophin (β-hCG), or carcinoembryonic antigen (CEA) (9). Levels of these substances, either in cerebrospinal fluid or blood, are useful in diagnosis as well as in monitoring response to treatment. Elevation of β-hCG must not be overinterpreted as evidence of choriocarcinoma since syncytiotrophoblastic cells are found in some germinomas and immature teratomas.

Microscopic Findings and Classification. Intracranial germ cell neoplasms are classified according to the widely used classification of Mostofi and Price for testicular tumors (14a), in which they are subdivided into either lesions exhibiting only one histologic pattern or those composed of two or more components. The former category includes the common germinoma

(seminoma), embryonal carcinoma, yolk sac tumor, teratomas (both mature and immature), and the rare choriocarcinoma. Various combinations of these elements comprise the mixed germ cell tumors: immature teratoma with embryonal carcinoma (teratocarcinoma) or yolk sac carcinoma with germinoma.

The *germinoma*, the most frequently occurring intracranial germ cell tumor, is composed of sheets and lobules of large cells with often indistinct, somewhat vacuolated, glycogen-rich cytoplasm; round vesicular nuclei with prominent nucleoli; and often brisk mitotic activity (fig. 8-2). Cohesion of cells may be evident and denotes prognostically insignificant early carcinomatous transformation (14). Germinomas often show an associated T-lymphocyte infiltrate, which, while scanty in some cases, can predominate in others, obscuring neoplastic cells and posing a diagnostic problem. Granulomas (fig. 8-3) and syncytiotrophoblastic giant cells may be seen in some cases. Taken out of context, such foci may suggest an erroneous diagnosis of sarcoidosis or tuberculosis (4,12). In

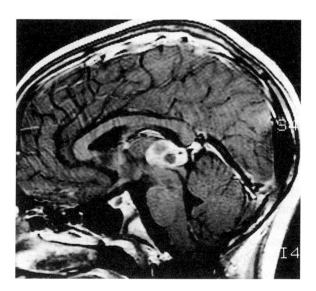

Figure 8-1
GERMINOMA

Intracranial germinomas occur most frequently as contrast-enhancing masses in the pineal region. As in this 12-year-old, boys are most often affected.

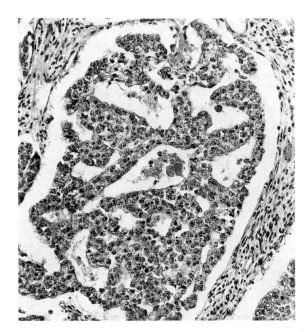

Figure 8-5
EMBRYONAL CARCINOMA
Embryonal carcinoma presents as sheets, thick cords, or gland-like arrangements of primitive-appearing epithelial cells.

is rare (6). This epithelial tumor consists variably of compact sheets, ribbons, cords, or papillae (28). Diagnostic Schiller-Duval bodies, when present, are identified as tufted epithelium covered vessels projecting into clear spaces lined by similar cells (fig. 8-6, left). A loose-knit vitelline pattern is also common (fig. 8-6, right). Also diagnostic of yolk sac carcinoma are PAS-positive, cytoplasmic and extracellular eosinophilic droplets immunoreactive for alpha-fetoprotein (fig. 8-7).

Teratomatous lesions are divided into mature and immature types. In most instances they contain tissues from each of the three germ cell layers. In mature examples, the components are fully differentiated. The intracranial "fetus-in-fetu" is the ultimate expression (1,30). The more frequently occurring immature teratomas are composed of fetal-appearing tissue of the type seen in "products of conception." In this melange, one regularly sees developing neuroectodermal structures such as embryonic medullary neuroepithelium (fig. 8-8), retina (fig. 8-9), and choroid plexus. Common mesenchymal elements include nondescript cellular or myxoid stroma, islands of cartilage occasionally undergoing ossification, and intersecting bands of striated

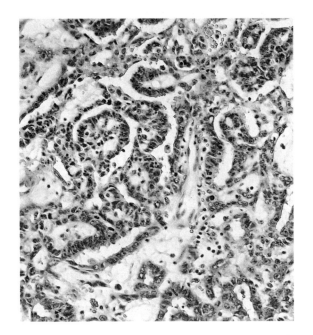

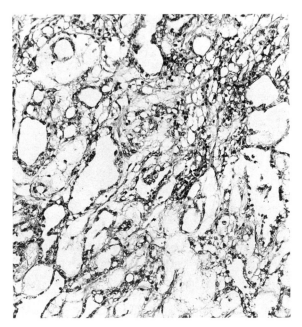

Figure 8-6
YOLK SAC TUMOR
Schiller-Duval bodies (left) and the loose-knit vitelline pattern (right) are common features of the intracranial yolk sac tumor.

muscle. Ectoderm and endoderm are represented by skin and adnexa as well as respiratory tract, pancreatic parenchyma, or intestinal epithelium. The last may be accompanied by a remarkably well-differentiated muscularis (fig. 8-10). Rare lesions contain both immature and mature elements. In such instances, we consider the designation *immature teratoma* most appropriate. Descriptive terms are preferable in cases in which teratomas are associated with malignant germ cell components. Thus, the term "embryonal carcinoma with teratoma" is more informative than the confusing designation "teratocarcinoma." Similarly, teratomas with frankly malignant tissues of conventional type, such as carcinoma or sarcoma, are better characterized as "teratoma with adenocarcinoma" or "teratoma with rhabdomyosarcoma" than simply "malignant teratoma" (20).

The rarest of the intracranial germ cell tumors, the pure *choriocarcinoma*, is composed of two cell types, syncytiotrophoblasts and cytotrophoblasts (5,11). The typical bilaminar arrangement of these constituents is an essential diagnostic feature since prognostically insignificant

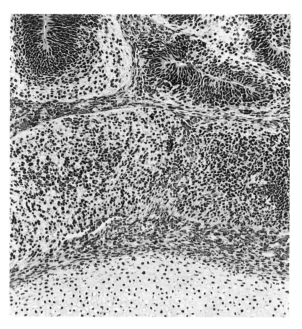

Figure 8-8
IMMATURE TERATOMA
Resembling the tissues of a fetus, this lesion combines mesenchyme in the form of cartilage, undifferentiated tissue, and elements of the developing central nervous system.

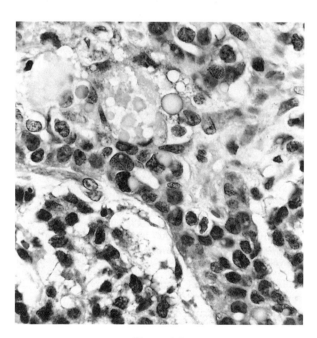

Figure 8-7
YOLK SAC TUMOR
Strands of epithelium as well as intracytoplasmic or stromal hyaline droplets are typical features of yolk sac tumor. The neoplasm's immunoreactivity for alpha-fetoprotein is shown in figure 8-12.

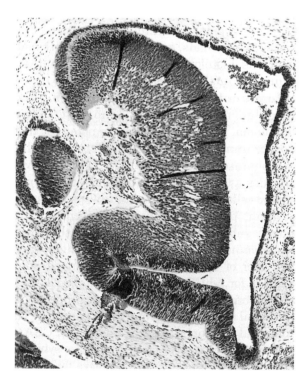

Figure 8-9
IMMATURE TERATOMA
A developing eye with retina and lens illustrates the complex differentiating potential of immature teratomas.

9
TUMORS OF MENINGOTHELIAL CELLS

Meningioma

Definition. A neoplasm derived from meningothelial (arachnoidal) cells.

General Comments. The term meningioma has been used in both broad and restrictive senses. The broad perspective, employed by Cushing and Eisenhardt in their classic monograph (17), considers as a meningioma almost any macroscopically discrete primary meningeal mass regardless of histologic type. The more narrow usage employed in this volume limits the designation to lesions clearly derived from meningothelial (arachnoidal) cells (9). As a result, tumors such as meningeal hemangiopericytoma and hemangioblastoma are not designated meningiomas and are described separately in chapters 10 and 7, respectively.

Although occasional meningiomas are the unwanted consequence of cranial irradiation (10,35,82), and rare examples have perhaps been the result of trauma (5), the etiology of most is unknown. Genetic influences underlie some: a locus on chromosome 22 in patients with the central form of neurofibromatosis (NF2) may be responsible for the occurrence of multiple meningiomas. Monosomy 22, with or without additional chromosomal abnormalities, is a common cytogenetic finding in the spontaneous types (93). Children may be affected (19,21, 25,36) but most meningiomas occur in adults. An association with other estrogen-dependent tumors including breast and endometrial cancers is noted in some cases (41,52). Rare meningiomas are host to metastatic carcinoma (22,97).

A rare form of "collision" tumor affecting the nervous system consists of meningioma either abutting or intermingled with a glioma (29,55, 68,81). While coincidence seems the basis of the association in most cases, induction of the glioma by the meningioma is suspected to underlie some cases. The issue is unresolved.

Clinical and Radiographic Features. *Meningiomas of the Intracranial Meninges.* In this most common location, symptoms of meningiomas represent nonspecific expressions of an expanding intracranial mass: focal neurologic deficits, increased intracranial pressure, and seizures. Seizures are less common than in patients with intraparenchymal tumors such as gliomas and metastases. Intracranial meningiomas exhibit a distinct predilection for females (approximately 3 to 2).

In radiographic terms, intracranial meningiomas are usually globular, highly vascular, contrast enhancing, and dura based (fig. 9-1). Although meningiomas are arachnoidal in origin, they are intimately related to, and often highly infiltrative of, the dura. A wedge-shaped cluster of small vessels or a tongue of neoplastic tissue lying within the angle between the tumor and the attached dura produces a radiographically useful, although nonspecific, focus of contrast enhancement known as the "dural tail sign" (figs. 9-1, 9-2) (2,90). Calcium can be detected by computerized tomography in some cases (see Appendix E). Occasional tumors, particularly those of the sphenoid ridge, diffusely carpet the

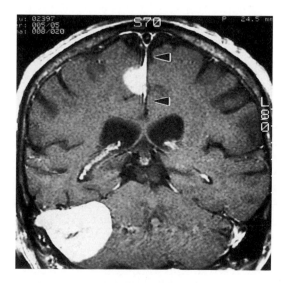

Figure 9-1
MENINGIOMAS

Meningiomas are generally dura based and contrast enhancing. Triangular areas of enhancement (arrows) extend along the dura from the edge of the falcine lesion and form the diagnostically helpful, albeit nonspecific, dural tail sign.

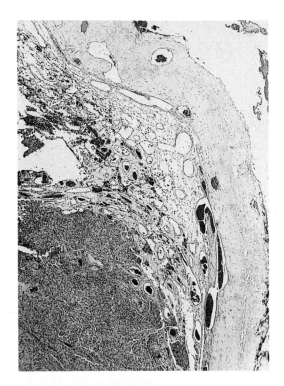

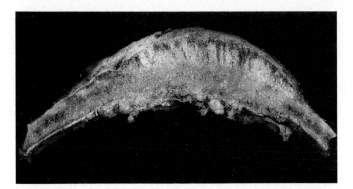

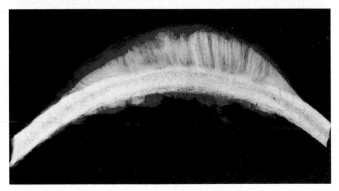

Figure 9-2
MENINGIOMA

As is typical, this meningioma is densely adherent to the dura at the right of the illustration. At the top left is a wedge-shaped area of loose vascular tissue, the "dural tail."

Figure 9-3
MENINGIOMA

As apparent both in cut section (top) and specimen radiograph (bottom), meningiomas that penetrate the skull often induce bony spicules which radiate from the outer and, to a lesser extent, the inner tables.

dura to form a lesion termed *meningioma en plaque*. Some meningiomas are associated with a large intratumoral or peritumoral cyst (54, 71,75) (see Appendix D).

On T2-weighted images, a correlation has been noted between the histologic subtype of the tumor and the signal characteristics (22a). Collagen-rich fibrous and transitional tumors are hypointense (dark) relative to the cerebral cortex, whereas the syncytial variants and hemangiopericytomas are hyperintense (bright) as a presumed consequence of lesser amounts of collagen and greater content of water (22a).

In contrast to intra-axial lesions such as gliomas, which rely primarily on branches of the internal carotid and vertebral arteries, meningiomas derive their blood supply largely from the external carotid system. Some meningiomas induce considerable vasogenic edema in the underlying brain. Although the pathogenesis of this effect is unclear, it appears to be related in part to the size (31), proliferative activity (16), and histologic type of the tumor (38). The extent of vascularization by the cerebral arteries also appears to be important (38). Malignant meningiomas invasive of the brain are often associated with marked cerebral edema (see fig. 9-39) (63a).

Intracranial meningiomas frequently induce cranial hyperostosis consisting of bony spicules radiating from the outer and, to a lesser extent, the inner tables of the skull (fig. 9-3). After penetrating the calvarium, such tumors elevate or penetrate the galea and produce a scalp mass which may be the first clinical expression of the neoplasm. Only rarely are meningiomas osteolytic (96).

Meningiomas of the Optic Nerve Sheath. These are considerably less common than intracranial or intraspinal examples (12,43,64). Children are rarely affected. Clinical signs include visual loss, strabismus, or ptosis. Whereas some tumors are primarily intradural, others lie largely free within orbital soft tissues.

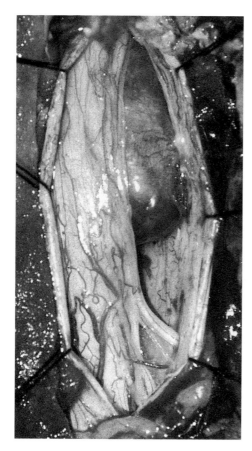

Figure 9-4
MENINGIOMA
Most spinal meningiomas are discrete, intradural, extramedullary, and laterally situated. (Courtesy of Dr. Allan H. Friedman, Durham, NC.)

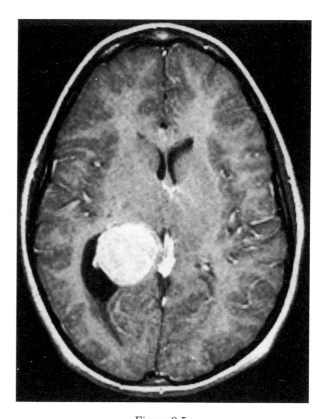

Figure 9-5
MENINGIOMA
Rare meningiomas are intraventricular.

Intraspinal Meningiomas. These tumors expand at the expense of the adjacent spinal cord and produce the expected segmental neurologic deficits (fig. 9-4). Radicular pain, a common symptom of the macroscopically similar schwannoma, is not usually a symptom. Women are far more often affected than men, in our experience, at a ratio approaching 10 to 1. Most tumors are ventrally or laterally situated near the nerve root exit zone, an area where meningothelial cells are normally concentrated. Schwannomas are usually dorsal. Most intraspinal meningiomas are intradural extramedullary lesions (see Appendix G). Only a very rare lesion is intramedullary (84). Cervicothoracic segments are most often affected; lumbosacral lesions are rare (23). Dense calcification is common (see Appendix E). In contrast to intracranial counter-

parts, intraspinal meningiomas rarely involve surrounding osseous structures. The differential diagnostic possibilities for intraspinal tumors are given in Appendix G.

Meningiomas of the Ventricular System. Since the choroid plexus originates as an invagination of vessels and meninges along the choroidal fissure, it is not surprising that meningothelial cells may be found within its stroma, or that they occasionally give rise to intraventricular meningiomas (fig. 9-5) (see Appendix F). The third (33,76), lateral (27,32), and fourth (74,91) ventricles may be affected.

Epidural Meningiomas. The principal component of these meningiomas lies outside the dura. Such tumors are uncommon, but occur both intracranially and intraspinally. Given the apposition of cranial dura to the inner table of the skull, the intracranial examples are often osteoinvasive. The spinal counterparts, in contrast, rarely involve bone, although they frequently demonstrate a minor intradural component.

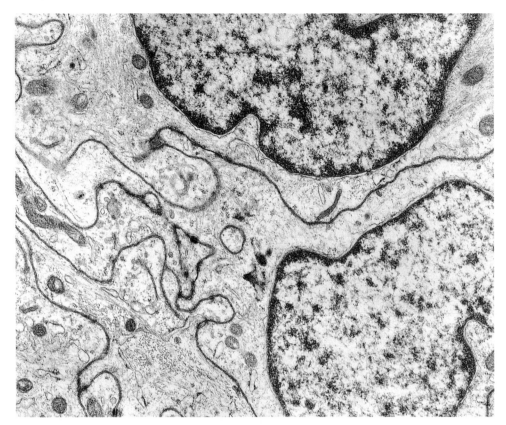

Figure 9-28
MENINGIOMA
Syncytial meningioma cells are noted for interdigitating cell borders, well-formed desmosomes, and abundant intermediate filaments.

Ultrastructural Findings. Classic meningiomas, particularly meningotheliomatous or transitional types, are noted for interdigitating processes, cytoplasmic intermediate filaments in varying number and distribution, and well-formed desmosomes and hemidesmosomes (fig. 9-28) (14,46). Desmosomes and interdigitating cytoplasmic processes are the most telling features of meningioma in cases in which electron microscopy is required for diagnosis.

The cells of fibrous meningiomas exhibit few intercellular junctions since they lack cohesion and interdigitation, being separated from one another by varying quantities of collagen. In addition, cytoplasmic filaments are often sparse and a vague condensation of intercellular matrix partially invests the cells. With the addition of abundant collagen, fibrous meningiomas gain a distinctly mesenchymal appearance. In contrast to fibroblasts, however, they lack highly developed rough endoplasmic reticulum and segmented nuclei.

Microcystic tumors are characterized by elongated, often fibril-poor cell processes joined terminally by well-formed desmosomes (fig. 9-29). Flocculent electron lucent material fills the intercellular spaces.

The pseudopsammoma bodies of secretory meningiomas are masses of minute vesicles and debris within an intracellular space whose luminal surface exhibits numerous short microvilli (fig. 9-30) (7,26,45,46). Multiple acini may be present within the same cell. Desmosomes connect adjacent cells.

Immunohistochemical Findings. The most diagnostically useful marker of meningioma is a membranous pattern of immunoreactivity for epithelial membrane antigen (fig. 9-31) (86). Not surprisingly, positivity is more marked in meningothelial and transitional lesions, which at the ultrastructural level show greater epithelial differentiation than fibrous variants. Staining is often focal at best in chordoid meningiomas. Unfortunately a number of meningiomas lack membrane staining, with reactivity being cytoplasmic instead. The latter can be difficult to interpret, particularly when focal and weak, since diffuse cytoplasmic staining may be

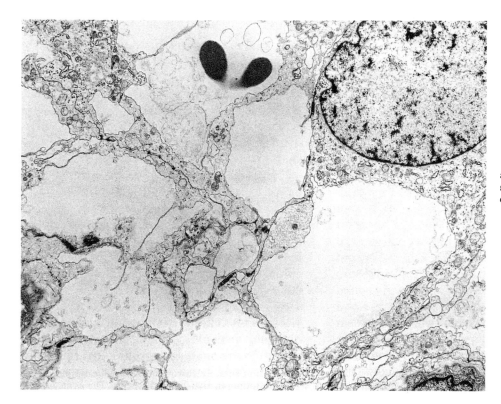

Figure 9-29
MICROCYSTIC
MENINGIOMA
Small circular spaces
are surrounded by desmo-
some-linked cytoplasmic
extensions.

Figure 9-30
SECRETORY
MENINGIOMA
The pseudopsam-
moma bodies are micro-
villous-lined spaces filled
with membranous de-
bris.

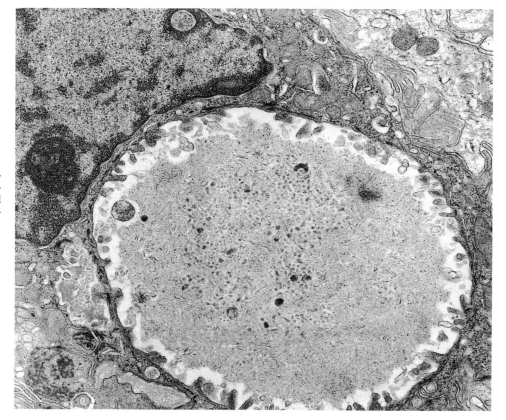

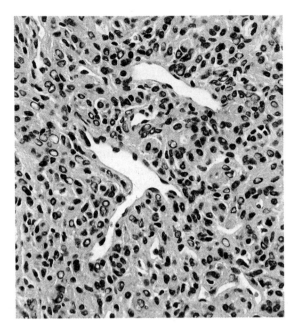

Figure 9-34
MENINGIOMA
In some cases, dense cellularity and staghorn vessels produce a histologic picture similar to that of hemangiopericytoma. Prominent intranuclear pseudoinclusions and tight whorls identify this lesion as a meningioma.

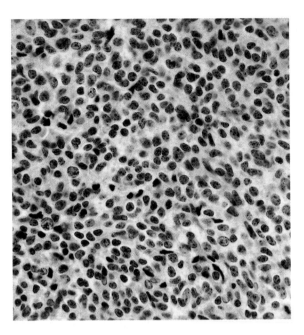

Figure 9-35
MENINGEAL NEOPLASM
Occasional meningeal neoplasms are densely cellular and lack the cytologic and architectural features of either meningioma or hemangiopericytoma. Such reticulin-poor tumors frequently behave in an aggressive fashion.

meningiomas. Some examples show focal artifactual papillae. We do not consider such tumors to be papillary meningiomas, nor do we regard them as a bridge linking hemangiopericytoma and meningioma.

Every attempt should be made to distinguish meningiomas from hemangiopericytomas since the latter are highly aggressive and prone to both frequent recurrences and late metastases. The distinction is aided by immunohistochemistry since hemangiopericytomas lack membranous staining for EMA. It is notable, however, that EMA positivity may be scant or absent in atypical cellular meningiomas that occasionally mimic hemangiopericytomas. Electron microscopy is helpful in this setting since hemangiopericytomas exhibit pericellular basal lamina-like material and lack both cellular interdigitation and desmosomal attachments.

Occasional cellular primary meningeal neoplasms lack specific architecture or cytologic features of either meningioma or hemangiopericytoma. These are usually locally aggressive and prone to recurrence (fig. 9-35). The classification of these lesions is problematic since they do not fit clearly into either the meningioma or hemangiopericytoma category.

As previously noted, the capillary hemangioblastoma can arise, albeit rarely, in the supratentorial space and resemble either microcystic meningioma or a more ordinary meningioma with a lobular pattern and cellular lipidization (see fig. 9-17). The similarity to microcystic meningioma results from a mutual content of vacuolated cells, conspicuous vascularity, and variable nuclear pleomorphism. In contrast to hemangioblastoma, most meningiomas lack high capillary density and exhibit a membraneous pattern of EMA staining. We find the application of the PAS stain for glycogen or fat stains on frozen sections to be of little or no diagnostic utility since meningiomas, hemangioblastomas, and metastatic renal cell carcinoma may all exhibit reactivity.

Though sometimes designated melanotic meningioma, nearly all extra-axial pigmented tumors represent proliferations of either Schwann cells or leptomeningeal melanocytes.

Meningiomas with prominent lymphoplasmacytic infiltrates need to be distinguished from a variety of inflammatory pseudotumors. Meningothelial cell–rich plaques of meningioangiomatosis can be misinterpreted as infiltrative meningioma (see Appendix A).

Treatment and Prognosis. Since most meningiomas lend themselves to gross total removal, surgery is the primary therapeutic modality. Resection is especially successful for lesions overlying the cerebral convexities and for those in the intraspinal compartment. Large tumors at the base of the skull, en plaque lesions, and meningiomas encompassing major vessels are obvious exceptions. Given the importance of location, it is difficult to make general statements about the recurrence rate of meningiomas. The oft-quoted figures for recurrences generally overestimate the incidence for lesions overlying the cerebral convexities and those within the spinal compartment, and underestimate the rate for skull base tumors or ones exhibiting diffuse or invasive growth.

Prognostication in specific cases is, therefore, imprecise and depends less upon histologic parameters than on factors such as tumor location, extent of resection, and radiographic as well as surgical findings (39,67). One study determined an overall recurrence rate of 19 percent during long follow-up for well-differentiated tumors that were felt to have been totally excised. Bone invasion and location upon the sphenoid ridge or within the olfactory groove were associated with a higher recurrence rate (39,42). In another study, histologic factors associated with a greater risk of recurrence included a sheet-like, rather than lobular, pattern of growth of tumor cells; nuclear pleomorphism; nucleolar prominence; mitoses; and single cell or focal necrosis (20). The point at which these features are sufficiently prominent to justify the designation "atypical meningioma" is not clear, and is discussed below. As was discussed briefly above, the chordoid papillary and clear cell variants may behave aggressively.

The assessment of the pathologist is necessarily limited, being based upon analysis of the brain-tumor interface, histologic and cytologic features, labeling indices, and perhaps ploidy determination. A greater propensity for recurrence has been noted in aneuploid tumors and in those with elevated labeling indices for dividing

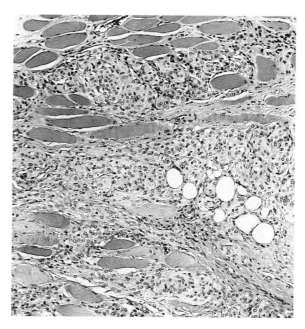

Figure 9-36
MENINGIOMA
Some meningiomas, even remarkably well-differentiated examples, are extensively invasive of bone and soft tissues.

or cycling cells (57). Invasion of the skull base and of course brain invasion are prognostically significant findings since they indicate a higher likelihood of recurrence (42). Death may result from mass effects, parenchymal destruction, or bacterial meningitis acquired through defects in the skull and dura.

Atypical and Malignant Meningiomas

The definition of malignancy in meningiomas is beset by frequent discordance between histologic and biologic features. For instance, whereas infiltration of bone and soft tissue is of little clinical importance in resectable lesions affecting the cranial vault (fig. 9-36), this same finding has a major, and unfavorable, effect upon the prognosis of tumors at the skull base. The significance of bone invasion thus varies with tumor geography. Although it is not necessarily predictive of recurrence, it is an ominous finding in certain locations. Alternatively, some meningiomas with histologic features of malignancy and obvious potential for aggressive behavior are sufficiently discrete to permit total resection. The definition of malignant meningioma, furthermore, includes

80. Russell DS, Rubinstein LS. Pathology of tumors of the nervous system. 5th ed. Baltimore: Williams & Wilkins, 1989.

81. Sackett JF, Stenwig JT, Songsirikul P. Meningeal and glial tumors in combination. Neuroradiology 1974; 7:153–60.

82. Saleh J, Silberstein HJ, Salner AL, Uphoff DF. Meningioma: the role of a foreign body and irradiation in tumor formation. Neurosurgery 1991;29:113–9.

83. Salibi SS, Nauta HJ, Brem H, Epstein JI, Cho KR. Lipomeningioma: report of three cases and review of the literature. Neurosurgery 1989;25:122–6.

84. Salvati M, Artico M, Lunardi P, Gagliardi FM. Intramedullary meningioma: case report and review of the literature. Surg Neurol 1992;37:42–5.

85. Scheithauer BW. Tumors of the meninges: proposed modifications of the World Health Organization classification. Acta Neuropathol (Berl) 1990;80:343–54.

86. Schnitt SJ, Vogel H. Meningiomas: diagnostic value of immunoperoxidase staining for epithelial membrane antigen. Am J Surg Pathol 1986;10:640–9.

87. Shiraishi K. Glycogen-rich meningioma. Case report and short review. Neurosurg Rev 1991;14:61–4.

88. Som PM, Sacher M, Strenger SW, Biller HF, Malis LI. "Benign" metastasizing meningiomas. AJNR Am J Neuroradiol 1987;8:127–30.

89. Theaker JM, Gatter KC, Esiri MM, Fleming KA. Epithelial membrane antigen and cytokeratin expression by meningiomas: an immunohistological study. J Clin Pathol 1986;39:435–9.

90. Tien RD, Yang PJ, Chu PK. "Dural tail sign": a specific MR sign for meningioma? J Comput Assist Tomog 1991;15:64–6.

91. Tsuboi K, Nose T, Maki Y. Meningioma of the fourth ventricle: a case report. Neurosurgery 1983;13:163–6.

92. Tsunoda S, Takeshima T, Sakaki T, et al. Secretory meningioma with elevated serum carcinoembryonic antigen level. Surg Neurol 1992;37:415–8.

93. Vagner-Capodano AM, Grisoli F, Gambarelli D, Sedan R, Pellet W, De Victor B. Correlation between cytogenetic and histopathological findings in 75 human meningiomas. Neurosurgery 1993;32:892–900.

94. Wilson AJ, Ratliff JL, Lagios MD, Aguilar MJ. Mediastinal meningioma. Am J Surg Pathol 1979;3:557–62.

95. Winek RR, Scheithauer BW, Wick MR. Meningioma, meningeal hemangiopericytoma (angioblastic meningioma), peripheral hemangiopericytoma, and acoustic schwannoma: a comparative immunohistochemical study. Am J Surg Pathol 1989;13:251–61.

96. Younis G, Sawaya R. Intracranial osteolytic malignant meningiomas appearing as extracranial soft-tissue masses. Neurosurgery 1992;30:932–5.

97. Zon LI, Johns WD, Stomper PC, et al. Breast carcinoma metastatic to a meningioma. Case report and review of the literature. Arch Intern Med 1989;149:959–62.

✧✧✧

10

TUMORS OF MESENCHYMAL TISSUE

VASCULAR TUMORS AND TUMOR-LIKE LESIONS

VASCULAR MALFORMATIONS

While it is impossible to assign all vascular malformations to precise categories, four divisions are generally recognized: arteriovenous malformation, cavernous angioma, venous malformation, and capillary telangiectasis (5,9,18).

Arteriovenous Malformation

Arteriovenous malformations (AVMs) are usually large, threatening, medusa-like lesions with a potential for imminent rupture (fig. 10-1). Occasional small, sometimes microscopic examples can cause a fatal hemorrhage. Most arise over the lateral hemispheric surfaces of the middle cerebral artery, although some lie deep within the brain where their effluent enlarges the deep venous or galenic system. In children, such arteriovenous shunting may produce enlargement of the great vein of Galen ("aneurysm" of the great vein of Galen) and cardiac decompensation. Multiple lesions are occasionally seen with hereditary hemorrhagic telangiectasia (Rendu-Osler-Weber disease) or Wyburn-Mason syndrome as is discussed in chapter 18.

AVMs are common in adults, producing seizures, focal neurologic deficits, progressive signs of increased intracranial pressure, or the sudden and catastrophic consequences of hemorrhage. One long-term follow-up study of unoperated cases suggested an annual rate of major hemorrhage of 4 percent (12).

Spinal arteriovenous lesions are subdivided into two types (17). The first is an intradural malformation which is morphologically identical to those of the brain. The second is a dural arteriovenous fistula in which the draining veins are distended to form ectatic, serpentine channels on the surface of the cord (fig. 10-2). Treatment is directed at obliterating the offending dural fistula rather than attacking the enlarged but otherwise innocent leptomeningeal veins (17). The back pressure from such lesions may

produce vascular enlargement and thickening of the intraparenchymal vessels as well. Resultant gliosis and parenchymal destruction may be responsible for some cases of the Foix-Alajoúanine syndrome (2,22a). Dura-based fistulae may also occur intracranially.

Microscopically, AVMs are composed of vessels that vary greatly in caliber and construction (fig. 10-3). Those at the core of the lesion are often more irregular in size and cross-sectional configuration and less sclerotic than those of the cavernous angioma. Muscularization is variable, ranging from the delicate laminae of myocytes in large veins to prominent, often irregular layers in abnormal arteries. Varying thickness of the medial coat, seen on trichrome or pentachrome stains as well as in immunostains for actin (8), is a particular characteristic. Also distinctive are large "cushions" of smooth muscle which project into the lumina of abnormal vessels.

Although the most central portion of an AVM may exclude preexisting brain parenchyma, the feeding and draining vascular channels are separated by parenchyma over most of the cross-sectional area of the malformation. The parenchyma may or may not be affected by gliosis or ferrugination. The prominence of oligodendroglia noted in some cases is due either to collapse of the white matter from myelin loss or to malformative-appearing nodules of white matter trapped within the lesion (6).

In an effort to reduce their vascularity and to facilitate surgical resection, arteriovenous malformations may be embolized preoperatively. As a result, synthetic material may be seen within the lumina where it elicits a foreign body response, the extent of which depends upon the nature of the substance and the postembolization interval (4,23).

Assisted by angiographic and intraoperative data, the diagnosis of a vascular malformation is usually obvious in histologic sections. Nonetheless, the normal vessels of the subarachnoid space may be artifactually so compacted by the biopsy procedure as to resemble a malformation (fig. 10-4). The problem is resolved by attention

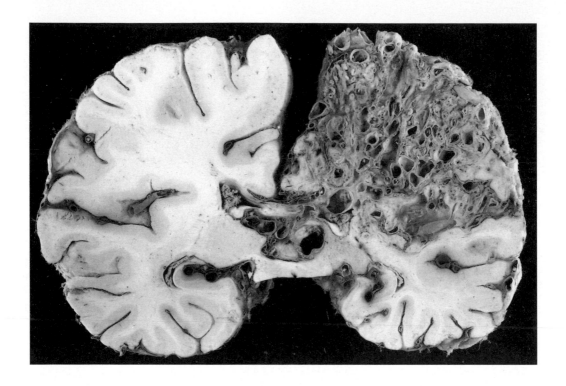

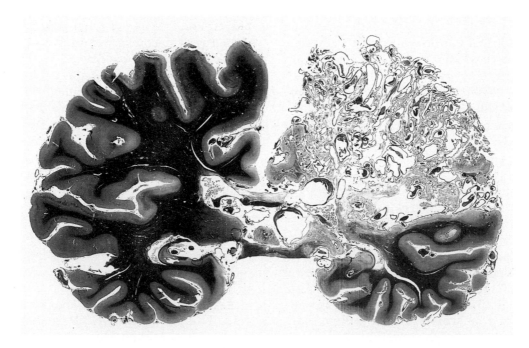

Figure 10-1

ARTERIOVENOUS MALFORMATION

As seen both grossly (top) and in a whole mount histologic section (bottom), this large arteriovenous malformation occupies much of the parietal lobe. There is little mass effect from this large lesion which has gradually replaced the regional brain.

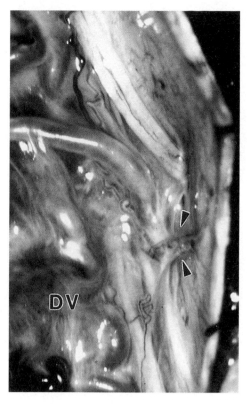

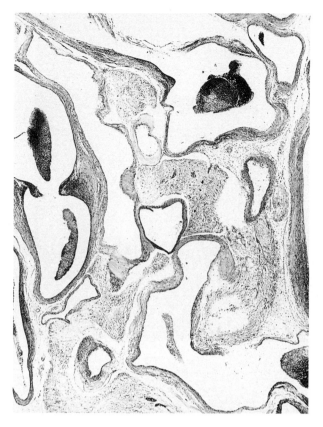

Figure 10-2
ARTERIOVENOUS MALFORMATION
The arteriovenous shunt in some spinal arteriovenous malformations lies within the dura (arrows). In this case, the bulk of the intradural lesion is formed of draining veins (DV). (Courtesy of Dr. Allan H. Friedman, Durham, NC.)

Figure 10-3
ARTERIOVENOUS MALFORMATION
The arteriovenous malformation consists of a jumble of abnormal vessels with varying degrees of muscularization. Small luminal protrusions or cushions are typical. In contrast to the cavernous angioma in figure 10-7, there is considerable parenchyma between the abnormal vessels.

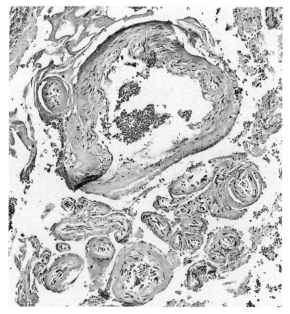

Figure 10-4
COMPRESSED NORMAL LEPTOMENINGEAL VESSELS
SIMULATING ARTERIOVENOUS MALFORMATION
Normal leptomeningeal vessels may be artifactually compressed in such a way as to resemble a vascular malformation.

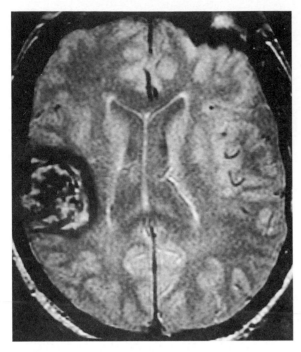

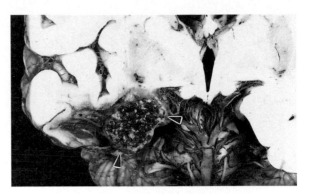

Figure 10-6
CAVERNOUS ANGIOMA
Some cavernous angiomas (arrows) arise in the lepto-meninges.

Figure 10-5
CAVERNOUS ANGIOMA
As seen in a proton density MRI, a central mass of vascular profiles surrounded by a dark rim of hemosiderin stained brain is characteristic of a cavernous angioma. (Courtesy of Dr. Linda Gray, Durham, NC.)

to the morphology of the component vessels since, in contrast to those of AVM, compressed subarachnoid vessels are individually normal. In general, AVM and cavernous angioma are easily differentiated. Although the noncommittal diagnosis of vascular malformation is appropriate in cases in which the histology is indeterminate, the presence of arterial shunting on angiography is strong clinical evidence for an AVM. Surgeons rightfully object to the diagnosis of cavernous angioma in the face of such shunting since cavernous angiomas are, as a rule, angiographically occult (21).

Cavernous Angioma

The archetypic cavernous angioma or *cavernoma* is a compact spherical mass that is more likely to present with seizures than with focal neurologic symptoms or signs of increased intracranial pressure (19,20). Hemorrhages are common but are usually small and unaccompanied by devastating mass effects or intraventricular rupture, both common features of AVMs.

The majority of cavernous angiomas affect the cerebrum, but the brain stem, cerebellum, spinal cord, and even the leptomeninges may be involved (13,19,20). Multiple lesions are frequent. Some cases are familial and, in the United States, an increased incidence has been noted among Mexican-Americans (14), but this may be an artifact of the population under study. A number of cavernous angiomas are incidental postmortem findings.

By computerized tomography (CT) the lesions are often calcified and exert little or no mass effect. In magnetic resonance images (MRIs) the compact mass, in which vascular profiles are resolved in some cases, is surrounded by a dark area of decreased signal intensity on T2-weighted images (fig. 10-5) (21). This combination of vascular profiles and a dark perilesional corona of iron-rich parenchyma is almost diagnostic of cavernous angioma. Due to extensive thrombosis, vascular thickening, and paucity of feeding vessels, the lesions are not angiographically evident, in contrast to AVMs (21), although an associated large vein similar to a venous angioma is occasionally observed. Calcification is common (see Appendix E).

The macroscopic appearance of cavernous angiomas mirrors the radiographic findings. The lesions are discrete and compact knots of vascular profiles. Most angiomas are less than several centimeters in diameter (fig. 10-6). Subacute hemorrhage, apparent as clotted blood, is frequently noted. Evidence of remote hemorrhage

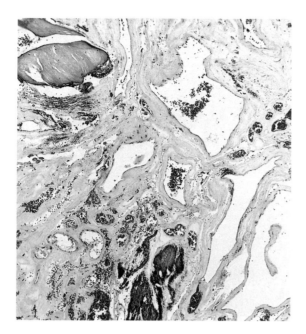

Figure 10-7
CAVERNOUS ANGIOMA
A compact mass of sclerotic, variably calcified, vessels characterizes the cavernous angioma. Little parenchyma is evident between the vessels. Hemosiderin is frequently deposited in surrounding tissue.

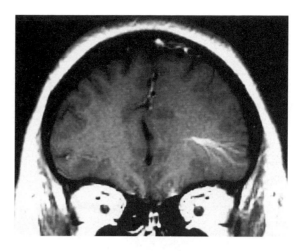

Figure 10-8
VENOUS MALFORMATION
As seen on the right in a gadolinium-enhanced scan, venous malformations are common incidental neuroradiologic findings. Here, the feeding vessels pass from right to left of the illustration, where they enter a draining vein. (Courtesy of Dr. Linda Gray, Durham, NC.)

is seen in virtually all lesions as evidenced by a rusty rim of gliotic hemosiderin stained brain.

Microscopically, cavernous angiomas consist of a honeycomb of compact vessels which vary considerably in caliber and degree of collagenization (fig. 10-7). The vessels are free of muscle and elastic lamellae (19,20). In contrast to those of telangiectasis and AVM, the vessels of a cavernous angioma are closely opposed, leaving little, if any, interstitial parenchyma. Hemosiderin discolors the surrounding parenchyma and burdens the cytoplasm of both macrophages and astrocytes. Even granulation tissue may be noted.

Although the distinction between cavernous angioma and capillary telangiectasis is not of immediate practical relevance to the surgical pathologist, there has been considerable debate concerning the relationship between these two lesions (15,18). Some suggest that cavernous angiomas evolve from telangiectases. Only a few lesions exhibit the characteristics of both (21). Thus, the evidence is not compelling that these two lesions represent the same entity, differing only in chronicity.

Vasculature identical to that of cavernous angioma need not form a compact mass. Indeed, racemose or compact and racemose malformations composed of these hyaline vessels are common among angiographically occult vascular malformations. Their clinical and neuroimaging characteristics are identical to those of typical cavernous angiomas (21).

Venous Malformation

Consisting solely of venous channels without the small but irregularly ectatic capillaries of telangiectasis, venous angiomas occur both in the brain and spinal cord. They are common incidental radiographic findings; only a rare example is symptomatic (5a,7). Angiographically, the lesions appear as veins with a "caput medusae" profile (figs. 10-7, 10-8) (16,22). In the spinal cord, serpentine enlargement of the constituent veins must be distinguished from the normally prominent venous channels occurring on the dorsal surface in the lumbar region, and the secondarily enlarged draining veins that accompany AVMs and dural arteriovenous fistulae.

On cross section the lesion is formed of ectatic channels without associated parenchymal degeneration (fig. 10-10). Histologically, the thin-walled channels lie within brain parenchyma unaffected by gliosis or hemosiderosis.

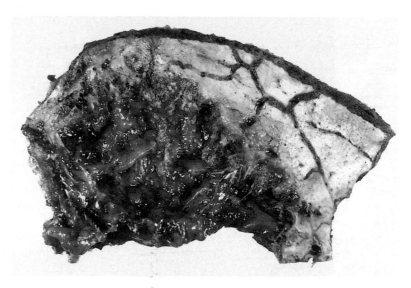

Figure 10-13
HEMANGIOPERICYTOMA
The aggressive behavior of the hemangiopericytoma is apparent in this destructive recurrent lesion.

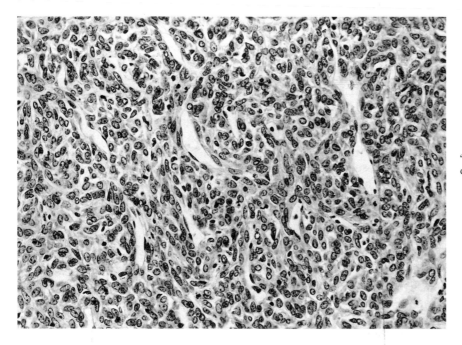

Figure 10-14
HEMANGIOPERICYTOMA
High cellularity and slit-like, "staghorn" vascular channels are common features.

highly destructive without the hyperostosis seen with meningiomas (fig. 10-13).

Microscopic Findings. Even a cursory macroscopic examination of the stained slides, with their intense and uniform blueness, often suggests the diagnosis. At low magnification, slit-like vascular spaces are apparent which, when large and branched, assume the classic "staghorn" pattern (fig. 10-14) (36). At higher magnification, the highly cellular lesions usually have a distinctive turbulent pattern, the cells appearing to writhe in a reticulin-rich stroma. Patches of hypocellularity frequently punctuate the tumor (fig. 10-15). Foci of necrosis are uncommon but may be seen in high-grade or anaplastic hemangiopericytomas of the type discussed under Treatment and Prognosis. Small whorl-like lobules are not uncommon (fig. 10-16), but the tight concentric whorls, psammoma bodies, and sclerotic vessels so common in meningiomas are lacking.

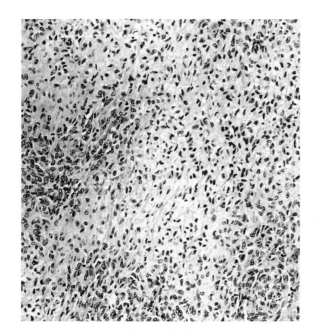

Figure 10-15
HEMANGIOPERICYTOMA
Pale zones of hypocellularity are frequent.

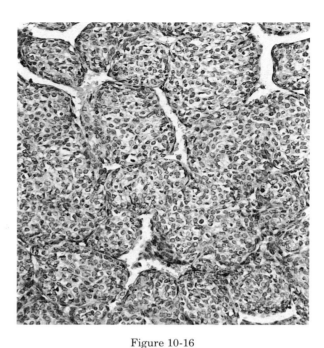

Figure 10-16
HEMANGIOPERICYTOMA
Lobules may resemble those of meningioma, although tight whorls, psammoma bodies, and immunoreactivity for epithelial membrane antigen are not observed.

Considerable morphologic variation exists in the degree of nuclear atypia and cellularity exhibited by hemangiopericytomas. Most often, the nuclei are oval, plump, and exhibit moderate chromatin density, although in some instances they are elongated or even uniformly spherical. Nucleoli are inconspicuous. Mitotic activity, although highly variable, is readily found in most examples. The characteristic intranuclear pseudoinclusions of meningiomas are absent, although freezing may induce a superficially similar nuclear clearing. Tumors with spindle cell components rich in collagen can be mistaken for meningioma (fig. 10-17).

Classically, reticulin is abundant and invests individual cells (fig. 10-18), but may be sparse in nodular (fig. 10-16) or fibrous lesions (fig. 10-17).

Electron Microscopic Findings. The neoplastic cells vary in differentiation from pericytic to myogenic and fibroblastic. In many cases they are surrounded by amorphous material somewhat resembling basal lamina (25,32). Rudimentary intercellular junctions may be seen, but neither well-formed desmosomes nor complex interdigitations of cell membranes are observed (fig. 10-19). Spherical whorled masses of intermediate filaments (vimentin) may be present.

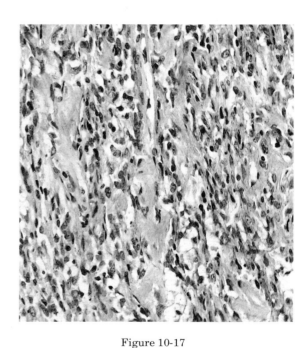

Figure 10-17
HEMANGIOPERICYTOMA
Cellular elongation and collagen production result in a "fibrous" pattern readily confused with fibrous meningioma.

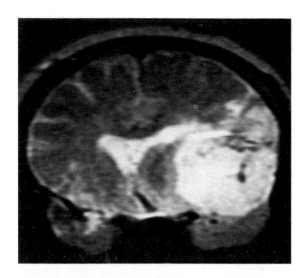

Figure 10-30
CHONDROMA
Intracranial chondromas usually arise from the dura.

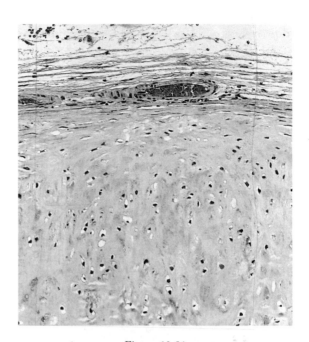

Figure 10-31
CHONDROMA
Chondromas are globular masses of cytologically benign hyaline cartilage.

normal tissue without aggressive infiltration of indigenous elements. Although lipomas of the internal auditory canal enlarge and resection has been suggested, they are more hamartomatous than neoplastic in nature.

Chondroma and Osteochondroma

Chondromas are benign, slow-growing tumors which generally arise from the skull base (59) or dura (fig. 10-30) (61–63,64a,65,67). In some cases, the tumors are a consequence of the systemic predisposition inherent in Ollier disease (66) or Mafucci syndrome (58). At any site, chondromas are circumscribed exophytic masses and are composed of well-differentiated, cytologically benign hyaline cartilage (fig. 10-31). Rare lesions containing both cartilage and bone are designated osteochondroma (57,60,64). Total excision may not be possible for lesions at the skull base and, although they are slow growing, delayed clinical recurrence has been described. Cure is possible for dura-based tumors.

Fibroma and Fibromatosis

Fibromas are rare, often bulky, discrete masses arising either from the meninges (73,75) or within the parenchyma of the brain (70,71). Paucicellular, they are composed of widely separated elongated

cells and an eosinophilic collagen-rich matrix. The observation of marked immunoreactivity for S-100 protein in one case (75) and the ultrastructural finding of desmosome-like junctions in another (69), leave the issue of histogenesis unresolved and permit some heterogeneity of the lesions grouped under the designation fibroma. Tumors that combine collagen and glia (gliofibroma) are discussed in chapter 3.

Fibromas must be distinguished from fibromatoses, which are reactive but infiltrative and potentially aggressive lesions. The latter may arise from the dura, either within the craniospinal space or may be epidural. Both spontaneous (68) and postoperative (72,74) examples have been reported. Although fibromatosis is less cellular and more collagenous, it is not always possible to make a sharp distinction between it and low-grade fibrosarcoma.

Other Benign Mesenchymal Lesions

Other uncommon benign mesenchymal lesions include *fibrous xanthoma* (76), *leiomyoma* (77), and *rhabdomyoma* (78).

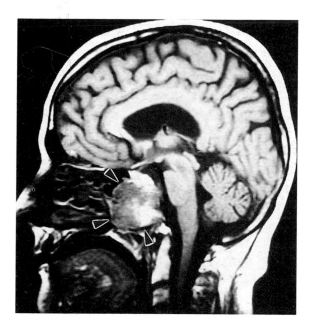

Figure 10-32
CHORDOMA
Cranial chordomas (arrows) typically arise from the clivus as bulky lesions which destroy bone, entrap cranial nerves, and compress the base of the brain.

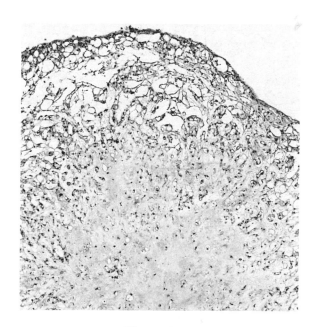

Figure 10-33
ECCORDOSIS PHYSALIPHORA
Small, incidental, chordoma-like masses are occasionally encountered projecting from the clivus or attached to the basilar artery. This example combines the cord and ribbon-like arrangement of epithelial cells, so common to chordomas, with chondroid differentiation, another feature frequently encountered in this neoplasm.

MALIGNANT NONVASCULAR TUMORS

Chordoma

Definition. A notochord-derived tumor of the skull and spine.

Clinical and Radiographic Features. Chordomas arise along an archipelago of notochordal remnants extending from their rostral reaches in the region of the sella turcica to their caudal extreme in the sacrum. The tumors are unevenly distributed along the craniospinal axis; approximately half arise in the sacrum, one third in the spheno-occipital region or clivus, and the remainder in the articulating vertebrae (fig. 10-32) (96). A notochordal origin seems inescapable in light of histologic, immunohistochemical, ultrastructural, and in vitro features common to both chordomas and notochordal remnants. Larger remnants, referred to as *ecchordosis physaliphora*, are sometimes seen at autopsy as small translucent nodules projecting from the clivus or delicately attached to the basilar artery (fig. 10-33). Sizable, occasionally symptomatic lesions unattached to bone have been likened to giant ecchordoses (106). Rare intracranial (104) or intraspinal (101) chordomas are also extraosseous. Their distinction from large symptomatic ecchordoses may be semantic.

Sacral chordomas are destructive intrasacral tumors which produce pain, sphincter disturbances, and neurologic symptoms from pressure upon regional nerve roots (85,96,101). Intracranial lesions, midline and often destructive of the clivus, generally produce headache and cranial nerve palsies, particularly diplopia (82,83,96, 97,105). Cranial nerve signs are often unilateral. Chordomas usually occur in adults, but pediatric cases have been reported (81a,99,105).

Macroscopic Findings. Chordomas are infiltrative, osseodestructive, often lobulated lesions that may be sufficiently rich in stromal mucopolysaccharide to be grossly mucoid. Intratumoral hemorrhage is rarely seen.

Microscopic Findings. The macroscopic lobularity is reflected at the microscopic level as round or oval lobules delineated by septate mesenchymal stroma. At higher magnification, great histologic variability can be expected. Commonly, the neoplastic cells are phenotypically

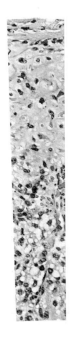

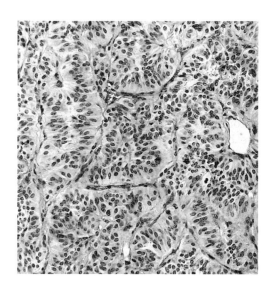
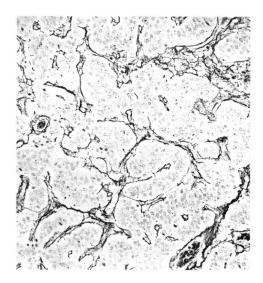

Figure 11-2
PARAGANGLIOMA

A nested "zellballen" pattern typical of paraganglioma is apparent in sections stained by the H&E method (left) and those prepared for reticulin (right).

In cont
chondroma
cellular an

Progn
· patient a
presence

Intra
ther the
large ba
termine
110–113
(109). I
guishe
chordor
hypocel
may be
ated ch
sarcom
sarcom

Give
ally, it
of pati
drosar
ularly
tially e

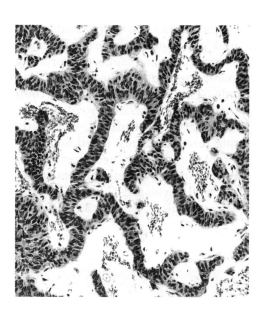

Figure 11-3
PARAGANGLIOMA

Ribbons of cells, found in many carcinoid tumors, are evident in some lesions.

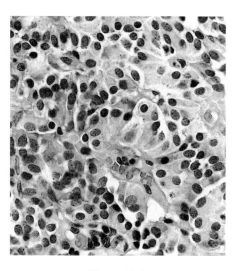

Figure 11-4
PARAGANGLIOMA

Discrete cell borders and an orderly relationship to blood vessels give cells of paragangliomas a distinctly epithelial appearance. The delicate nuclei with "salt and pepper" chromatin are typical of neuroendocrine neoplasms.

intermediate filament whorls may also be present, as are intercellular junctions and basal lamina in areas where cells abut stroma. The elongated processes of agranular, electron-dense sustentacular cells surround zellballen and occasionally embrace small groups of chief cells.

Histochemical and Immunohistochemical Findings. Paragangliomas typically exhibit argyrophilia on Grimelius stain (fig. 11-6). In contrast, argentaffin-reactive cells are few. Immunoreactivity for neuron-specific enolase (NSE) is the rule, as is staining for chromogranin (fig. 11-7). Neurofilament stains often show

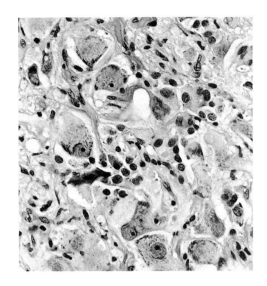

Figure 11-5
GANGLIOCYTIC PARAGANGLIOMA
Ganglion cells here commingle singly with chief cells but may also aggregate in a fibrillar, Schwann cell–containing matrix.

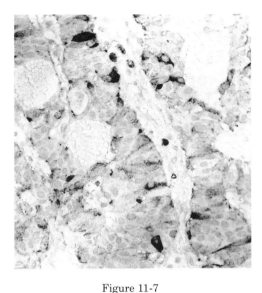

Figure 11-7
PARAGANGLIOMA
Immunostains for chromogranin decorate the granule-containing chief cells.

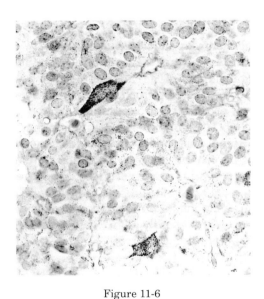

Figure 11-6
PARAGANGLIOMA
Scattered argyrophilic (Grimelius-positive) cells are regularly encountered. Argentaffin reaction is usually scant.

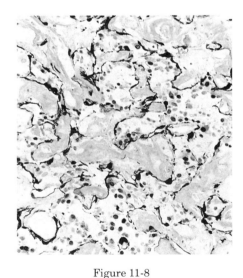

Figure 11-8
PARAGANGLIOMA
The sustentacular cells surrounding lobules of chief cells are immunoreactive for S-100 protein.

paranuclear globular reactivity corresponding in distribution to the above noted intermediate filament whorls. Sustentacular cells are uniformly reactive for S-100 protein (fig. 11-8) and often show glial fibrillary acidic protein (GFAP) positivity as well. In tumors occurring within the filum terminale, trapped astrocytes, usually perivascular or subcapsular in location, may be seen. The latter are positive for GFAP.

Although primary spinal paragangliomas are unassociated with endocrine symptoms, a variety of hormones and neurotransmitter substances including somatostatin, serotonin, and metenkephalin may be demonstrated immunohistochemically (3,6).

319

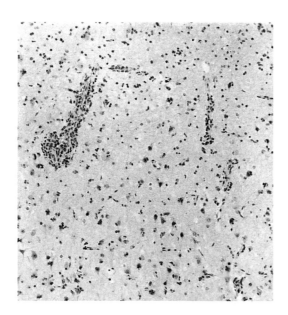
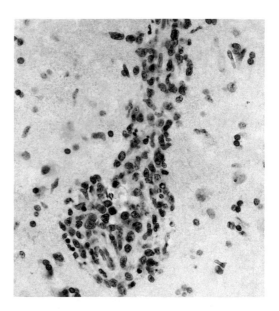

Figure 12-9
PRIMARY CENTRAL NERVOUS SYSTEM LYMPHOMA
Left: Some surgical specimens with only slight perivascular involvement may at first glance mimic an inflammatory process.
Right: Confusion is often furthered by scattered microglia among tumor cells and in the surrounding parenchyma. The diagnosis of lymphoma is usually apparent at higher magnification given the cytologic atypia of perivascular cells.

be used to determine the T- versus B-cell nature of lymphomas. As indicated above, most are B-cell lesions. The uncommon Ki-1 lymphoma may be LCA negative and is often epithelial membrane antigen (EMA)-positive; overinterpretation may therefore result in an erroneous diagnosis of carcinoma.

Ultrastructural Findings. Lymphomas are noted for their lack of specific ultrastructural features: the absence of intermediate filaments, specific organelles, and intercellular junctions (10). Nonetheless, "nuclear pockets" are a common feature of large cell lymphomas. In addition, plasmacytoid differentiation is accompanied by a characteristic pattern of chromatin aggregation and by prominence of the paranuclear Golgi apparatus and rough endoplasmic reticulum.

Differential Diagnosis. The differential diagnosis of PCNSL revolves around two issues. If a lesion is recognized as unequivocally neoplastic, other tumors need to be excluded. If the hematopoietic nature of the lesion is apparent, the distinction between an inflammatory and neoplastic process must be resolved.

In most cases, the distinction between the lymphoma and other neoplasms is achieved at the time of frozen section. If not, routine perma-

nent sections generally suffice, often without the need for immunohistochemistry. With hematoxylin and eosin (H&E) staining alone, the distinctive cytologic features of lymphoma, coupled with its angiocentricity, usually brings the diagnosis to mind. Unlike metastatic carcinoma, primary cerebral lymphoma behaves like gliomas, diffusely invading and incorporating rather than displacing host tissue. Trapped neurons and reactive astrocytes may, therefore, be encountered. In contrast to glioblastoma, palisading around necrosis and vascular proliferation are lacking in lymphoma.

Although the diagnosis of lymphoma may be made on frozen section coupled with smear preparations, prudence suggests that fresh and frozen tissue be reserved for cytogenetic/molecular and marker studies, respectively.

In light of the marked cytologic atypia of most lymphomas, their distinction from chronic inflammatory lesions is usually not difficult. Exceptions include uncommon cases of well-differentiated lymphoma and situations in which the neoplastic cells of a higher-grade lesion are obscured by an inflammatory, often T-cell, infiltrate (fig. 12-9). Idiopathic inflammatory lesions composed of dense lymphoplasmacytic infiltrates exhibit

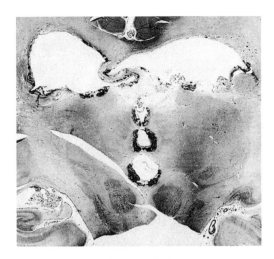

Figure 12-10
PRIMARY CENTRAL NERVOUS
SYSTEM LYMPHOMA
Lymphomas, especially in recurrent or terminal phases,
often disseminate to the periventricular regions.

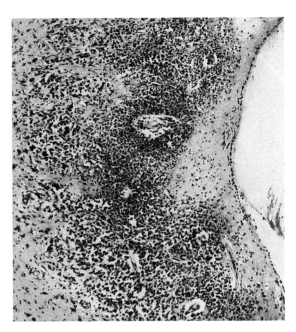

Figure 12-11
PRIMARY CENTRAL NERVOUS
SYSTEM LYMPHOMA
A section from the lesion illustrated in figure 12-10 shows
subependymal involvement as well as angiocentricity.

minor, but definite, atypia. These may be difficult to distinguish from lymphoma in H&E stained sections, but are often polyclonal and usually contain mature plasma cells. More problematic are polyclonal inflammatory infiltrates occurring in normal and immunocompromised patients, lesions that exhibit many atypical nuclei. These often contain a prominent component of mature plasma cells, an element contrasting with the less well-differentiated plasmacytoid lymphocytes seen in many lymphomas.

Immunohistochemically, most inflammatory CNS lesions contain both B and T cells, T cells being predominant. Most lymphomas also contain a number of reactive T cells. They are generally overshadowed by obviously neoplastic B cells.

Stereotactic needle biopsy is commonly employed in the diagnosis of cerebral lymphomas. The small specimens obtained may not be representative and may include only a mixed, reactive-appearing infiltrate rather than the dense perivascular populations composed primarily of lymphoma cells. Assessment of such small biopsies is difficult since immunotyping reveals a polyclonal cell population, one in which neoplastic cells are absent or present in such small numbers as to make the identification of a neoplasm difficult or impossible. This difficulty can be usually avoided by frozen section examination to insure that overtly neoplastic tissue is obtained.

Treatment and Prognosis. Although lymphomas are often exquisitely sensitive to corticosteroids, and may vanish from radiologic images for weeks, months, or even years following treatment, this dramatic effect is temporary. Treatment by radiotherapy or chemotherapy has a similar lytic effect (5,8,11,15,18). The majority of patients with PCNSL die within 2 years (8,11). A longer course from presentation to death has been noted for patients with better differentiated tumors (11). As a consequence of the diffuse nature of the disease, failure is often multicentric in meninges and parenchyma (17). A diffuse subependymal pattern is often seen (figs. 12-10, 12-11). Occasional patients are long-term survivors, but cures are rare.

Plasmacytoma

Intracranial involvement by solitary plasmacytoma is rare but well documented (25,27,29). Most are attached to the dura and radiographically and macroscopically resemble meningioma (figs. 12-12, 12-13). A few have been intrasellar and have mimicked pituitary adenoma, both grossly and microscopically (28). Rare examples arise within the substance of the brain (31).

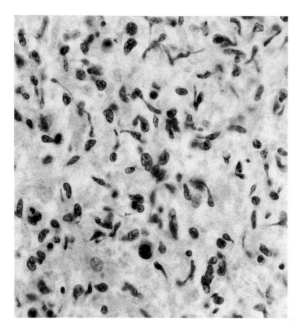

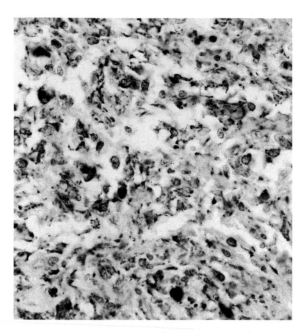

Figure 12-15
MICROGLIOMATOSIS
Both plump and markedly elongated nuclei are seen, an appearance easily confused with diffuse glioma or reactive microglial proliferation.

Figure 12-16
MICROGLIOMATOSIS
Immunoreactivity for macrophage markers, such as HAM-56, is the basis for the identification of this lesion.

cortex, exhibit neuronal satellitosis to create a form of microglial nodule. Distinguishing between these processes may be difficult in very small specimens, but should be possible on the basis of cell density, pattern of infiltration, disposition of cells, nuclear characteristics, and the presence or absence of reactive lymphocytes and astrocytes.

Subpial aggregation is typical of infiltrative neoplasia but not of inflammatory states.

Cases of microgliomatosis are too few to permit conclusions regarding biologic behavior. The intrinsic highly infiltrative nature of the lesion and its seemingly well-differentiated state make it unlikely that either surgery or conventional therapies will be effective.

REFERENCES

Primary Central Nervous System Lymphoma

1. Ashby MA, Barber PC, Holmes AE, Freer CE, Collins RD. Primary intracranial Hodgkin's disease. A case report and discussion. Am J Surg Pathol 1988;12:294–9.
2. Baumgartner JE, Rachlin JR, Beckstead JH, et al. Primary central nervous system lymphomas: natural history and response to radiation therapy in 55 patients with acquired immunodeficiency syndrome. J Neurosurg 1990;73:206–11.
3. Bednar MM, Salerni A, Flanagan ME, Pendlebury WW. Primary central nervous system T-cell lymphoma. Case report. J Neurosurg 1991;74:668–72.
4. Clark WC, Callihan T, Schwartzberg L, Fontanesi J. Primary intracranial Hodgkin's lymphoma without dural attachment. Case report. J Neurosurg 1992;76:692–5.
5. DeAngelis LM, Yahalom J, Heinemann MH, Cirrincione C, Thaler HT, Krol G. Primary CNS lymphoma: combined treatment with chemotherapy and radiotherapy. Neurology 1990;40:80–6.
6. Eby NL, Grufferman S, Flannelly CM, Schold SC Jr, Vogel FS, Burger PC. Increasing incidence of primary brain lymphoma in the US. Cancer 1988;62:2461–5.

7. Geppert M, Ostertag CB, Seitz G, Kiessling M. Glucocorticoid therapy obscures the diagnosis of cerebral lymphoma. Acta Neuropathol (Berl) 1990;80:629–34.

8. Grant JW, Isaacson PG. Primary central nervous system lymphoma. Brain Pathol 1992;2:97–109.

9. Gray RS, Abrahams JJ, Hufnagel TJ, Kim JH, Lesser RL, Spencer DD. Ghost-cell tumor of the optic chiasm. Primary CNS lymphoma. J Clin Neuro Ophthalmol 1989;9:98–104.

10. Hirano A. A comparison of the fine structure of malignant lymphoma and other neoplasms in the brain. Acta Neuropathol (Berl) 1975;6(Suppl):141–5.

11. Hochberg FH, Miller DC. Primary central nervous system lymphoma. J Neurosurg 1988;68:835–53.

12. Jellinger K, Radaskiewicz TH, Slowik F. Primary malignant lymphomas of the central nervous system in man. Acta Neuropathol (Berl) 1975;6(Suppl):95–102.

13. Kobayashi H, Sano T, Ii K, Hizawa K. Primary Burkitt-type lymphoma of the central nervous system. Acta Neuropathol (Berl) 1984;64:12–4.

14. Mauney M, Sciotto CG. Primary malignant lymphoma of the cauda equina. Am J Surg Pathol 1983;7:185–90.

15. O'Neill BP, Illig JJ. Primary central nervous system lymphoma. Mayo Clin Proc 1989;64:1005–20.

16. _____, Kelly PJ, Earle JD, Scheithauer BW, Banks PM. Computer-assisted stereotaxic biopsy for the diagnosis of primary central nervous system lymphoma. Neurology 1987;37:1160–4.

17. _____, O'Fallon J, Jack C, Banks P, Colgan J, Earle J. Patterns of failure in primary central nervous system non-Hodgkin's lymphoma (PCNSL) [Abstract]. Proc Am Soc Clin Oncol 1989;8:87.

18. Pollack IF, Lunsford LD, Flickinger JC, Dameshek HL. Prognostic factors in the diagnosis and treatment of primary central nervous system lymphoma. Cancer 1989;63:939–47.

19. Roman-Goldstein SM, Goldman DL, Howieson J, Belkin R, Neuwelt EA. MR of primary CNS lymphoma in immunologically normal patients. AJNR Am J Neuroradiol 1992;13:1207–13.

20. Sherman ME, Erozan YS, Mann RB, et al. Stereotactic brain biopsy in the diagnosis of malignant lymphoma. Am J Clin Pathol 1991;95:878–83.

21. Slager UT, Kaufman RL, Cohen KL, Tuddenham WJ. Primary lymphoma of the spinal cord. J Neuropathol Exp Neurol 1982;41:437–45.

22. Slowik F, Mayer Á, Áfra D, Deák G, Hável J. Primary spinal intramedullary malignant lymphoma. A case report. Surg Neurol 1990;33:132–8.

23. Vaquero J, Martinez R, Rossi E, Lopez R. Primary cerebral lymphoma: the "ghost" tumor. Case report. J Neurosurg 1984;60:174–6.

Plasmacytoma

24. Du Preez JH, Branca EP. Plasmacytoma of the skull: case reports. Neurosurgery 1991;29:902–6.

25. Kohli CM, Kawazu T. Solitary intracranial plasmacytoma. Surg Neurol 1982;17:307–12.

26. Krivoy S, González JE, Céspedes G, Walzer I. Solitary cerebral falx plasmacytoma. Surg Neurol 1977;8:222–4.

27. Krumholz A, Weiss HD, Jiji VH, Bakal D, Kirsh MB. Solitary intracranial plasmacytoma: two patients with extended follow-up. Ann Neurol 1982;11:529–32.

28. Losa M, Terreni MR, Tresoldi M, et al. Solitary plasmacytoma of the sphenoid sinus involving the pituitary fossa: a case report and review of the literature. Surg Neurol 1992;37:388–93.

29. Mancardi GL, Mandybur TI. Solitary intracranial plasmacytoma. Cancer 1983;51:2226–33.

30. Scully RE. Case records of the Massachusetts General Hospital. Case 21–1992. N Engl J Med 1992;326:1417–24.

31. Wisniewski T, Sisti M, Inhirami G, Knowles DM, Powers JM. Intracerebral solitary plasmacytoma. Neurosurgery 1990;27:826–9.

Microgliomatosis

32. Hulette CM, Downey BT, Burger PC. Macrophage markers in diagnostic neuropathology. Am J Surg Pathol 1992;16:493–9.

33. Russell DS, Rubinstein LJ. Pathology of tumours of the nervous system. 5th ed. Baltimore: Williams & Wilkins, 1989:592–3.

❖❖❖

13
TUMORS OF THE PERIPHERAL NERVE SHEATH

Schwannoma

Definition. A benign tumor composed entirely of Schwann cells.

General Comments. Schwannomas, also termed *neurilemmomas*, are common, and are important lesions in the differential diagnoses of para-axial masses. Most arise from cranial or spinal nerve roots; only rarely do they occur within the substance of the brain or spinal cord.

Clinical and Radiographic Features. Intracranial schwannomas, at one time referred to as neurinomas or neuromas, most often involve the eighth cranial nerve, but occasionally arise from others, especially the fifth. In their classic location on the eighth nerve, schwannomas arise from the vestibular division, lying near or within the vestibular ganglion. They are, therefore, not technically acoustic lesions, although hearing loss is the common initial symptom. The reason for this preference for the vestibular division is not clear since the density of Schwann cells is no greater than in the acoustic division (52). Finding little resistance to enlargement along the course of the nerve, the tumors mushroom into the intracranial compartment to occupy the cerebellopontine angle. At this point, they may be large enough to produce cerebellar dysfunction as well as cranial nerve deficits, particularly of the fifth and seventh nerves (53). Bilaterality is a feature of the central or type 2 variant of neurofibromatosis. Schwannomas are rare in children (2).

Radiographically, acoustic schwannomas appear as discrete contrast-enhancing masses; larger examples are associated with enlargement or flaring of the entry of the internal auditory canal (fig. 13-1). Such meatal expansion is rare in other extra-axial tumors, such as meningioma, and provides strong presumptive evidence of the diagnosis. Smaller intracanalicular lesions are now being detected by magnetic resonance imaging. Intratumoral or extratumoral cysts are found in a minority of lesions (51a). Calcification is rare.

Intraspinal schwannomas, like their cranial counterparts, tend to involve sensory nerves to produce intradural extramedullary masses (see

Appendix G). As a result, dorsal roots are primarily affected (fig. 13-2). Most tumors occur as solitary sporadic lesions, but multiplicity may be seen in neurofibromatosis 2 (see fig. 18-4). In that setting, symptomatic masses are often accompanied by small subclinical intraneural Schwann cell proliferations collectively termed *schwannosis*. Intraspinal schwannomas may occur at any level but most affect the lumbosacral and cauda equina regions. Expanding freely in the intraspinal and extraspinal compartments, but not within the confines of the dural root sleeve or nerve foramen, many lesions take on the classic "dumbbell" configuration (37). Lesions arising from lumbosacral nerve roots can become extremely large (giant sacral schwannomas), erode bone, and displace the rectum (1).

Uncommonly, schwannomas occur within the parenchyma of the spinal cord (30,41,50) or brain (4,12,21,25,49,54). These presumably arise either from small myelinated peripheral nerve fibers that accompany blood vessels into the parenchyma or from Schwann cells near the dorsal

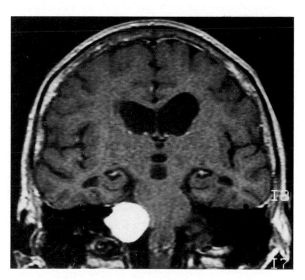

Figure 13-1
ACOUSTIC SCHWANNOMA
The nipple-like projection of the contrast-enhancing mass at the left represents the original intracanalicular portion of this tumor, which is now largely intracranial and compressive of the pons.

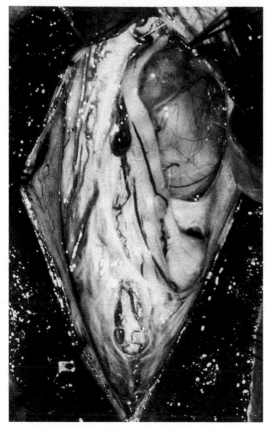

Figure 13-2
SPINAL NERVE ROOT SCHWANNOMA
This intraspinal schwannoma is discrete, laterally situated, and attached to a nerve root. (Courtesy of Dr. Allan H. Friedman, Durham, NC.)

root entry zone (35). In practice, a distinction between intramedullary and extramedullary spinal schwannomas is not always easy since nerve root tumors invaginating the cord may become partially intramedullary. Conversely, intramedullary lesions may traverse the pia to become partially extramedullary (26). Both extramedullary and intramedullary schwannomas may, infrequently, be melanotic.

Schwannomas arising within brain substance are rare, but all regions including cerebrum, cerebellum, and brain stem have been affected. Although their source remains obscure, the presence of aberrant peripheral nerve fibers has been documented in the medulla oblongata of occasional patients (13). The normal vasomotor nerves discussed above represent another potential source of parenchymal schwannomas. A

plexus of nerves somewhat resembling traumatic neuroma also accompanies some brain stem infarcts (47). A rare variant of intraparenchymal schwannoma of the brain stem, noted for perivascular tongues of neoplastic Schwann cells accompanied by a proliferation of astrocytes, resembles a pilocytic astrocytoma (5). *Spinal schwannosis*, a proliferation of nerve fibers and accompanying Schwann cells, affects the spinal cord after trauma. Some intraparenchymal schwannomas of the brain or spinal cord morphologically resemble and, in nosologic terms, overlap with the gliofibroma or glioneurofibroma.

Macroscopic Findings. Schwannomas arising from cranial or spinal nerve roots are typically well circumscribed and more often globular than fusiform in configuration. The parent nerve may be detected within the substance of small or early lesions, but this relationship soon becomes obscured as the nerve assumes an eccentric superficial location when a tumor becomes large. The discrete appearance of schwannomas is attributed to the presence of a thick, complete, collagenous capsule. Internally, schwannomas are often yellow, a reflection of lipid deposition. Cystic degeneration is a common feature of large tumors but even small lesions, particularly in the cauda equina region, may be largely thin walled and translucent. Melanotic lesions vary from gray to black. Compressive atrophy of the nerve is a common feature.

Microscopic Findings. The classic schwannoma is a biphasic lesion exhibiting alternating areas of compact fascicular tissue and loose textured spongy tissue with a distinctive, somewhat degenerative appearance (fig. 13-3). The former, or Antoni A pattern, consists of elongated bipolar cells disposed in fascicles; the cell borders are obscured at the light microscopic level. Long club-shaped nuclei are typical (fig. 13-4). Intraspinal, and to a much lesser extent, intracranial schwannomas may show striking palisades resulting from stacked arrays of nuclei alternating with anuclear fibrillar zones composed of cell processes (fig. 13-5). The term Verocay body has been applied to such cell arrangements. The loose textured, degenerative-appearing tissue comprises the Antoni B pattern in which neoplastic cells with round condensed nuclei and indistinct cytoplasm may superficially resemble lymphocytes (fig. 13-6). Xanthoma cells often

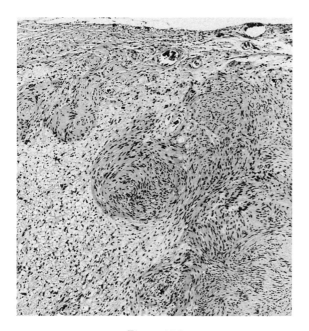

Figure 13-3
SCHWANNOMA
Seen at low magnification is the typical biphasic architecture of a schwannoma, with both compact (Antoni A) and loose-knit (Antoni B) regions.

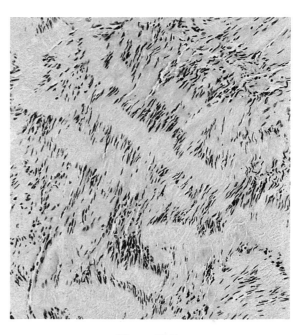

Figure 13-5
SCHWANNOMA
Although seen in only occasional intracranial schwannomas, rows of cells with nuclear palisading (Verocay bodies) are often prominent in spinal examples.

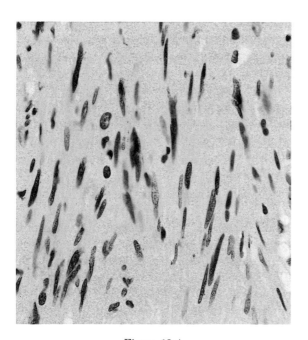

Figure 13-4
SCHWANNOMA
Long club-shaped nuclei are a distinctive feature in compact Antoni A regions. The length of these nuclei generally exceeds that in other spindle cell neoplasms, such as fibrous meningioma.

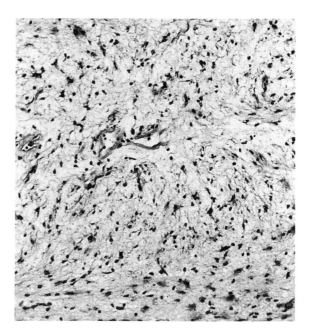

Figure 13-6
SCHWANNOMA
Antoni B tissue is loose textured and composed of uniform, small, somewhat stellate cells, whose nuclei resemble lymphocytes.

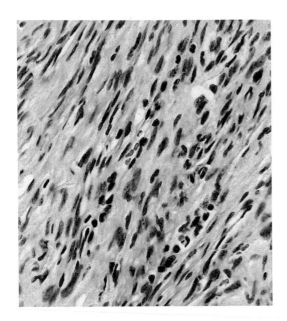

Figure 13-11
MENINGIOMA SIMULATING SCHWANNOMA
Some fibrous meningiomas closely resemble schwannomas.

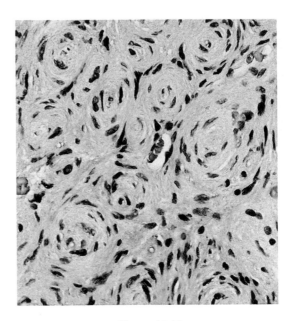

Figure 13-12
SCHWANNOMA SIMULATING MENINGIOMA
The occasional schwannoma with perivascular whorls can resemble a meningioma.

schwannoma exhibits perivascular whorl-like structures (fig. 13-12).

In contrast to meningiomas, most schwannomas have long club-shaped nuclei, some element of an Antoni B component, and vascular hyalinization associated with hemosiderin deposition. In addition, they demonstrate strong generalized staining for S-100 protein. Meningiomas may be S-100 positive but the reaction is often weak and patchy (57). Meningiomas also show a membranous pattern of immunoreaction for epithelial membrane antigen (EMA), although it is often weak in the fibrous variant, the only subtype likely to be confused with a schwannoma. The occasional EMA reactivity seen in schwannomas is often cytoplasmic rather than membranous (57). Meningiomas are rare in the lumbosacral region where schwannomas are common.

Schwannomas arising within brain and spinal cord parenchyma represent a diagnostic problem, largely because the diagnosis of a Schwann cell tumor does not come to mind. Once considered, the lesion is often readily recognized on the basis of its histologic and immunohistochemical features. In some schwannomas, the prominence of loose textured Antoni B tissue, composed as it is of stellate cells, resembles a glioma.

Reticulin staining as well as reactivity for S-100 protein unaccompanied by GFAP reactivity usually resolves the diagnostic problem. Schwannomas, however, may express GFAP reactivity (44). In some instances, electron microscopy may demonstrate pericellular basal lamina and the relative paucity of microfilaments in schwannomas.

A schwannoma with dense fascicular cellularity and mitotic activity must be distinguished from MPNST. The correct diagnosis rests in part upon noting the typical features of a schwannoma in other portions of the specimen. MPNSTs often lack a thick fibrous capsule, hyaline vessels, and hemosiderin deposits; usually show only patchy or minimal S-100 protein reactivity; and are far less differentiated at the ultrastructural level.

Distinguishing pigmented schwannomas from melanocytic neoplasms (melanoma and melanocytoma) is not always possible without special studies including electron microscopy, since both are immunoreactive for S-100 protein and often for melanocytic markers such as HMB-45. Ultrastructurally, schwannomas exhibit a uniform pericellular basal lamina whereas melanocytic neoplasms do not.

Treatment and Prognosis. Most craniospinal nerve root Schwann cell tumors are cured by

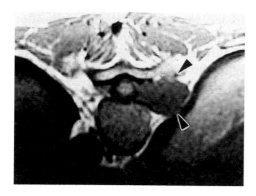

Figure 13-13
NEUROFIBROMA
Some examples enter (arrows), or arise within, the intraspinal compartment and compress the spinal cord.

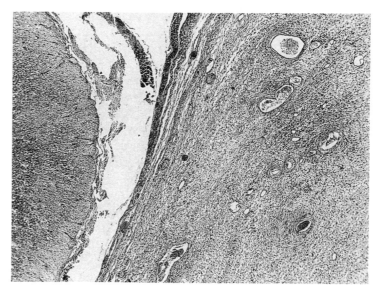

Figure 13-14
NEUROFIBROMA
This expanded nerve root has a delicate "capsule" representing the perineurium and epineurium. The spinal cord is seen at the left.

surgery alone. Malignant examples, arising in transition from previously well-differentiated lesions, are extremely rare. Exceptions are found primarily among melanocytic schwannomas, a small minority of which are mitotically active and biologically malignant. Such tumors occasionally seed the cerebrospinal space or even metastasize systemically. A small proportion of cellular schwannomas have recurred, but none have metastasized (50a).

Neurofibroma

Definition. A well-differentiated nerve sheath tumor composed predominantly of Schwann cells and, to a lesser extent, fibroblasts and perineural cells.

Clinical and Radiographic Features. Neurofibromas occur both as cutaneous lesions that infiltrate the dermis, sometimes producing pedunculated masses, and as intraneural tumors arising from larger nerves. The latter may be solitary or plexiform. Plexiform tumors involve multiple fascicles within a nerve, extending proximally and distally along its length. Ropy enlargement of numerous branches of a nerve result. Solitary neurofibromas form globular discrete masses with a fusiform configuration.

Neurofibromas rarely impinge upon the central nervous system (figs. 13-13, 13-14). Most involve multiple or single dorsal spinal nerve roots and occur in patients with neurofibromatosis 1 (see fig. 18-1). Neurofibromas of cranial nerves are extremely rare.

Macroscopic Findings. The tumors are soft to mucoid in consistency and appear as fusiform expansions of the involved nerves; the parent nerve is overrun rather than peripherally displaced. Unlike schwannomas, neurofibromas have only a thin capsule, do not undergo cystic change, and are not yellow.

Microscopic Findings. Neurofibromas consist in large part of Schwann cells arrayed in short wavy bundles separated by a loose, mucoid interstitial matrix (fig. 13-15). Axons, retaining or having lost their myelin sheaths, pass through the tumor, a reflection of the neoplasm's intimate relation to the parent nerve. Tactile-like bodies are seen occasionally (51). A rare neurofibroma is melanotic (3,48).

Immunohistochemical Findings. Neurofibromas are at least partially immunoreactive for S-100 protein, in keeping with their significant Schwann cell content (34). The fibroblastic component exhibits a vimentin reaction alone, whereas occasional perineural cells are positive for EMA but lack S-100 protein reactivity.

7. Brooks JS, Freeman M, Enterline HT. Malignant "triton" tumors: natural history and immunochemistry of nine new cases with literature review. Cancer 1985;55:2543–9.

8. Carney JA. Psammomatous melanotic schwannoma. A distinctive, heritable tumor with special associations, including cardiac myxoma and the Cushing syndrome. Am J Surg Pathol 1990;14:206–22.

9. Christensen WN, Strong EW, Bains MS, Woodruff JM. Neuroendocrine differentiation in the glandular peripheral nerve sheath tumor. Pathologic distinction from the biphasic synovial sarcoma with glands. Am J Surg Pathol 1988;12:417–26.

10. Coffin CM, Dehner LP. Peripheral neurogenic tumors of the soft tissues in children and adolescents: a clinicopathologic study of 139 cases. Pediatr Pathol 1989;9:387–407.

11. Cras P, Ceuterick-de Groote C, Van Vyve M, Vercruyssen A, Martin JJ. Malignant pigmented spinal nerve root schwannoma metastasizing in the brain and viscera. Clin Neuropathol 1990;9:290–4.

12. Cruz-Sanchez F, Cervos-Navarro J, Kashihara M, Ferszt R. Intracerebral neurinomas in a case of von Recklinghausen's disease (neurofibromatosis). Clin Neuropathol 1987;6:174–8.

13. Demyer W. Aberrant peripheral nerve fibers in the medulla oblongata of man. J Neurol Neurosurg Psychiatry 1965;28:121–3.

14. Deruaz JP, Janzer RC, Costa J. Cellular schwannomas of the intracranial and intraspinal compartment: morphological and immunological characteristics compared with classical benign schwannomas. J Neuropathol Exp Neurol 1993;52:114–8.

15. DiCarlo EF, Woodruff JM, Bansal M, Erlandson RA. The purely epithelioid malignant peripheral nerve sheath tumor. Am J Surg Pathol 1986;10:478–90.

16. Ducatman BS, Scheithauer BW. Malignant peripheral nerve sheath tumors with divergent differentiation. Cancer 1984;54:1049–57.

17. _____, Scheithauer BW. Postirradiation neurofibrosarcoma. Cancer 1983;51:1028–33.

18. _____, Scheithauer BW, Piepgras DG, Reiman HM. Malignant peripheral nerve sheath tumors in childhood. J Neurooncol 1984;2:241–8.

19. _____, Scheithauer BW, Piepgras DG, Reiman HM, Ilstrup DM. Malignant peripheral nerve sheath tumors: a clinicopathologic study of 120 cases. Cancer 1986;57:2006–21.

20. Erlandson RA, Woodruff JM. Peripheral nerve sheath tumors: an electron microscopic study of 43 cases. Cancer 1982;49:273–87.

21. Ezura M, Ikeda H, Ogawa A, Yoshimoto T. Intracerebral schwannoma: case report. Neurosurgery 1992;30:97–100.

22. Fletcher CD, Davies SE, McKee PH. Cellular schwannoma: a distinct pseudosarcomatous entity. Histopathology 1987;11:21–35.

23. Foley KM, Woodruff AM, Ellis FT, Posner JB. Radiation induced malignant and atypical peripheral nerve sheath tumors. Ann Neurol 1980;7:311–8.

24. Giangaspero F, Fratamico FC, Ceccarelli C, Brisigotti M. Malignant peripheral nerve sheath tumors and spinal clear cell sarcomas: an immunohistochemical analysis of multiple markers. Appl Pathol 1989:7:134–44.

25. Gökay H, Izgi N, Barlas O, Ervesen G. Supratentorial intracerebral schwannomas. Surg Neurol 1984;22:69–72.

26. Gorman PH, Rigamonti D, Joslyn JN. Intramedullary and extramedullary schwannoma of the cervical spinal cord—case report. Surg Neurol 1989;32:459–62.

27. Gregorios JB, Chou SM, Bay J. Melanotic schwannoma of the spinal cord. Neurosurgery 1982;11:57–60.

28. Guccion JG, Enzinger FM. Malignant schwannoma associated with von Recklinghausen's neurofibromatosis. Virchows Arch [A] 1979;383:43–57.

29. Han DH, Kim DG, Chi JG, Park SH, Jung HW, Kim YG. Malignant triton tumor of the acoustic nerve. Case report. J Neurosurg 1992;76:874–7.

30. Herregodts P, Vloeberghs M, Schmedding E, Goossens A, Stadnik T, D'Haens J. Solitary dorsal intramedullary schwannoma. Case report. J Neurosurg 1991;74:816–20.

31. Hirose T, Sano T, Hizawa K. Heterogeneity of malignant schwannomas. Ultrastruct Pathol 1988;12:107–16.

32. _____, Sano T, Hizawa K. Ultrastructural localization of S-100 protein in neurofibroma. Acta Neuropathol (Berl) 1986;69:103–10.

33. Hisaoka M, Ohta H, Haratake J, Horie A. Melanocytic schwannoma in the spinal cord. Acta Pathol Jpn 1991;41:685–8.

34. Johnson MD, Glick AD, Davis BW. Immunohistochemical evaluation of Leu-7, myelin basic-protein, S100-protein, glial-fibrillary acidic-protein, and LN3 immunoreactivity in nerve sheath tumors and sarcomas. Arch Pathol Lab Med 1988;112:155–60.

35. Kamiya M, Hashizume Y. Pathological studies of aberrant peripheral nerve bundles of spinal cords. Acta Neuropathol (Berl) 1989;79:18–22.

36. Levy WJ, Ansbacher L, Byer J, Nutkiewicz A, Fratkin J. Primary malignant nerve sheath tumor of the gasserian ganglion: a report of two cases. Neurosurgery 1983;13:572–6.

37. _____, Latchaw J, Hahn JF. Spinal neurofibromas: a report of 66 cases and a comparison with meningiomas. Neurosurgery 1986;18:331–4.

38. Liwnicz BH. Bilateral trigeminal neurofibrosarcoma. Case report. J Neurosurg 1979;50:253–6.

39. Lodding P, Kindblom LG, Angervall L. Epithelioid malignant schwannoma: a study of 14 cases. Virchows Arch [A] 1986;409:433–51.

40. _____, Kindblom LG, Angervall L, Stenman G. Cellular schwannoma. A clinicopathologic study of 29 cases. Virchow Arch [A] 1990;416:237–48.

41. Marchese MJ, McDonald JV. Intramedullary melanotic schwannoma of the cervical spinal cord: report of a case. Surg Neurol 1990;33:353–5.

42. McGavran WL III, Sypert GW, Ballinger WE. Melanotic schwannoma. Neurosurgery 1978;2:47–51.

43. Meis JM, Enzinger FM, Martz KL, Neal JA. Malignant peripheral nerve sheath tumors (malignant schwannomas) in children. Am J Surg Pathol 1992;16:694–707.

44. Memolli VA, Brown EF, Gould VE. Glial fibrillary acidic protein (GFAP) immunoreactivity in peripheral nerve sheath tumors. Ultrastruct Pathol 1984;7:269–75.

45. Mennemeyer RP, Raisis JE, Hammar SP, Hallman KO, Tytus JS, Bockus D. Melanotic schwannoma. Clinical and ultrastructural studies of three cases with evidence of intracellular melanin synthesis. Am J Surg Pathol 1979;3:3–10.

46. Miller RT, Sarikaya H, Sos A. Melanotic schwannoma of the acoustic nerve. Arch Pathol Lab Med 1986;110:153–4.

47. Payan H, Levine S. Focal axonal proliferation in pons (central neurinoma). Arch Pathol 1965;79:501–4.

48. Payan MJ, Gambarelli D, Keller P, et al. Melanotic neurofibroma: a case report with ultrastructural study. Acta Neuropathol (Berl) 1986;69:148–52.

49. Redekop G, Elisevich K, Gilbert J. Fourth ventricular schwannoma. Case report. J Neurosurg 1990;73:777–81.

50. Ross DA, Edwards MS, Wilson CB. Intramedullary neurilemomas of the spinal cord: report of two cases and review of the literature. Neurosurgery 1986;19:458–64.

50a. Scheithauer BW, Casadei GP, Manfrini M, Wood MB. Cellular schwannoma: a clinicopathologic study of 56 cases [Abstract]. J Neuropathol Exp Neurol 1993;52:329.

50b. Seppälä MT, Haltia MJ. Spinal malignant nerve-sheath tumor or cellular schwannoma? A striking difference in prognosis. J Neurosurg 1993;79:528–32.

51. Smith TW, Bhawan J. Tactile-like structures in neurofibromas: an ultrastructural study. Acta Neuropathol (Berl) 1980;50:233–6.

51a. Tali ET, Yuh WT, Nguyen HD, et al. Cystic acoustic schwannomas: MR characteristics. AJNR Am J Neuroradiol 1993;14:1241–7.

52. Tallan EM, Harner SG, Beatty CW. Does the distribution of schwann cells correlate with the observed occurrence of acoustic neuromas? Am J Otol 1993;14:131–4.

53. Thomsen J, Tos M. Acoustic neuroma: clinical aspects, audiovestibular assessment, diagnostic delay, and growth rate. Am J Otol 1990;11:12–19.

54. Tran-Dinh HD, Soo YS, O'Neil P, Chaseling R. Cystic cerebellar schwannoma: case report. Neurosurgery 1991;29:296–300.

55. White, W, Shiu MH, Rosenblum MK, Erlandson RA, Woodruff JM. Cellular schwannoma: a clinicopathologic study of 57 patients and 58 tumors. Cancer 1990;66:1266–75.

56. Wick MR, Swanson PE, Scheithauer BW, Manivel JC. Malignant peripheral nerve sheath tumor: an immunohistochemical study of 62 cases. Am J Clin Pathol 1987;87:425–33.

57. Winek RR, Scheithauer BW, Wick MR. Meningioma, meningeal hemangiopericytoma (angioblastoma meningioma), peripheral hemangiopericytoma, and acoustic schwannoma. A comparative immunohistochemical study. Am J Surg Pathol 1989;13:251–61.

58. Woodruff JM. Peripheral nerve tumors showing glandular differentiation (glandular schwannomas). Cancer 1976;37:2399–413.

59. _____, Chernik NL, Smith MC, Millet WB, Foote FW Jr. Peripheral nerve tumors with rhabdomyosarcomatous differentiation (malignant "triton" tumors). Cancer 1973;32:426–39.

60. _____, Godwin TA, Erlandson RA, Susin M, Martin N. Cellular schwannoma: a variety of schwannoma sometimes mistaken for malignant tumor. Am J Surg Pathol 1981;5:733–44.

Granular Cell Tumor

61. Chimelli L, Symon L, Scaravilli F. Granular cell tumor of the fifth cranial nerve: further evidence for Schwann cell origin. J Neuropathol Exp Neurol 1984;43:634–42.

62. Rao TV, Puri R, Reddy GN. Intracranial trigeminal granular cell myoblastoma. Case report. J Neurosurg 1983;59:706–9.

14

MELANOCYTIC TUMORS

Melanocytoma and Malignant Melanoma

The central nervous system is host to a wide variety of melanocytic neoplasms including the common metastatic malignant melanoma and the relatively benign, as well as overtly malignant, primary neoplasms of leptomeningeal melanocytes. This section is devoted to the primary tumors presumed to arise from normally occurring leptomeningeal melanocytes which are most numerous at the base of the brain and in the upper cervical region. Melanotic neoplasms derived from Schwann cells, i.e., melanotic schwannomas, are discussed separately, but are also described below in the context of differential diagnosis since their distinction from neoplasms of melanocytes may be difficult. Rare melanocytic tumors arise in the pineal gland (20a).

Clinical Features. Primary melanocytic tumors occur both as diffuse leptomeningeal proliferations and discrete masses (fig. 14-1). Patients of all ages are affected. Diffuse lesions, which usually affect children, are occasionally associated with multiple or extensive pigmented lesions of the skin (see fig. 18-20). This complex is known as neurocutaneous melanosis. It may be difficult in malignant examples to rule out the possibility of a small extracranial primary as its source.

Macroscopic Findings. Diffuse lesions vary from a faint dusky clouding of the leptomeninges to dense black replacement of the subarachnoid space.

Discrete lesions occur within the cranial or spinal compartments, but the posterior fossa is the preferred site. Most tumors are either obviously meningeal in location or are so superficially situated within parenchyma that an origin from the meninges is assumed. Spinal melanocytomas are often situated near nerve exit zones. The degree of pigmentation of the spectrum of discrete melanocytic lesions ranges from shades of gray to jet black.

Microscopic Findings. Diffuse lesions vary in cytologic appearance from well-differentiated lesions with nevoid cytologic features to unequivocally malignant proliferations for which the term malignant melanoma is appropriate (2,6, 7,8,16). Some diffuse tumors, despite biologic aggressiveness, are morphologically intermediate in their cytologic appearance and defy precise classification as either benign or malignant.

Discrete melanocytic neoplasms vary from a well-differentiated unique lesion termed *melanocytoma* (5,12,17,22) to frankly malignant tumors designated *malignant melanoma* (1,4,7,9,13, 15,18–20). Given the considerable variation in the histologic appearance of both melanocytoma and melanoma, consideration of clinical, topographic, gross, and other microscopic features is essential in distinguishing one from the other.

Melanocytomas show a proclivity for the spinal and, to a lesser extent, the basilar leptomeninges of adult patients. The tumors are solitary, discrete, variably pigmented masses which, as previously noted, vary in cytologic appearance and have few if any mitoses. Lesions can, however, be intimately attached to the brain by superficial extension along the Virchow-Robin spaces, or to the surface of the spinal cord. They

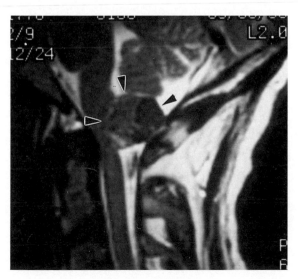

Figure 14-1
PRIMARY MENINGEAL MALIGNANT MELANOMA

Note the heterogeneous but overall dark signal intensity of melanotic neoplasms seen in T2-weighted MRIs. This meningioma-like mass arose without a recognized extra-CNS primary in a 52-year-old woman. (Courtesy of Dr. Cheryl M. Harris, Birmingham, AL.)

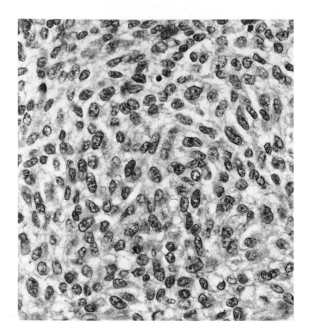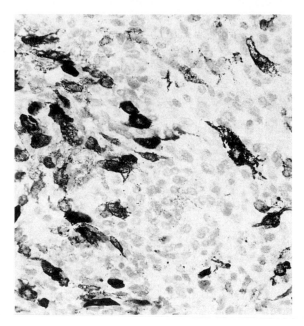

Figure 14-2
MELANOCYTOMA
Left: In an H&E stained section, the cells are somewhat spindle shaped, markedly uniform, and free of mitotic activity.
Right: The dendritic nature of some cells is readily apparent after staining for melanin.

vary histologically from spindle cell tumors resembling "spindle A melanoma of the eye," to neoplasms more epithelioid in appearance (figs. 14-2, 14-3). Nests and small lobules are not uncommon (fig. 14-3). Melanocytomas of the spindle cell type have been likened to blue nevi since they vary in pigmentation and possess nuclei that are elongated and often delicate (12). Epithelioid lesions may show a lobular low-power pattern. Their cells tend to have large vesicular nuclei with prominent nucleoli but, given the absence or paucity of mitoses, are not considered frankly malignant. In some instances, nuclear features are so obscured by pigment that bleaching is required to permit cytologic assessment. A rare association with Mongolian spot suggests the lesion may be part of a neurocutaneous melanosis syndrome (11).

Primary malignant melanomas of the central nervous system vary in cytologic features much like those at other sites (fig. 14-4). Mitoses range from scant to numerous. Necrosis may be extensive, producing perivascular pseudopapillae. Transition to a diffuse growth pattern, satellite nodule formation in surrounding meninges, and irregular invasion of spinal cord substance is common in melanoma.

It is difficult in some cases to decide whether the tumor is best classified as melanocytoma or melanoma. Unfortunately, little information is available regarding histologic features of prognostic importance in this spectrum of lesions. These uncertainties are reflected in reports of series of "melanomas" in which no attempt is made to distinguish the two.

Immunohistochemical Findings. Melanocytic tumors are vimentin reactive but lack epithelial markers. Staining for S-100 protein varies, but is often strong. Though not melanoma specific, the HMB-45 stain is usually positive.

Ultrastructural Findings. As expected, the cells lack junctions and contain melanosomes in varying stages of pigmentation (1,3,10,14,16,21, 22). Too few melanocytomas have been systematically studied to formulate criteria for their firm distinction from melanoma. Although, in contrast to Schwann cell tumors, a well-formed pericellular basal lamina is lacking, groups of melanocytoma cells may be ensheathed.

Differential Diagnosis. Historically, an issue was often made of distinguishing discrete melanocytic neoplasms from so-called pigmented meningiomas. In that the latter are melanocytic

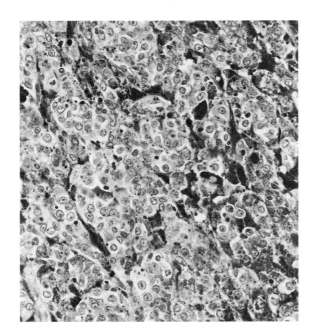 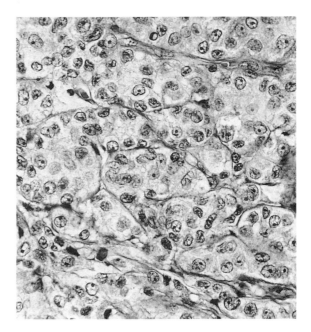

Figure 14-3
MELANOCYTOMA

Left: The cells of some melanocytomas are more polygonal or epithelioid, as in this well-demarcated, coal black spinal lesion in a middle-aged female.

Right: The clustering of cells, their prominent nucleoli, and the absence of mitotic figures are well seen in a bleached section of this same tumor.

at both the immunohistochemical and ultrastructural levels, it is unlikely that a truly melanotic meningioma exists (14). Most reported cases represent melanocytomas. Melanocytic neoplasms further differ from meningioma in their lack of immunoreactivity for epithelial membrane antigen, membrane interdigitations, and desmosomes.

A more difficult problem is distinguishing melanocytic tumors from pigmented schwannomas, and many published cases leave uncertainty as to whether the neoplasm was melanocytic or schwannian. The distinction is most likely to be an issue in the intraspinal compartment, a site where melanotic Schwann cell tumors are more common. The cells of melanocytic schwannoma often have a more spindled appearance and exhibit a greater ratio of cytoplasm and extracellular material to nuclear volume than is apparent in melanocytic tumors. Attention to surgical findings is of diagnostic importance since most pigmented schwannomas arise from spinal nerve roots. Extensive pericellular basal laminae, characteristic ultrastructural features of Schwann cell tumors, are light microscopically highlighted by reticulin or periodic acid–Schiff

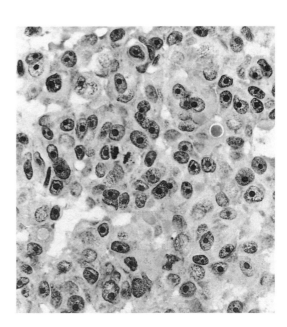

Figure 14-4
MALIGNANT MELANOMA

Large nucleoli, coarse chromatin, and mitotic figures all attest to the malignancy of this meningeal lesion which was widely disseminated in the patient with a "bathing trunk nevus" illustrated in figure 18-20. Emphasizing the value of melanin stains in the assessment of leptomeningeal neoplasms, marked pigmentation was seen only focally.

staining. Since pigmented schwannomas may exhibit HMB-45 staining, it remains doubtful whether the demonstration of other melanoma-associated antigens are useful in distinguishing melanocytic neoplasms from the morphologically similar pigmented Schwann cell tumors.

Treatment and Prognosis. Experience with melanocytic lesions indicates that to some extent the prognosis is related to cytologic findings, with overtly malignant lesions behaving as expected. More problematic are the melanocytomas that undergo multiple local recurrences, a not surprising occurrence given the tendency of some for limited diffuse spread or superficial infiltration of adjacent parenchyma. Rare cases show transformation to melanoma (5).

REFERENCES

1. Aichner F, Schuler G. Primary leptomeningeal melanoma. Diagnosis by ultrastructural cytology of cerebrospinal fluid and cranial computed tomography. Cancer 1982;50:1751–6.
2. Bergdahl L, Boquist L, Liliequist B, Thulin CA, Tovi D. Primary malignant melanoma of the central nervous system. A report of 10 cases. Acta Neurochir (Wien) 1972;26:139–49.
3. Botticelli AR, Villani M, Angiari P, Peserico L. Meningeal melanocytoma of Meckel's cave associated with ipsilateral Ota's nevus. Cancer 1983;51:2304–10.
4. Bouton J. Primary melanoma of the leptomeninges. J Clin Pathol 1958;11:122–7.
5. Cordoba A, Tunon T, Vasquez JJ. Meningeal melanocytoma. Presentation of a case and review of the literature. Arch Neurobiol (Madr) 1989;52:93–9.
6. Gibson JB, Burrows D, Weir WP. Primary melanoma of the meninges. J Pathol Bacteriol 1957;74:419–38.
7. Haddad FS, Jamali AF, Rebeiz JJ, Fahl M, Haddad GF. Primary malignant melanoma of the gasserian ganglion associated with neurofibromatosis. Surg Neurol 1991;35:310–6.
8. Iglesias-Rozas JR, Kroh H, Sauer E, Sarioglu N. Disseminated melanomatosis of the central nervous system and other organs: a case report. Clin Neuropathol 1989;8:11–5.
9. Iizuka H, Nakamura T, Kurauchi M. Primary intracranial melanoma. Case report. Neurol Med Chir (Tokyo) 1990;39:698–702.
10. Jellinger K, Böck F, Brenner H. Meningeal melanocytoma. Report of a case and review of the literature. Acta Neurochir (Wien) 1988;94:78–87.
11. Kawara S, Takata M, Hirone T, Tomita K, Hamaoka H. A new variety of neuroectocutaneous melanosis: benign leptomeningeal melanocytoma associated with extensive Mongolian spot on the back. Nippon Hifuka Gakkai Zasshi 1989;99:561–6.
12. Lach B, Russell N, Benoit B, Atack D. Cellular blue nevus ("melanocytoma") of the spinal meninges: electron microscopic and immunohistochemical features. Neurosurgery 1988;22:773–80.
13. Larson TC III, Houser OW, Onofro BM, Piepgras DG. Primary spinal melanoma. J Neurosurg 1987;66:47–9.
14. Limas C, Tio FO. Meningeal melanocytoma ("melanotic meningioma"). Its melanocytic origin as revealed by electron microscopy. Cancer 1972;30:1286–94.
15. Morris LL, Danta G. Malignant cerebral melanoma complicating giant pigmented naevus: a case report. J Neurol Neurosurg Psychiatry 1968;31:628–32.
16. Nakamura Y, Becker LE. Meningeal tumors of infancy and childhood. Pediatr Pathol 1985;3:341–58.
17. Naul LG, Hise JH, Bauserman SC, Todd FD. CT and MR of meningeal melanocytoma. AJNR Am J Neuroradiol 1991;12:315–6.
18. Pappenheim E, Bhattacharji SK. Primary melanoma of the central nervous system. Arch Neurol 1962;7:101–33.
19. Pasquier B, Couderc P, Pasquier D, Panh MH, Arnould JP. Primary malignant melanoma of the cerebellum. A case with metastases outside the nervous system. Cancer 1978;41:344–51.
19a. Prabhu SS, Lynch PG, Keogh AJ, Parekh HC. Intracranial meningeal melanocytoma: a report of two cases and a review of the literature. Surg Neurol 1993;40:516–21.
20. Rodriquez y Baena R, Gaetani P, Danova M, Bosi F, Zappoli F. Primary solitary intracranial melanoma: case report and review of the literature. Surg Neurol 1992;38:26–37.
20a. Rubino GJ, King WA, Quinn B, Marroquin CE, Verity MA. Primary pineal melanoma: case report. Neurosurgery 1993;33:511–5.
21. Uematsu Y, Yukawa S, Yokote H, Itakura T, Hayashi S, Komai N. Meningeal melanocytoma: magnetic resonance imaging characteristics and pathologic features. J Neurosurg 1992;76:705–9.
22. Winston KR, Sotrel A, Schnitt SJ. Meningeal melanocytoma. Case report and review of the clinical and histological features. J Neurosurg 1987;66:50–7.

15
CRANIOPHARYNGIOMAS

Craniopharyngiomas are complex epithelial neoplasms arising in the sellar and third ventricular regions. Although discussions of craniopharyngiomas have generally focused on the classic adamantinomatous type, a more squamous or papillary variety is increasingly recognized. Occasional cases appear to bridge these tumors, but the two are distinct enough in clinical, radiologic, and histologic terms to warrant separate discussions.

The histogenesis of craniopharyngiomas is unresolved and remains a subject of interest. The adamantinomatous variant closely resembles the adamantinoma of the jaw and is even more similar to a close relative of the latter, the keratinizing and calcifying odontogenic cyst (4). Misplaced odontogenic epithelium is, therefore, a reasonable source of craniopharyngioma. If the papillary lesion is accepted as a distinct entity, then the similarities between it and the Rathke cleft cyst, a lesion that may show extensive squamous metaplasia, must be considered. The finding of occasional goblet cells in papillary craniopharyngiomas further strengthens the association (8,10).

Adamantinomatous Craniopharyngioma

Clinical and Radiographic Features. This most frequent form of craniopharyngioma presents most commonly during the first two decades of life as a calcified cystic suprasellar mass (fig. 15-1) (see Appendices D, E). Intranasal (5) and third ventricle examples occur occasionally (see Appendix F), as do rare but convincing examples in the pineal (12) and infratentorial (1,7) regions. Hypopituitarism and visual abnormalities are the usual complications of suprasellar lesions. Occasional lesions rupture and spill the cholesterol-rich, irritating contents into the cerebrospinal fluid (11a).

Macroscopic Findings. At the time of presentation, adamantinomatous lesions are typically adherent to structures at the base of the brain and frequently indent the floor of the third ventricle. Recurrent tumors are often widely and densely adherent to regional structures, partic-

ularly the vasculature and pituitary stalk. Longstanding untreated craniopharyngiomas may attain massive size.

Adamantinomatous lesions are almost always cystic and are filled with a dark brown "machinery oil" fluid. Floating within this turbid liquid are minute glistening crystals of cholesterol, whose characteristic multilaminar construction and "state of Utah" outline are evident under polarized light (fig. 15-2). They are distinctive and aesthetically pleasing in the extreme.

Gray-yellow flecks of "wet keratin," the microscopic features of which are discussed below, are diagnostic findings readily seen through the operating microscopic. Recurrent lesions often consist primarily of fibrous tissue and grumous debris.

Microscopic Findings. In its full expression, the adamantinomatous craniopharyngioma is an unmistakable entity, its recognition requiring but a glance at low magnification (fig. 15-3). The prominent epithelial lobules, when grouped in a multinodular clover leaf configuration, are highly distinctive. Cells at the periphery of the lobules are palisaded whereas internally situated cells are loosely textured (fig. 15-4); they readily

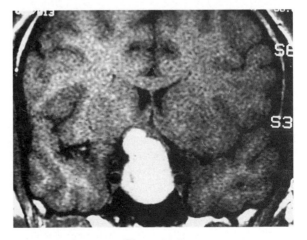

Figure 15-1
ADAMANTINOMATOUS CRANIOPHARYNGIOMA
This typical craniopharyngioma is a lobular suprasellar mass with an intrinsically high signal intensity as in this T1-weighted image.

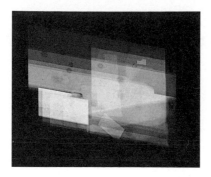

Figure 15-2
ADAMANTINOMATOUS CRANIOPHARYNGIOMA
Cholesterol crystals, a typical finding in the cyst fluid,
are readily identified by examination under polarized light.

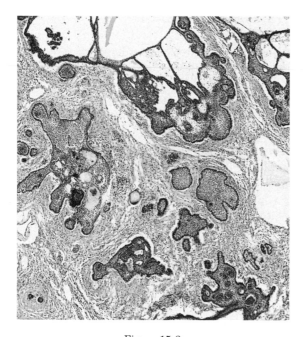

Figure 15-3
ADAMANTINOMATOUS CRANIOPHARYNGIOMA
The "clover-leaf" architecture, cystic spaces, and periph-
eral palisading of nuclei are distinctive features.

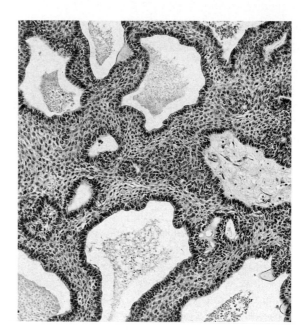

Figure 15-4
ADAMANTINOMATOUS CRANIOPHARYNGIOMA
The cells abutting cyst-like spaces or connective tissue
stroma assume a palisaded pattern. The remaining cells
have a somewhat stellate configuration.

dehisce to create a somewhat stellate myxoid appearance ("stellate reticulum"). Progression of the lesion, in concert with degeneration about the blood vessels, produces cystic spaces filled with fluid or amorphous debris (11). The neoplastic cells surrounding the cysts often assume the same palisaded profiles as those on the periphery.

A highly significant and diagnostic finding is wet keratin. These are nodules of plump, eosinophilic, keratinized cells with a necrobiotic nature apparent from their ghost nuclei (fig. 15-5).

Calcium is frequently deposited dystrophically on nodules of wet keratin. A rare lesion is so fully odontogenic as to form teeth (2).

In addition to the epithelial components, extensive fibrosis, chronic inflammation, and cholesterol clefts abound, particularly in recurrent tumors where they often constitute the bulk of the lesion. Extensive calcification is common.

In macrocystic regions the epithelium often becomes flattened and may, due to cell stratification, focally approximate the histologic appearance of epidermoid cyst or papillary craniopharyngioma (fig. 15-6). Although such areas generally retain some peripheral palisading, in some attenuated regions even this helpful diagnostic feature is lost.

Craniopharyngiomas are locally invasive, with tongues of tumor projecting into adjacent brain. The response of the brain to this intrusion is a remarkably dense gliosis. Specimens obtained from the immediate periphery of a craniopharyngioma consist in large part of Rosenthal fiber–rich gliosis which closely simulates pilocytic astrocytoma. (fig. 15-7).

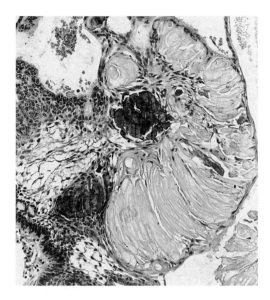

Figure 15-5
ADAMANTINOMATOUS CRANIOPHARYNGIOMA
Stacked arrays of plump, necrobiotic squames (wet keratin) are a classic feature of the adamantinomatous variant. Note the dystrophic calcification as well as the loose, degenerative-appearing tissue at the left and bottom of the illustration ("stellate reticulum").

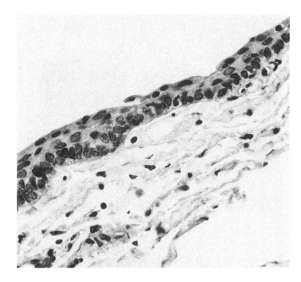

Figure 15-6
ADAMANTINOMATOUS CRANIOPHARYNGIOMA
The peripheral palisading of epithelial cells may be inapparent or lost in cystic regions of the tumor.

Ultrastructural Findings. The epithelial cells contain bundles of tonofilaments and are joined by well-formed desmosomes. While epithelial cells that abut the stroma are covered by a basal lamina, those situated internally or lining microcysts have microvilli but lack basement membranes (6,13).

Differential Diagnosis. Usually, adamantinomatous craniopharyngiomas are so distinctive that no other diagnosis is considered. In recurrent or irradiated tumors, much of the mass may be degenerative and only a small proportion diagnostic. In such instances, the finding of epithelial tissue with peripherally palisaded cells or wet keratin is sufficient for the diagnosis.

Distinguishing adamantinomatous from papillary craniopharyngiomas is not always simple since some cases show transitional features. Findings that exclude papillary tumors are palisading of peripheral epithelial cells, nodules of wet keratin, calcification, and, to a lesser extent, extensive fibrosis and cholesterol deposition.

The attenuated epithelium in large cystic craniopharyngiomas must not be confused with that of the epidermoid cyst. In most cases, this is not a problem given the architectural complexity of

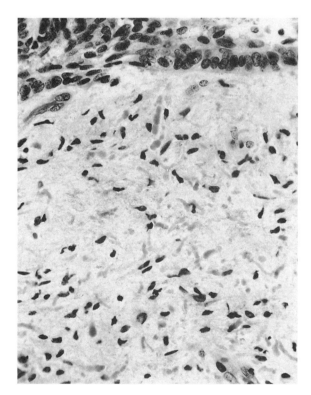

Figure 15-7
ADAMANTINOMATOUS CRANIOPHARYNGIOMA
Gliosis with often striking Rosenthal fiber formation is a prominent feature of brain abutting or invaded by craniopharyngioma.

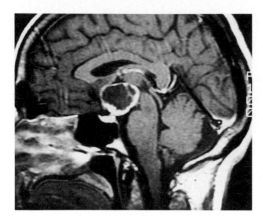

Figure 15-8
PAPILLARY CRANIOPHARYNGIOMA
In contrast to the adamantinomatous variety, papillary craniopharyngiomas usually occur in adults and are often intraventricular.

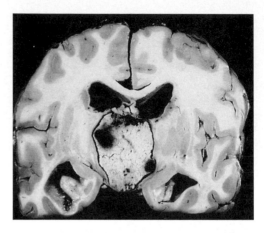

Figure 15-9
PAPILLARY CRANIOPHARYNGIOMA
This solid lesion fills the third ventricle.

the craniopharyngioma. Craniopharyngiomas also lack keratohyaline granules and the uniform surface maturation that generates thin anuclear squames of the sort that characterize epidermoid cysts. The latter lack palisaded cells, wet keratin, calcification, and fibrodegenerative changes.

Although the gliosis induced by invasive craniopharyngiomas may infrequently be misinterpreted as pilocytic astrocytoma, the specimen includes the distinctive palisaded epithelium in most cases. The reactive gliosis accompanying craniopharyngioma is paucicellular, compacted, piloid, and lacking the cellularity and microcystic architecture present in most pilocytic neoplasms.

Treatment and Prognosis. Ideally, the treatment of craniopharyngioma is surgical; radiotherapy is reserved for incompletely excised or recurrent lesions. The degree to which these tumors are amenable to total excision, and the vigor with which resection should be attempted, remains controversial (3,9,14). Most recurrences are seen within 5 years of initial surgery.

Papillary Craniopharyngioma

Clinical and Radiographic Features. In contrast to the classic adamantinomatous lesion, papillary craniopharyngiomas are usually encountered in adults as solid noncalcified masses often within the third ventricle (fig. 15-8) (15–18)(see Appendix F).

Macroscopic Findings. The tumors are generally encapsulated solid masses lacking the cholesterol-rich, machinery oil content of adamantinomatous craniopharyngioma (fig. 15-9). In many instances the lesion can be separated readily from surrounding brain tissue because papillary tumors are smooth surfaced.

Microscopic Findings. Papillary craniopharyngiomas are composed of solid sheets of remarkably well-differentiated epithelial cells interrupted by prominent cores of fibrovascular stroma (fig. 15-10). The cellular sheets typically dehisce, either by nature or due to specimen processing, to form prominent pseudopapillae. Absent are the features so characteristic of the adamantinomatous lesion: conspicuous palisading of cells, well-formed keratin pearls, nodules of wet keratin, inflammatory response, and cholesterol deposition. Unlike the epithelium of epidermoid cysts, that of papillary craniopharyngiomas exhibits neither diffuse surface maturation nor keratohyaline granule formation. As in Rathke cleft cysts, papillary craniopharyngiomas may focally exhibit goblet or ciliated cells (fig. 15-11).

Immunohistochemical Findings. Immunoreactivities for cytokeratins and epithelial membrane antigen are a regular feature of papillary craniopharyngioma.

Ultrastructural Findings. The cells maintain a high degree of squamous differentiation, being interconnected by desmosomes and internally trussed with bundles of tonofilaments (17).

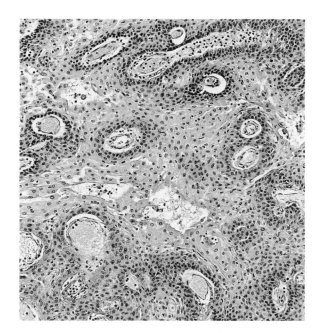 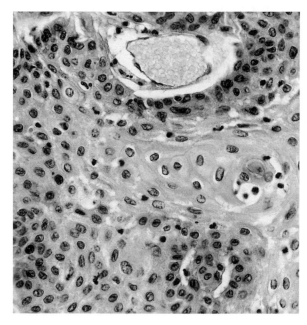

Figure 15-10
PAPILLARY CRANIOPHARYNGIOMA

The overt squamous character of this papillary craniopharyngioma is apparent at both low (left) and high (right) magnification. The lesion lacks the well-developed nuclear palisades, microcystic degeneration, calcification, and wet keratin formation that characterizes the adamantinomatous variant.

Surface microvillous-like projections are frequently seen.

Differential Diagnosis. The principal differential diagnostic consideration is the adamantinomatous craniopharyngioma discussed in detail in the previous section. The high degree of squamous differentiation also raises the issue of epidermoid and dermoid cysts. These latter lesions, however, have a surface layer of highly organized squamous cells methodically generating anucleate squames which come to form the bulk of the mass. In further contrast, the epithelium of epidermoid and dermoid cysts also exhibits prominent keratohyaline granule formation. Also, the papillary lesion shows little in the way of keratin pearl formation and lacks extensive squamous maturation and the cutaneous adnexa seen in dermoid cysts.

Treatment and Prognosis. As in the case of adamantinomatous craniopharyngioma, surgical excision is the treatment of choice; total excision is more often possible for papillary than for adamantinomatous tumors (15,16). In one series, there were no recurrences in 12 patients followed for a mean of 7.5 years (15).

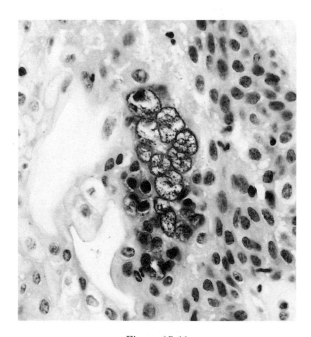

Figure 15-11
PAPILLARY CRANIOPHARYNGIOMA

Goblet cells, seen here stained by the mucicarmine method, are occasionally encountered.

REFERENCES

Adamantinomatous Craniopharyngioma

1. Altinörs N, Senveli E, Erdogan A, Arda N, Pak I. Craniopharyngioma of the cerebellopontine angle. Case report. J Neurosurg 1984;60:842–4.
2. Alvarez-Garijo JA, Froufé A, Taboada D, Vila M. Successful surgical treatment of an odontogenic ossified craniopharyngioma. Case report. J Neurosurg 1981; 55:832–5.
3. Baskin DS, Wilson CB. Surgical management of craniopharyngiomas. A review of 74 cases. J Neurosurg 1986;65:22–7.
4. Bernstein ML, Buchino JJ. The histologic similarity between craniopharyngioma and odontogenic lesions: a reappraisal. Oral Surg Oral Med Oral Pathol 1983;56:502–11.
5. Cooper PR, Ransohoff J. Craniopharyngioma originating in the sphenoid bone. Case report. J Neurosurg 1972;36:102–6.
6. Ghatak NR, Hirano A, Zimmerman HM. Ultrastructure of a craniopharyngioma. Cancer 1971;21:1465–75.
7. Gökalp HZ, Egemen N, Ildan F, Bacaci K. Craniopharyngioma of the posterior fossa. Neurosurgery 1991;29:446–8.
8. Goodrich JT, Post KD, Duffy P. Ciliated craniopharyngioma. Surg Neurol 1985;24:105–11.
9. Hoffman HJ, De Silva M, Humphreys RP, Drake JM, Smith ML, Blaser SI. Aggressive surgical management of craniopharyngiomas in children. J Neurosurg 1992;76:47–52.
10. Matsushima T, Fukui M, Ohta M, Yamakawa Y, Takaki T, Okano H. Ciliated and goblet cells in craniopharyngioma. Light and electron microscopic studies at surgery and autopsy. Acta Neuropathol (Berl) 1980; 50:199–205.
11. Petito CK, DeGirolami U, Earle KM. Craniopharyngiomas. A clinical and pathological review. Cancer 1976;37:1944–52.
11a. Satoh H, Uozumi T, Arita K, et al. Spontaneous rupture of craniopharyngioma cysts. A report of five cases and review of the literature. Surg Neurol 1993;40:414–9.
12. Solarski A, Panke ES, Panke TW. Craniopharyngioma in the pineal gland [Letter]. Arch Pathol Lab Med 1978;102:490–1.
13. Vilches J, Lopez A, Martinez MC, Gomez J, Barbera J. Scanning and transmission electron microscopy of a craniopharyngioma: x-ray microanalytical study of the intratumoral mineralized deposits. Ultrastruct Pathol 1981;2:343–56.
14. Yasargil MG, Curcic M, Kis M, Siegenthaler G, Teddy PJ, Roth P. Total removal of craniopharyngiomas. Approaches and long-term results in 144 patients. J Neurosurg 1990;73:3–11.

Papillary Craniopharyngioma

15. Adamson TE, Wiestler OD, Kleihues P, Yasargil MG. Correlation of clinical and pathological features in surgically treated craniopharyngiomas. J Neurosurg 1990;73:12–7.
16. Crotty T, Scheithauer BW, Young WF, Jr, Davis D, Miller G, Burger PC. Papillary craniopharyngiomas: a morphological and clinical study of 46 cases. Endocrine Pathol 1992;3(Suppl 1):S6.
17. Giangaspero F, Burger PC, Osborne DR, Stein RB. Suprasellar papillary squamous epithelioma ("papillary craniopharyngioma"). Am J Surg Pathol 1984; 8:57–64.
18. Kahn EA, Gosch HH, Seeger JF, Hicks SP. Forty-five years experience with the craniopharyngiomas. Surg Neurol 1973;1:5–12.

16

BENIGN CYSTIC LESIONS

Colloid Cyst of the Third Ventricle

Definition. A mucus-filled, epithelial-lined cyst occurring in the anterosuperior third ventricle.

General Comments. Although colloid cysts have long been assumed to be derived from neuroectodermal tissue, such as the paraphysial remnants in the region of the third ventricle, evidence now favors an endodermal origin (1–3,5–7). Short of its location, the colloid cyst is identical to bronchial epithelium and resembles enterogenous cysts. Histologically, Rathke cleft cysts also closely resemble colloid cysts. Unlike bronchial mucosa and these other related cysts, however, the colloid cyst shows no tendency to squamous metaplasia. Proponents of the endodermal origin theory need to explain the lesion's heterotopic third ventricle location. An endodermal designation must also be reconciled with the ectodermal (stomodeum) origin of the Rathke pouch.

Clinical and Radiographic Features. Intermittent obstruction of cerebrospinal fluid flow, a natural consequence of the cyst's position near the foramen of Monro, produces classic symptoms including headache, sudden transient paralysis of the lower extremities ("drop attacks"), incontinence, personality changes, and, occasionally, dementia. Young to middle-aged adults are primarily affected.

In view of their stereotypic intraventricular location (see Appendix F), cystic nature, smooth-surfaced contours, and signal characteristics, colloid cysts are radiologically diagnosed with considerable confidence. The mucoid protein-rich contents often have an intrinsically bright (white) signal on nonenhanced T1-weighted magnetic resonance images (MRIs) (fig. 16-1) (9). These same imaging characteristics are shared by the closely related Rathke cleft cysts.

Macroscopic Findings. The thin-walled cyst is impacted in the anterosuperior third ventricle in the region of the fornices and foramen of Monro (figs. 16-2, 16-3). It is generally loosely attached to these structures as well as to choroid plexus which snakes through the adjacent interventricular foramina (fig. 16-4). Colloid cysts contain a turbid, tenacious material which solidifies upon formalin fixation.

Microscopic Findings. In the absence of pressure atrophy or degenerative changes, the lining epithelium is a simple layer of columnar cells, both goblet and ciliated (figs. 16-4, 16-5). Occasional basal cells may also be seen. The cyst contents are largely amorphous, but scattered cell ghosts and masses of filamentous material representing degenerate nucleoprotein may be seen (fig. 16-6) (11). The latter resemble organisms of the *Actinomyces* group. In longstanding lesions, a xanthogranulomatous reaction may fill the cyst and replace its degenerating epithelium (10,12).

Immunohistochemical Findings. The epithelium of the colloid cyst exhibits a distinctive pattern of immunoreactivity: individual cells are positive for cytokeratins or epithelial membrane antigen (3,4,6,8) and scattered cells are reactive for Clara cell–specific antigens (6). Reactivity for carcinoembryonic antigen and focal S-100 reactivity has been seen (8).

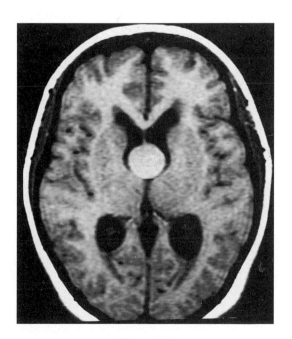

Figure 16-1
COLLOID CYST

Colloid cysts are spherical midline masses situated near the foramen of Monro. As a consequence of the mucoid, protein-rich contents, nearly all colloid cysts have an intrinsically bright magnetic resonance imaging signal in T1-weighted images.

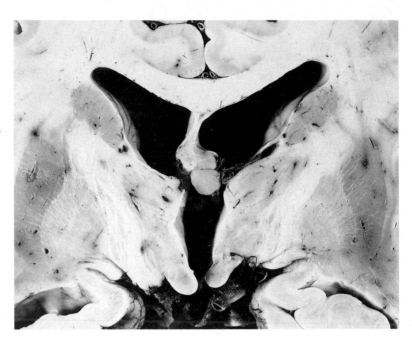

Figure 16-2
COLLOID CYST
This colloid-filled lesion, lying immediately below the fornices, was an incidental finding.

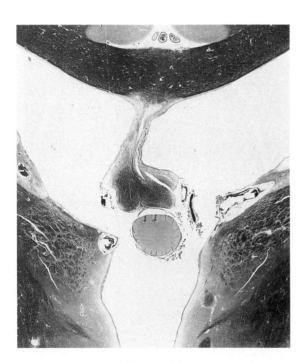

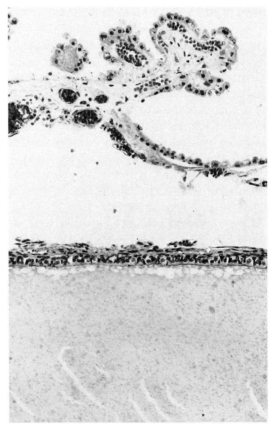

Figure 16-3
COLLOID CYST

A whole mount histologic section of the lesion illustrated in figure 16-2 shows the spherical mass immediately below the fornices. Segments of choroid plexus pass over its surface.

Figure 16-4
COLLOID CYST

The specimens of colloid cyst wall with its mucin-producing epithelium (bottom) is often accompanied by adherent choroid plexus epithelium (top).

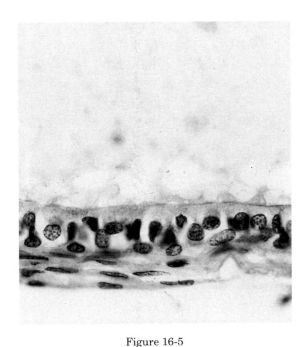

Figure 16-5
COLLOID CYST
Remarkably well-differentiated, columnar, mucin-producing ciliated epithelium is typical of colloid cysts.

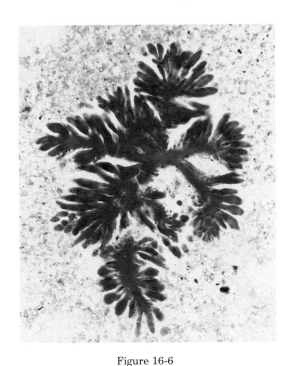

Figure 16-6
COLLOID CYST
Filamentous masses of nucleoprotein can closely resemble fungi or other organisms.

Ultrastructural Findings. The architecture of colloid cysts has been compared to bronchial epithelium, and as many as six cell types have been described (1,2,6,7). These include ciliated cells, nonciliated cells with surface microvilli, goblet cells, basal cells, occasional electron-lucent basal horizontal cells with neurosecretory granules analogous to Kulchitsky cells, and small cells without specific features of differentiation (2,6,7). The epithelial cells are seated squarely upon a well-formed basal lamina covered with a finely granular surface coating, and are interconnected by desmosomes and apical junctional complexes (1,2,6). On scanning electron microscopy, the lining of the cyst is formed both of ciliated cells and nonciliated cells with bleb-like apical projections (7).

Differential Diagnosis. The macroscopic and radiographic characteristics of colloid cysts are so stereotypical that, with an adequate specimen, little consideration need be given to other entities. Although only scant epithelium may be observed in small specimens, its identification is usually sufficient for a diagnosis. The fragments of normal choroid plexus, often attached to the outer surface of the cyst, must not be interpreted as neoplastic (fig. 16-4). In contrast to the epithelium of colloid cyst, that of choroid plexus has a cobblestoned surface profile. It is not ciliated, mucin producing, or subject to pressure atrophy.

Treatment and Prognosis. Excision is curative. Incompletely resected, marsupialized, or aspirated cysts may slowly reform (9a).

Rathke Cleft Cyst

Definition. An intrasellar or suprasellar cyst lined by cuboidal to columnar epithelium.

General Comments. In embryologic terms, the adenohypophysis is derived from proliferating elements lining the cranial termination of the hypophyseal duct (13). As the duct regresses, its distal lumen remains a slit-like space which, within the substance of the pituitary, involutes to form a series of microcysts. Situated at the interface of the anterior and posterior lobes, these small hollow structures persist throughout life as Rathke cleft remnants or, when approaching macroscopic dimension, cysts of the intermediate lobe. On occasion, their symptomatic enlargement leads to the formation of a Rathke cleft cyst.

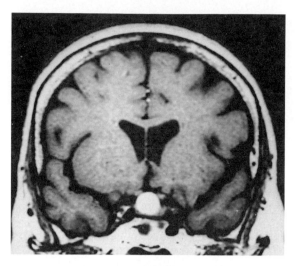

Figure 16-7
RATHKE CLEFT CYST
Rathke cleft cysts generate variable signal characteristics on magnetic resonance imaging. The white or "bright" T-1 signal in this case reflects its protein-rich cyst contents. The lesion involves both the sellar and suprasellar region.

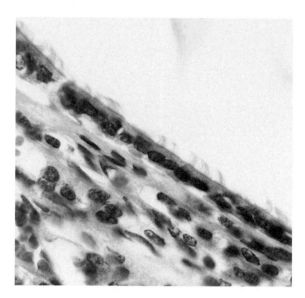

Figure 16-8
RATHKE CLEFT CYST
A delicate, highly ciliated columnar epithelium is characteristic of Rathke cleft cyst, but mucin-producing or endocrine cells may also be encountered.

Rare pituitary adenomas are accompanied by cysts with ciliated columnar epithelium identical in appearance to that of a Rathke cleft cyst (14,17,21,23). In some such cases, transitions have been reported between the cells of the cyst and those of the adenoma, thus suggesting that these are true transitional tumors reflecting the primordial potential of the hypophyseal duct to produce both hypophyseal and intermediate lobe cells. This entity, referred to as transitional cell tumor of the pituitary, remains controversial.

Clinical and Radiographic Features. Rathke cleft cysts are often incidental postmortem findings. Larger lesions, usually ones measuring 1 cm or more, are symptomatic, producing disturbances of vision or hypothalamic/pituitary function (22). Adults are most often affected.

Radiologically, Rathke cleft cysts vary considerably in their MRI appearance (18,22,22a). Although all are well-circumscribed intrasellar or suprasellar masses (22), some exhibit an extrasellar component. In one study, the signal intensity varied with the architectural lining and character of the cyst contents (18). Those lined by simple epithelium and containing clear fluid had a MRI density similar to cerebrospinal fluid, whereas those more solid or mucus-filled produced heterogeneous signal characteristics. Some, as a pre-

sumed consequence of high protein content, have a hyperintense (white) signal on nonenhanced T1-weighted images (fig. 16-7). In contrast to the adamantinomatous variant of craniopharyngioma, Rathke cleft cysts are not calcified.

Macroscopic Findings. Rathke cleft cysts are thin-walled structures with a content that varies considerably. In surgical specimens, the diagnostic epithelium may be elusive. It may be either fragmented and found in association with the mucoid content, or present as scant strips adherent to fragments of pituitary tissue. An occasional specimen consists largely, if not entirely, of mucin.

Microscopic Findings. In its native state, the classic lesion is composed of tall, well-differentiated columnar epithelium with both ciliated and goblet cells (fig. 16-8). Endocrine cells containing pituitary hormones may also be present in small number. Frequently, this typical pattern is altered by the presence of squamous metaplasia, presumably the product of proliferating reserve cells beneath the surface epithelium (fig. 16-9). In some instances, the metaplastic component predominates and the superficial columnar element becomes inconspicuous or undetectable. Like its close relative, the colloid cyst of the third

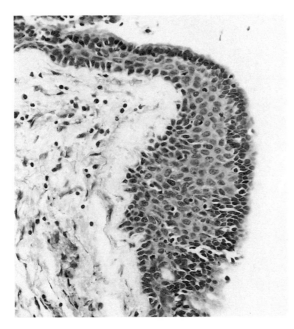

Figure 16-9
RATHKE CLEFT CYST
The columnar epithelium, best seen at the top of the illustration, is being lifted off the basement membrane by a proliferation of metaplastic squamous cells. (Courtesy of Dr. Robert L. Shelper, Iowa City, IA.)

ventricle, xanthomatous degeneration may predominate in some larger examples and obscure the epithelial nature of the lesion (24).

Cytology. The ciliated mucin-contained cells are readily seen in cytologic preparations (pl. IXC, p. 325).

Immunohistochemical Findings. The columnar cells are variably positive for cytokeratins and epithelial membrane antigen (15,16), as are proliferating or metaplastic squamous cells. Scattered endocrine cells, often containing one or several pituitary hormones, and chromogranin, may also be present (15). Reactivity for carcinoembryonic antigen has been reported (16,19a).

Ultrastructural Findings. As anticipated, highly differentiated ciliated and goblet cells with desmosomes and apical junctional complexes are seen (19). A deeper layer of basal and relatively undifferentiated cells is also present. As immunostains would suggest, scattered pale cells with secretory granules identical to those seen in the adenohypophysis are found in some cases. Squamous metaplasia adds cells exten-

sively interconnected by well-formed desmosomes and rich in tonofilament bundles.

Differential Diagnosis. The diagnosis is self-evident when well-differentiated columnar epithelium and mucin are found in a specimen from a discrete intrasellar or suprasellar cyst. Squamous metaplasia can confuse the issue, although not seriously, if its presence is viewed as a secondary or metaplastic change. In certain cases the metaplasia becomes so prominent as to obscure the columnar epithelium. The possible relationship of such squamous lesions to papillary craniopharyngioma is discussed in the previous chapter.

Treatment and Prognosis. Rathke cleft cysts are benign and are cured by excision, although partial removal and drainage may be sufficient (20,22).

Endodermal Cyst

Definition. A cyst lined by columnar epithelium of presumed endodermal derivation.

General Comments. Cysts lined by a simple columnar ciliated or goblet cell–containing epithelium have been variably designated as endodermal (34), enterogenous (43), neurenteric (28, 33,36,37), enterogenic (39), foregut (27), respiratory (42), bronchogenic (26,30,44), epithelial (29), epithelial-lined (38), or teratomatous (41). The term endodermal encompasses these geographically varied lesions which presumably arise from misplaced epithelium of the nasopharynx, respiratory tree, or intestinal tract. Endodermal lesions occur intracranially and throughout the length of the spinal column. Although analogous to colloid cyst and Rathke cleft cyst, we treat these as individual lesions, given their distinctive radiographic, clinical, and therapeutic aspects.

Clinical and Radiographic Features. Endodermal cysts occur at all ages. Many intraspinal lesions are accompanied by abnormalities of the spine anterior to the lesion. Uncommonly, such cysts connect with a cyst or with normal structures within the thorax or abdomen.

Macroscopic Findings. Most endodermal cysts are simple thin-walled sacs filled with gray-white viscous or mucoid material. They are usually intradural and extramedullary, although occasional lesions are intramedullary. Some intraspinal cysts are posterior to the spinal cord (33).

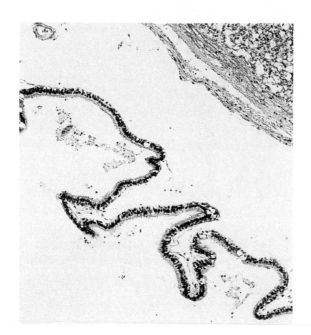
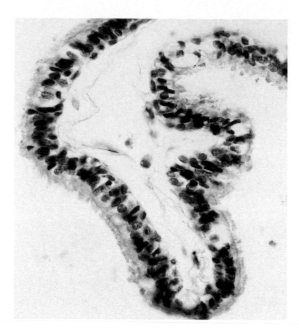

Figure 16-10
ENDODERMAL CYST
A leptomeningeal endodermal cyst in the basal leptomeninges is illustrated at low (left) and high (right) magnification. A high degree of differentiation and prominent cilia are evident on the right. (Courtesy of Dr. Robert L. Shelper, Iowa City, IA.)

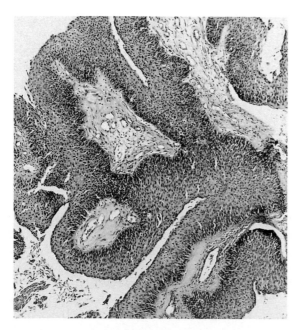

Figure 16-11
ENDODERMAL CYST
Extensive squamous metaplasia may be present in these cysts. (Courtesy of Dr. Robert L. Shelper, Iowa City, IA.)

Microscopic Findings. The most common form of endodermal cyst consists of a simple epithelium resting on a delicate fibrovascular capsule (fig. 16-10). Although columnar in its native state, the epithelium may be converted to a low cuboidal state by chronic pressure. Ciliation is a variable feature, but many cells contain globules of mucus. Squamous metaplasia is occasionally encountered as in the related Rathke cleft cyst (fig. 16-11) (26,34,42).

Certain endodermal cysts are more histologically intriguing in that they are convincing replicas of the respiratory or gastrointestinal tract. So-called "bronchogenic" lesions in the cervical region exhibit cartilaginous plates surrounding miniature "bronchi" with pseudostratified, ciliated, goblet cell–containing epithelium (30,44). Lesions reproducing the gastrointestinal tract are composed not only of gastric or intestinal mucosa but often possess a well-defined muscularis mucosa (32,35, 39,40). More complicated posterior lesions are associated with an overt embryologic abnormality, the split notochord syndrome (25).

Immunohistochemical Findings. The epithelial cells are typically reactive for epithelial membrane antigen, cytokeratin, and carcinoembryonic antigen (31,32a,34). Reactivity of some

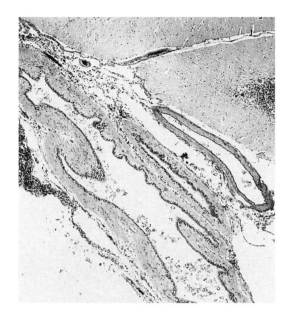
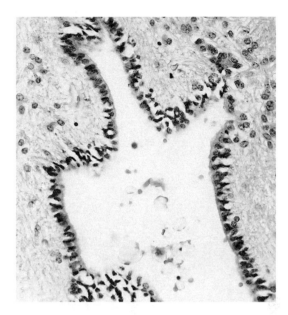

Figure 16-12
GLIOEPENDYMAL CYST
As seen at low (left) and high (right) magnification, this glioependymal cyst, which overlies the cerebellum, contains columnar epithelium resting upon a glial stroma. (Courtesy of Dr. Robert L. Shelper, Iowa City, IA.)

cells for S-100 protein has also been noted and underscores the similarity between endodermal cyst and colloid cyst of the third ventricle (31,34).

Ultrastructural Findings. Ultrastructural studies disclose an epithelium with ciliated cells, nonciliated goblet cells, and, in the case of bronchogenic-type cysts, neuroendocrine cells (Kulchitsky cells) as well as cartilage. The ultrastructural features of most endodermal cysts are essentially those of colloid cysts of the third ventricle (29,30). A surface coating of granulofibrillar material, a typical feature of endoderm, may be seen also (30,36,37). Fine "claw-like" projections from the tips of cilia have also been noted, as they have in other types of ciliated epithelia (36).

Differential Diagnosis. The presence of a well-differentiated epithelium abutting brain or spinal cord parenchyma understandably prompts consideration of a neuroectodermal cyst, e.g., ependymal cyst. Most lesions with abundant cilia or mucus-containing cells can be relegated to the neurenteric category on the basis of their microscopic appearance alone. While immunoreactivity for epithelial membrane antigen may be seen in ependyma and cytokeratins in choroid plexus epithelium, reactivity for both is indicative of enterogenous cyst. Conceptually, some

ependymal cysts contain some cells positive for glial fibrillary acidic protein (GFAP), whereas choroid plexus epithelium tends to show S-100, transthyretin, and vimentin staining.

Treatment and Prognosis. These slow-growing malformative lesions are cured by simple excision.

Ependymal (Glioependymal) Cyst

The increasing perception that simple ciliated or goblet cell–containing intracranial or intraspinal cysts are endodermal rather than ependymal in nature has tightened the diagnostic criteria for the latter. The diagnosis of ependymal cyst is appropriate for benign intraparenchymal, and often paraventricular, cysts with a ciliated epithelial lining (45–47,49) or for leptomeningeal cysts with a similar epithelium as long as both rest directly upon brain parenchyma or a layer of astroglia rather than a basement membrane and connective tissue (fig. 16-12) (48). Cysts remote from the ventricular system or lacking a direct astroglial interface are now largely assigned to the endodermal category. This seems especially appropriate if the epithelium demonstrates squamous metaplasia or, ultrastructurally, a fine apical surface coating.

361

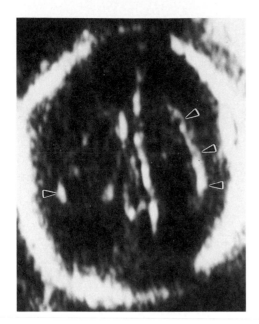

Figure 16-13
CHOROID PLEXUS CYST
Hypoechoic areas are common within the choroid plexus of the normal developing fetus. Uncommonly, and usually in patients with chromosomal defects, such lesions persist postnatally as symptomatic masses (arrows).

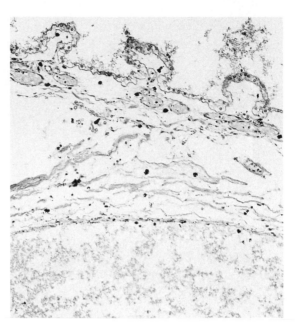

Figure 16-14
CHOROID PLEXUS CYST
The cyst illustrated in figure 16-13 is filled with granular material. No distinct epithelial lining is present. Choroid plexus epithelium is seen at the top of the illustration.

Choroid Plexus Cysts

Small cysts of the choroid plexus lined by a cuboidal epithelium are occasionally encountered as incidental postmortem findings. Symptomatic lesions are rare (53,54,56). The lining of reported cysts has varied from connective tissue to columnar epithelium. The lining of those with choroid plexus–type epithelium is understandably positive for transthyretin (prealbumin) (55).

A presumably distinct form of choroid plexus cyst is commonly encountered in utero as a hypoechoic focus which usually resolves spontaneously by birth (50,51). Histopathologic studies of these common lesions are few but those reported record the presence of a loose stroma surrounding a cyst without an epithelial lining (52), technically removing these lesions from the true cyst category. Markedly flattened cells can be found around the cyst but it is not clear whether these represent compressed epithelium or simply fibroblasts. Other cysts discovered during prenatal ultrasonography are associated with chromosomal defects (trisomy 18) and congenital malformations (figs. 16-13, 16-14).

Epidermoid and Dermoid Cysts

Definition. Cysts lined by benign keratinizing squamous epithelium. Cutaneous adnexa are present in the dermoid cyst.

Clinical and Radiographic Features. Epidermoid cysts occur throughout the neuraxis, but most are intracranial and lie within the cerebellopontine angle (fig. 16-15) (70). Intraspinal examples are less common (68). Because these cysts tend to surround and envelop, rather than displace, regional structures, symptoms typically occur late in the course when the cyst has attained considerable size. Epidermoid cysts may also arise in the cranial diploë where they present as a lytic defect with a sclerotic margin.

Due to the discrete nature of epidermoid cysts, their extra-axial position, and the neuroradiologic signal characteristics of keratinous debris, a confident preoperative diagnosis is often made. Depending upon the amount of lipid, the lesions exhibit a variable signal by MRI, appearing in T1-weighted images as either bright or white (when lipid content is high) or black (if lipid content is low) (fig. 16-15) (63). Although most epidermoid cysts have presumed developmental

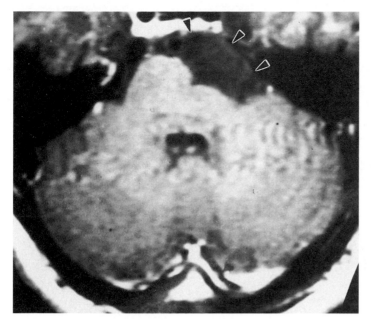

Figure 16-15
EPIDERMOID CYST
In this T1-weighted magnetic resonance image, the epidermoid cyst is the dark mass (arrows) compressing the pons.

origins, the transfer of fragments of cutaneous epithelium to the subarachnoid space during diagnostic procedures such as lumbar puncture has been implicated in the pathogenesis of rare intraspinal and intracranial examples (58,62).

Dermoid cysts are more restricted than epidermoid cysts in terms of patient age and location. Most present in childhood and lie in the midline, being related to a fontanelle, the fourth ventricle, or the spinal canal (66). In some, a sinus tract from the cutaneous surface provides a potential portal of entry for infectious organisms (65).

The hair and sebaceous content of a dermoid cyst give it a heterogeneous MRI signal, but the abundant lipid produces a high signal intensity in T1-weighted images (57,61,69). Rupture of both dermoid and epidermoid cysts can produce chemical meningitis (67,69).

Macroscopic Findings. The uniloculate thin-walled epidermoid cyst has an unmistakable pearly quality due to its thin wall and compact contents of keratin (fig. 16-16). The connective tissue–rich wall of the dermoid cyst is thicker, and its greasy, rather than flaky, content is often matted with hair.

Microscopic Findings. Microscopically, the overwhelming bulk of an epidermoid cyst consists of the layered anucleate squames produced by its thin, well-differentiated squamous epithelium. Keratohyaline granules are seen (fig. 16-17).

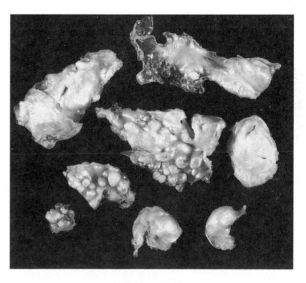

Figure 16-16
EPIDERMOID CYST
As surgical specimens, epidermoid cysts are commonly received as multiple fragments with a typical "mother-of-pearl" sheen.

The often irregularly thickened wall of the dermoid cyst is essentially dermis with adnexal structures such as hair follicles and sebaceous glands and supportive fibroadipose tissue (fig. 16-18). Mature bone is present in some cases. A foreign body reaction to the cyst contents is not infrequent.

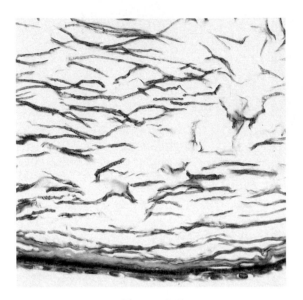

Figure 16-17
EPIDERMOID CYST
A remarkably thin, well-differentiated squamous epithelium generates the anucleate squames that are largely responsible for the lesion's mass.

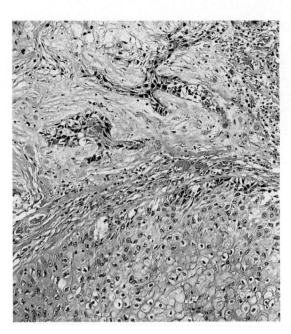

Figure 16-19
EPIDERMOID CYST
WITH MALIGNANT DEGENERATION
Malignant degeneration is rare in epidermoid cysts.

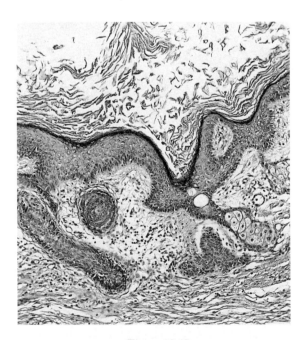

Figure 16-18
DERMOID CYST
The wall of this dermoid cyst is cutaneous-type epithelium with hair follicles and sebaceous glands.

Immunohistochemical Findings. The lining epithelium of both epidermoid and dermoid cysts is immunoreactive for cytokeratins and epithelial membrane antigen. The immunophenotypes of the adnexa in dermoid cysts are similar to those of their cutaneous counterparts.

Malignant Degeneration. Although epidermoid and dermoid cysts are benign, rare transformation to squamous carcinoma has been reported for both (fig. 16-19) (59,60,64).

Differential Diagnosis. In most locations, the epidermoid cyst is so distinctive that no troublesome diagnostic issues arise. In the suprasellar region, the practical distinction between this cyst and craniopharyngioma must be addressed, but is largely a semantic rather than practical problem since the delicate epithelium of epidermoid cysts is readily distinguished from the thicker, complex, and palisaded growth pattern of adamantinomatous craniopharyngioma. In addition, light microscopically apparent keratohyaline granules are limited to epidermoid cysts. The extensive secondary inflammatory reaction, cholesterol cleft formation, calcification, and machinery oil content typical of

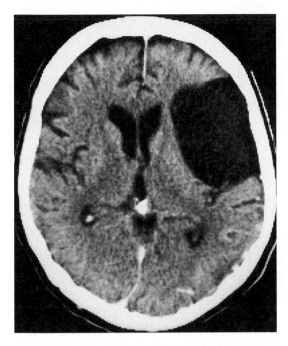

Figure 16-20
ARACHNOID CYST
The cerebrospinal fluid density of the arachnoid cyst illustrated in figure 16-21 is evident in this CT scan. Note the minimal mass effect despite the lesion's large size. (Courtesy of Dr. Donald P. Mueller, Iowa City, IA.)

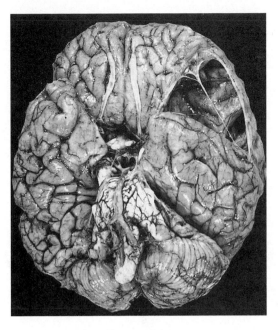

Figure 16-21
ARACHNOID CYST
Arachnoid cysts most commonly arise near the Sylvian fissure. Although the adjacent brain is indented there is little shift of midline structures. (Courtesy of Dr. Michael N. Hart, Iowa City, IA.)

adamantinomatous craniopharyngiomas are lacking in epidermoid cysts. The epithelium of the often solid papillary craniopharyngioma is well differentiated and squamous, but is generally thick and disposed in crude papillae with fibrovascular cores. Despite its high degree of differentiation, surface maturation in papillary craniopharyngiomas does not generally progress to the formation of anucleate squames, and certainly not to the extent that these hypermature elements are formed in epidermoid cysts.

A related differential diagnosis includes an endodermal or Rathke cleft cyst that has undergone extensive squamous metaplasia. These lack the generation of squames typical of the epidermoid cyst and the adnexa of the dermoid cyst. In addition, scattered residual columnar cells are usually present on the surface.

In concept, dermoid cysts must be distinguished from well-differentiated teratomas, such as those arising in the sellar and pineal regions. Dermoid cysts lack endodermal components or highly specialized mesenchyme such as muscle.

Treatment and Prognosis. Many epidermoid and dermoid cysts lend themselves to gross total excision. In some instances, however, the cysts cling to vital structures such as cranial nerves and major blood vessels, thus frustrating attempts at total resection. Cystic recurrences can result (70).

Arachnoid Cyst

Definition. A loculated collection of cerebrospinal fluid within a non-neoplastic reduplication of the arachnoidal membrane.

Clinical and Radiographic Features. Arachnoid cysts arise within both the cranial and spinal meninges, although the subarachnoid space in the region of the temporal lobe is a favored site (71,74). Large cysts in the latter location necessarily expand at the expense of the adjacent brain, thus producing a largely spherical indentation (figs. 16-20, 16-21). Some are symptomatic mass lesions whereas others are incidental postmortem findings. Curiously, many sizable arachnoid cysts are not associated with herniation or displacement of midbrain structures, leading to controversy

365

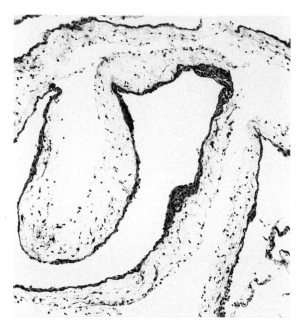

Figure 16-22
ARACHNOID CYST
Arachnoid cysts are lined by meningothelial cells focally aggregated into small clusters.

over whether the basic lesion is a cyst displacing the brain or a regional agenesis of the brain, with the defect passively filled by a compensatory expansion of the adjacent subarachnoid space. Comparison of the weights and volumes of the indented and nonindented hemispheres suggests that there is no agenesis (74,75).

Radiographically, the cerebrospinal fluid content is clearly seen by either computerized tomography (CT) or MRI, and can be easily distinguished from the solid, lipid-rich, keratinous or sebaceous debris of an epidermoid or dermoid cyst.

Macroscopic Findings. The watery content of an arachnoid cyst is readily seen through its delicate translucent wall. When the wall is punctured, the contents spill to expose the flattened gyri of the adjacent brain. Thereafter, the delicate membrane may be hard to find, its thin substance being almost inapparent.

Microscopic Findings. The wall of an arachnoid cyst consists of a delicate fibrous connective tissue membrane to which a thin layer of meningothelial cells is closely applied (fig. 16-22) (73,76).

Immunohistochemical Findings. The nature of the lining can be established by immunoreactivity for epithelial membrane antigen. As expected, the cysts are negative for markers found in other intracranial and intraspinal cysts such as GFAP, carcinoembryonic antigen, and transthyretin (72).

Treatment and Prognosis. Symptoms are relieved by release of the trapped fluid.

Pineal Cyst

Since they may be confused with pineocytomas, pineal cysts are described in chapter 6.

Nerve Root Cyst

Non-neoplastic meningeal diverticula that occur principally about the roots of the lower spinal cord are described either as nerve root cysts or as perineural cysts. The eponym Tarlov cyst has gained popularity (77–79). The lesions are generally of no clinical significance and are detected as incidental radiologic or surgical findings; only a minority produce pain (77a,80). The cysts consist of arachnoidal diverticulum free of inflammation. Occasional lesions that require decompression are effectively cured.

Synovial Cyst of Spine

Synovial cysts, sometimes referred to as *ganglion cysts*, are common intradural/extramedullary lesions, particularly at the L4-L5 level where they are associated with degenerative joint disease (81–83). Such cysts can also occur in the cervical region. The lesions are similar in their clinical presentation to the far more common herniated disc. Radiologically, they have a low density center and a denser fibrotic and sometimes calcified rim.

Macroscopically, a fibrous tissue capsule surrounds the contents of gelatinous fluid. Microscopically, the specimen is characterized only by fibrous connective tissue without an epithelial lining. Excision is curative.

Other Cysts

Uncommon cysts that defy ready classification include intraparenchymal ones without an epithelial lining (85,89), radiographically lucent lesions in the medial temporal lobe along the choroidal fissure (88), and a thick-walled sac protruding from the spinal dura, in essence a dural meningocele (84,86,87,90).

REFERENCES

Colloid Cyst of the Third Ventricle

1. Hirano A, Ghatak NR. The fine structure of colloid cysts of the third ventricle. J Neuropathol Exp Neurol 1974;33:333–41.
2. Ho KL, Garcia JH. Colloid cysts of the third ventricle: ultrastructural features are compatible with endodermal derivation. Acta Neuropathol (Berl) 1992;83:605–12.
3. Inoue T, Matsushima T, Fukui M, Iwaki T, Takeshita I, Kuromatsu C. Immunohistochemical study of intracranial cysts. Neurosurgery 1988;23:576–81.
4. Kondziolka D, Bilbao JM. An immunohistochemical study of neuroepithelial (colloid) cysts. J Neurosurg 1989;71:91–7.
5. Lach B, Scheithauer BW. Colloid cyst of the third ventricle: a comparative ultrastructural study of neuraxis cysts and choroid plexus epithelium. Ultrastruct Pathol 1992;16:331–49.
6. _____, Scheithauer BW, Gregor A, Wick MR. Colloid cyst of the third ventricle: a comparative immunohistochemical study of neuraxis cysts and choroid plexus epithelium. J Neurosurg 1993;78:101–11.
7. Leech RW, Freeman T, Johnson R. Colloid cyst of the third ventricle. A scanning and transmission electron microscopic study. J Neurosurg 1982;57:108–13.
8. MacKenzie IR, Gilbert JJ. Cysts of the neuraxis of endodermal origin. J Neurol Neurosurg Psychiatry 1991;54:572–5.
9. Maeder PP, Holtas SL, Basibüyük LN, Salford LG, Tapper UA, Brun A. Colloid cysts of the third ventricle: correlation of MR and CT findings with histology and chemical analysis. AJNR Am J Neuroradiol 1990;11:575–81.
9a. Mathiesen T, Grane P, Lindquist C, von Holst H. High recurrence rate following aspiration of colloid cysts in the third ventricle. J Neurosurg 1993;78:748–52.
10. Montaldi S, Deruaz JP, Cai ZT, de Tribolet N. Symptomatic xanthogranuloma of the third ventricle: report of two cases and review of the literature. Surg Neurol 1989;32:200–5.
11. Powers JM, Dodds HM. Primary actinomycoma of the third ventricle—the colloid cyst. A histochemical and ultrastructural study. Acta Neuropathol (Berl) 1977;37:21–6.
12. Shuangshoti S, Phonprasert C, Suwanwela N, Netsky MG. Combined neuroepithelial (colloid) cyst and xanthogranuloma (xanthoma) in the third ventricle. Neurology 1975;25:547–52.

Rathke Cleft Cyst

13. Ikeda H, Suzuki J, Sasano N, Niizuma H. The development and morphogenesis of the human pituitary gland. Anat Embryol (Berl) 1988;178:327–36.
14. _____, Yoshimoto T, Katakura R. A case of Rathke's cleft cyst within a pituitary adenoma presenting with acromegaly—do "transitional cell tumors of the pituitary gland" really exist? Acta Neuropathol (Berl) 1992;83:211–5.
15. _____, Yoshimoto T, Suzuki J. Immunohistochemical study of Rathke's cleft cyst. Acta Neuropathol (Berl) 1988;77:33–8.
16. Inoue T, Matsushima T, Fukui M, Iwaki T, Takeshita I, Kuromatsu C. Immunohistochemical study of intracranial cysts. Neurosurgery 1988;23:576–81.
17. Kepes JJ. Transitional cell tumor of the pituitary gland developing from a Rathke's cleft cyst. Cancer 1978;41:337–43.
18. Kucharczyk W, Peck WW, Kelly WM, Norman D, Newton TH. Rathke cleft cysts: CT, MR imaging, and pathologic features. Radiology 1987;165:491–5.
19. Lach B, Scheithauer BW. Colloid cyst of the third ventricle: a comparative ultrastructural study of neuraxis cysts and choroid plexus epithelium. Ultrastruct Pathol 1992;16:331–49.
19a. _____, Scheithauer BW, Gregor A, Wick MR. Colloid cyst of the third ventricle: a comparative immunohistochemical study of neuraxis cysts and choroid plexus epithelium. J Neurosurg 1993;78:101–11.
20. Midha R, Jay V, Smyth HS. Transsphenoidal management of Rathke's cleft cysts. A clinicopathological review of 10 cases. Surg Neurol 1991;35:446–54.
21. Nishio S, Mizuno J, Barrow DL, Takei Y, Tindall GT. Pituitary tumors composed of adenohypophysial adenoma and Rathke's cleft cyst elements: a clinicopathological study. Neurosurgery 1987;21:371–7.
22. Ross DA, Norman D, Wilson CB. Radiologic characteristics and results of surgical management of Rathke's cysts in 43 patients. Neurosurgery 1992;30:173–9.
22a. Sumida M, Uozumi T, Mukada K, Arita K, Kurisu K, Eguchi K. Rathke cleft cysts: correlation of enhanced MR and surgical findings. AJNR Am J Neuroradiol 1994;15:525–32.
23. Swanson SE, Chandler WF, Latack J, Zis K. Symptomatic Rathke's cleft cyst with pituitary adenoma: case report. Neurosurgery 1985;17:657–9.
24. Wolfsohn AL, Lach B, Benoit BG. Suprasellar xanthomatous Rathke's cleft cyst. Surg Neurol 1992;38:106–9.

Endodermal Cyst

25. Bentley JF, Smith JR. Developmental posterior enteric remnants and spinal malformations. The split notochord syndrome. Arch Dis Child 1960;35:476–86.
26. Del Bigio MR, Jay V, Drake JM. Prepontine cyst lined by respiratory epithelium with squamous metaplasia: immunohistochemical and ultrastructural study. Acta Neuropathol (Berl) 1992;83:564–8.
27. Dorsey JF, Tabrisky J. Intraspinal and mediastinal foregut cyst compressing the spinal cord. Report of a case. J Neurosurg 1966;24:562–7.
28. Harris CP, Dias MS, Brockmeyer DL, Townsend JJ, Willis BK, Apfelbaum RI. Neurenteric cysts of the posterior fossa: recognition, management, and embryogenesis. Neurosurgery 1991;29:893–8.

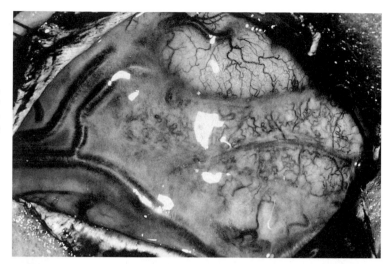

Figure 17-6
MENINGIOANGIOMATOSIS
As seen at surgery, the occasionally prominent surface vascularity of this lesion may suggest a vascular malformation. Upon dissection, the intracortical plaque-like lesion was firm and discrete.

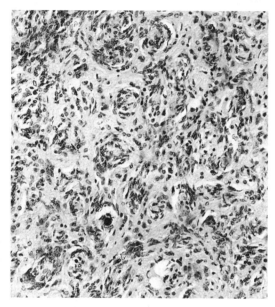

Figure 17-7
MENINGIOANGIOMATOSIS
Psammoma bodies within some examples lend a decidedly meningothelial appearance.

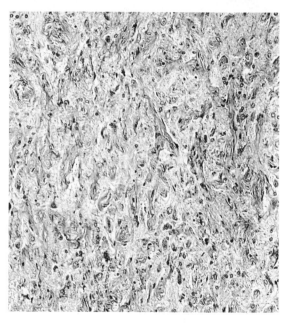

Figure 17-8
MENINGIOANGIOMATOSIS
Some examples are largely sclerotic and exhibit vascular thickening which encroaches on the surrounding parenchyma.

lesions, the connective tissue element becomes more prominent and large bands of dense collagen, with or without associated meningothelial cells, entrap and encroach upon islands of distorted parenchyma (fig. 17-8). Such lesions may be heavily calcified and more fibrous than meningiomatous or angiomatous. Neurons within or immediately around the lesion may demonstrate neurofibrillary tangles or even granulovacuolar degeneration. Osseous metaplasia may be seen in advanced lesions (fig. 17-9).

In some cases, the cortical component of meningioangiomatosis is associated with an overlying densely calcified mass in the leptomeninges (fig. 17-10) (16). When positioned within a sulcus, some of these "rocks" may appear partially buried within the substance of the brain. The same markedly calcified meningeal nodule appears in other patients as an ostensibly isolated finding without a recognizable underlying meningioangiomatous plaque (fig. 17-11). It is not clear whether such lesions are separate entities unrelated to meningioangiomatosis or whether a subjacent meningioangiomatous component is undetected. It seems unlikely that such a component is missed in all cases since the calcified meningeal lesions often occur in adults without any past history to suggest meningioangiomatosis. MRI studies may help resolve this issue by documenting the presence or absence of a meningioangiomatous focus in the cortex below these calcified leptomeningeal nodules.

The densely calcified nodules have a curious microscopic appearance resembling a cross between a gouty tophus, osteoma, and rheumatoid nodule (fig. 17-12). It is not surprising that they have been variably designated as "unusual fibro-osseous lesions" (14,17,19) and "calcifying pseudotumors of the neuraxis" (13). It is not clear whether all of these lesions represent the same entity, since some occur extra-axially (13).

Immunohistochemical Findings. Meningothelial cells exhibit reactivity for epithelial membrane antigen (EMA) and may, to a lesser

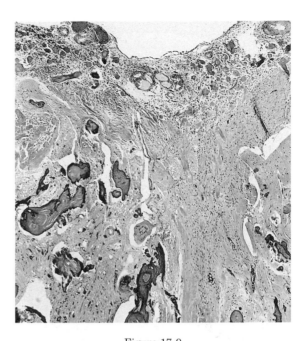

Figure 17-9
MENINGIOANGIOMATOSIS
Dense connective tissue and extensive osseous metaplasia may be noted in longstanding examples.

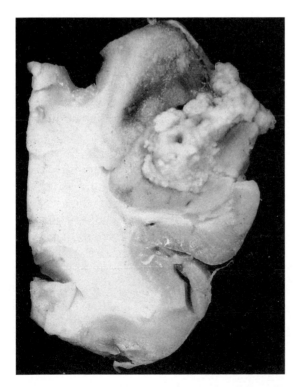 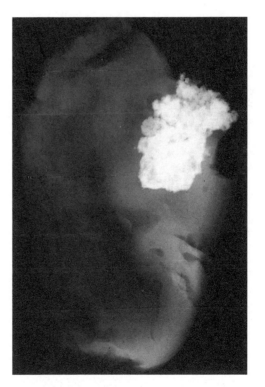

Figure 17-10
MENINGIOANGIOMATOSIS
The cortical lesions of meningioangiomatosis (left) are, in some instances, associated with an overlying, hard, densely calcified mass (right).

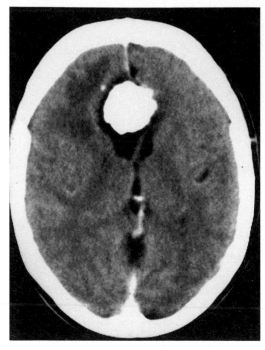

Figure 17-11
CALCIFIED LEPTOMENINGEAL LESION

Calcified leptomeningeal lesions such as that illustrated in figure 17-10, right can occur without a recognized underlying cortical plaque.

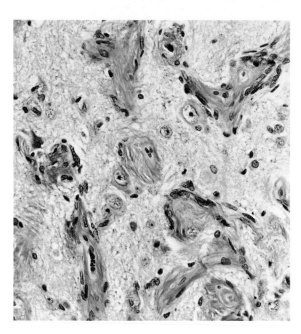

Figure 17-13
MENINGIOANGIOMATOSIS

Preexisting neurons trapped by the intricate vasculature should not be interpreted as those of a ganglion cell neoplasm, nor should the hyalinized vessels be misconstrued as evidence of a vascular malformation.

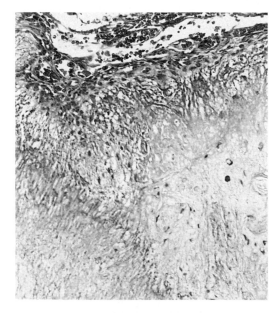

Figure 17-12
CALCIFIED LEPTOMENINGEAL LESION

Microscopically, the distinctive calcific mass noted in figure 17-11 consists of paucicellular, somewhat fibrillar tissue with an ill-defined fibro-chondro-myxoid appearance. Peripheral palisading creates a distinctive appearance.

extent, show S-100 or cytokeratin positivity. Reactivity for EMA is scant or absent in cases in which the cells are more spindled and fibroblastic than meningothelial (15).

Ultrastructural Findings. The meningothelial nature of the cortical perivascular proliferation is evidenced by cellular interdigitation, scattered cytoplasmic intermediate filaments, and well-formed desmosomes. Paired helical filaments may fill the trapped or adjacent neurons with neurofibrillary change (15,16).

Differential Diagnosis. In a large well-oriented specimen, the meningothelial/fibroblastic character of the intracortical lesion is readily apparent and the diagnosis depends only on recognition of the entity. In smaller specimens, particularly the more collagenized examples, a diagnosis is more difficult and one must consider the possibility of another slow-growing and often calcified epileptogenic mass, the ganglion cell tumor (fig. 17-13) (see Appendix A). An invasive meningioma also becomes a suspect if meningothelial cells are prominent. Vascular malformation is an additional diagnostic possibility. In contrast to meningioangiomatosis, ganglion cell tumors are generally less collagenized, contain clearly abnormal neurons, and do not demonstrate intracortical meningothelial cells. Interestingly, both of these chronic lesions may be associated with neurofibrillary tangles. In very small specimens, a nonspecific fibrotic lesion is a possibility.

Treatment and Prognosis. Most cases of meningioangiomatosis have been cured by surgical resection (16). Seizures may persist if surgical attention is given only to the superficial calcified nodule.

REFERENCES

Hypothalamic Hamartoma

1. Albright AL, Lee PA. Neurosurgical treatment of hypothalamic hamartomas causing precocious puberty. J Neurosurg 1993;78:77–82.
1a. Asa SL, Scheithauer BW, Bilbao JM, et al. A case for hypothalamic acromegaly: a clinicopathologic study of six patients with hypothalamic gangliocytomas producing growth hormone-releasing factors. J Clin Endocrinol Metab 1984;58:796–803.
2. Berkovic SF, Andermann F, Melanson D, Ethier RE, Feindel W, Gloor P. Hypothalamic hamartomas and ictal laughter: evolution of a characteristic epileptic syndrome and diagnostic value of magnetic resonance imaging. Ann Neurol 1988;23:429–39.
3. Boyko OB, Curnes JT, Oakes WJ, Burger PC. Hamartomas of the tuber cinereum: CT, MR, and pathologic findings. AJNR Am J Neuroradiol 1991;12:309–14.
4. Nishio S, Fujiwara S, Aiko Y, Takeshita I, Fukui M. Hypothalamic hamartoma. Report of two cases. J Neurosurg 1989;70:640–5.
5. Sato M, Ushio Y, Arita N, Mogami H. Hypothalamic hamartoma: report of two cases. Neurosurgery 1985; 16:198–206.
6. Sherwin RP, Grassi JE, Sommers SC. Hamartomatous malformation of the posterolateral hypothalamus. Lab Invest 1962;11:89–97.

Nasal Cerebral Heterotopia ("Nasal Glioma")

7. Barkovich AJ, Vandermarck P, Edwards MS, Cogen PH. Congenital nasal masses: CT and MR imaging features in 16 cases. AJNR Am J Neuroradiol 1991;12:105–16.
8. Bossen EH, Hudson WR. Oligodendroglioma arising in heterotopic brain tissue of the soft palate and nasopharynx. Am J Surg Pathol 1987;11:571–4.
9. Gorenstein A, Kern EB, Facer GW, Laws ER Jr. Nasal gliomas. Arch Otolaryngol 1980;106:536–40.
10. Kindblom LG, Angervall L, Haglid K. An immunohistochemical analysis of S-100 protein and glial fibrillary acidic protein in nasal glioma. Acta Pathol Microbiol Immunol Scand [A] 1984;92:387–9.
11. Mirra SS, Pearl GS, Hoffman JC, Campbell WG Jr. Nasal "glioma" with prominent neuronal component. Report of a case. Arch Pathol Lab Med 1981;105:540–1.
12. Patterson K, Kapur S, Chandra RS. "Nasal gliomas" and related brain heterotopias: a pathologist's perspective. Pediatr Pathol 1986;5:353–62.

Meningioangiomatosis

13. Bertoni F, Unni KK, Dahlin DC, Beabout JW, Onofrio BM. Calcifying pseudo-neoplasms of the neural axis. J Neurosurg 1990;72:42–8.
14. Garen PD, Powers JM, King JS, Perot PL Jr. Intracranial fibro-osseous lesion: case report. J Neurosurg 1989; 70:475–7.
15. Goates JJ, Dickson DW, Horoupian DS. Meningioangiomatosis: an immunocytochemical study. Acta Neuropathol (Berl) 1991;82:527–32.
16. Halper J, Scheithauer BW, Okazaki H, Laws ER Jr. Meningioangiomatosis: a report of six cases with special reference to the occurrence of neurofibrillary tangles. J Neuropathol Exp Neurol 1986;45:426–46.
17. Jun C, Burdick B. An unusual fibro-osseous lesion of the brain: case report. J Neurosurg 1984;60:1308–11.
18. Ogilvy CS, Chapman PH, Gray M, de la Monte SM. Meningioangiomatosis in a patient without von Recklinghausen's disease: case report. J Neurosurg 1989; 70:483–5.
19. Rhodes RH, Davis RL. An unusual fibro-osseous component in intracranial lesions. Hum Pathol 1978; 9:309–19.
20. Tien RD, Osumi A, Oakes JW, Madden JF, Burger PC. Meningioangiomatosis: CT and MR findings. J Comput Assist Tomogr 1992;16:361–5.

18

DYSGENETIC SYNDROMES

NEUROFIBROMATOSIS (VON RECKLINGHAUSEN DISEASE)

This important genetic disorder occurs in two somewhat overlapping but generally distinct clinicopathologic variants: neurofibromatosis 1 and 2. The term von Recklinghausen disease is often used, especially for neurofibromatosis 1.

Neurofibromatosis 1

Neurofibromatosis 1, the peripheral variant, is inherited in an autosomal dominant fashion from a locus on chromosome 17 (2). A high rate of spontaneous mutation adds to the genetic pool of this disease making it a common disorder. The complex includes café-au-lait spots, axillary freckling, multiple cutaneous neurofibromas, neurofibromas of spinal nerve roots, plexiform neurofibromas, localized hypertrophic neuropathy, pigmented iris hamartomas (Lisch nodules), and a variety of intracranial and intraorbital gliomas. Other features include skeletal changes such as scoliosis and thoracic meningomyelocele (12,14,15).

Lisch nodules are pigmented melanocytic neoplasms of the iris whose incidence increases with age. In one series they appeared in all individuals by the age of 21 years (10). Intraspinal nerve root tumors are common and consist of neurofibromas (fig. 18-1). In neurofibromatosis 2, by contrast, the peripheral nerve tumors at this site are schwannomas (see fig. 18-4) (5a,6). Gliomas in neurofibromatosis 1 are usually pilocytic astrocytomas of the visual system and are often bilateral (8,16–18). These same lesions also affect the hypothalamus, brain stem, thalamus, cerebellum, cerebrum, and the spinal cord. Less often seen are diffuse fibrillary astrocytomas or astrocytomas of varying histologic grade (3,8). Magnetic resonance imaging (MRI) studies have demonstrated foci of high signal intensity in T2-weighted images throughout much of the nervous system; the significance of these sometimes transient lesions is unclear (1,4,11a,20a,20b,21).

Of the peripheral neurofibromas, the plexiform type is the best known and is considered pathognomonic of the syndrome. This neoplasm produces unmistakable ropy enlargement of large nerve roots, trunks, and their branches, and may also affect small nerves such as those of the skin. Separate status is given a segmental variant of neurofibromatosis in which the neurofibromas are confined to one extremity or body region (5,13). A small proportion of peripheral neurofibromas, particularly those of plexiform type, undergo malignant transformation. The resulting malignant peripheral nerve sheath tumors (MPNSTs) are high-grade aggressive neoplasms.

An unusual central nervous system lesion in some cases of neurofibromatosis 1 is the subependymal nodule (fig. 18-2). Composed of elongated glial cells, this minute asymptomatic excrescence generally projects into the lateral ventricles. In the narrow confines of the Sylvian aqueduct such a nodule can obstruct the flow of cerebrospinal fluid and produce hydrocephalus (16,18).

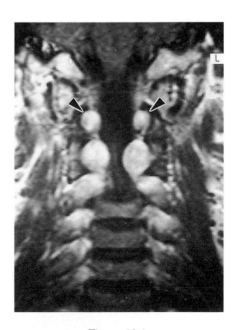

Figure 18-1
NEUROFIBROMATOSIS 1
Beginning at the C2-C3 level, multiple white contrast-enhancing neurofibromas impinge on the spinal cord of this 10-year-old boy. A histologic section from a similar lesion in another patient with neurofibromatosis 1 is shown in figure 10-19. (Courtesy of Dr. Steven N. Breiter, Baltimore, MD.)

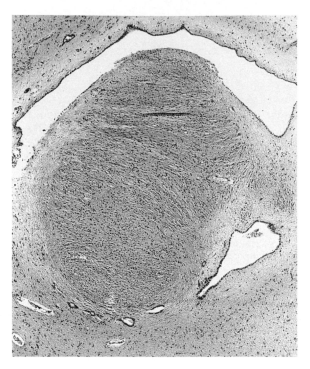

Figure 18-2
NEUROFIBROMATOSIS 1
Subependymal nodules of elongated glia are occasionally encountered. Lesions such as this example in the aqueduct of Sylvius may obstruct the flow of cerebrospinal fluid and produce hydrocephalus.

Neurofibromatosis 2

The central variant of neurofibromatosis is an autosomal dominant disorder linked to chromosome 22 (20). It is considerably less common than neurofibromatosis 1. It is classically noted for multiple schwannomas of cranial and spinal nerves (figs. 18-3, 18-4) (9,11,12,14,15,18). Bilateral acoustic nerve tumors are typical, but schwannomas of other cranial nerves, particularly the trigeminal, also occur. Intraspinal schwannomas are frequent and usually affect multiple dorsal roots (fig. 18-4) (5a,6). Completing the spectrum of this syndrome are multiple meningiomas (fig. 18-5) and multiple spinal cord ependymomas (16,18). Associated vascular abnormalities include aneurysms and arteriovenous fistulae (19).

Given the genetic abnormality in neurofibromatosis, it is not surprising that systematic microscopic study of the central nervous system expands the spectrum of lesions occurring in this disorder (16,18). This includes proliferations of Schwann cells in spinal roots (schwannomatosis) (fig. 18-6), aberrant clusters of ependymal cells in the spinal cord, and, most typically, minute clusters of pleomorphic amitotic cells resembling glial heterotopias within cerebral gray matter

Figure 18-3
NEUROFIBROMATOSIS 2
Bilateral schwannomas are readily apparent in this patient. The schwannoma on the left is encased by a plaque-like meningioma.

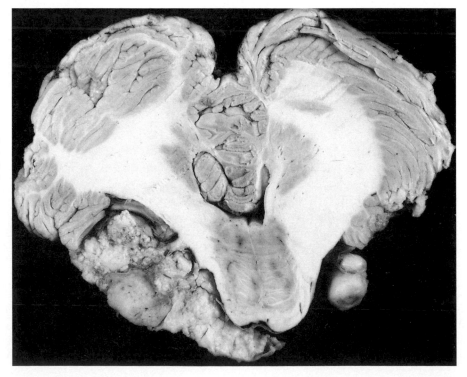

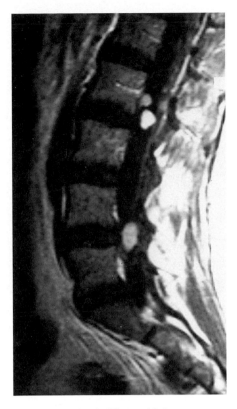

Figure 18-4
NEUROFIBROMATOSIS 2

As seen in this contrast-enhanced MRI, multiple bright intradural-extramedullary schwannomas are common in this dysgenetic disorder. (Courtesy of Dr. Roland Lee, Baltimore, MD.)

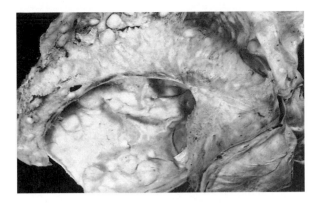

Figure 18-5
NEUROFIBROMATOSIS 2

Multiple meningiomas are common in advanced stages of this genetic disorder.

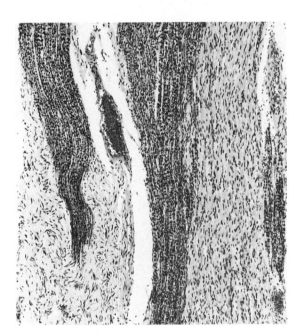

Figure 18-6
NEUROFIBROMATOSIS 2

Multiple focal proliferations of Schwann cells are commonly encountered within intraspinal nerve roots. The dark tissues in this H&E/Luxol fast blue stained section are the roots formed of myelinated nerve fibers. The lighter areas are the Schwann cell proliferations.

(fig. 18-7). The eosinophilic cytoplasm of the cells within these foci suggests an astrocytic derivation, but the cells are generally negative for glial fibrillary acidic protein (GFAP). Reactivity for S-100 protein has been noted (22).

Meningioangiomatosis may be associated with neurofibromatosis 2, as is discussed in chapter 17 (7,23).

OTHER DYSGENETIC SYNDROMES

Von Hippel-Lindau Syndrome

In its consummate form, this complex syndrome consists of hemangioblastomas of the central nervous system (CNS) (fig. 18-8) including the optic nerve and retina (figs. 18-9, 18-10) (27, 30a); renal cell carcinoma; pheochromocytoma; cysts or cystadenomas of the kidneys, liver, pancreas, and epididymis; and aggressive papillary middle ear tumors (26). The disorder is inherited in an autosomal dominant fashion (29,30). The defective gene resides on the short arm of chromosome 3 (28,32).

The hemangioblastoma is by far the most common CNS manifestation of the disease (30a,31), with metastases from renal cell carcinoma a

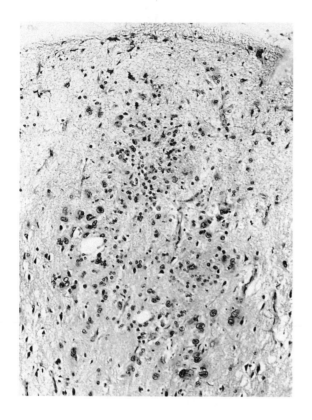

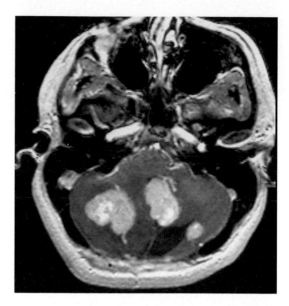

Figure 18-8
**MULTIPLE CEREBELLAR HEMANGIOBLASTOMAS
IN VON HIPPEL-LANDAU SYNDROME**

Multiple hemangioblastomas are a common expression of this genetic disease. Both eyes of this 35-year-old woman had been removed surgically because of retinal hemangioblastomas.

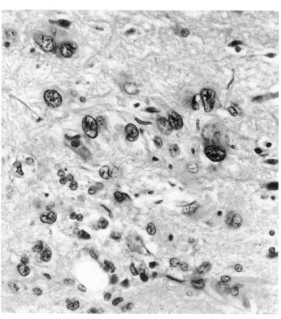

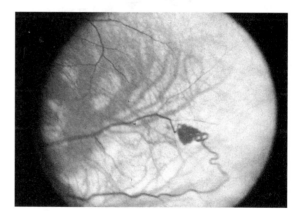

Figure 18-9
**OCULAR HEMANGIOBLASTOMA IN
VON HIPPEL-LINDAU SYNDROME**

As seen in this retinal angiogram, ocular hemangioblastomas are a common component of this multiorgan disorder. (Courtesy of Dr. Stephen C. Pollack, Durham, NC.)

Figure 18-7
NEUROFIBROMATOSIS 2

Top: Small heterotopia-like aggregates of atypical cells are widely scattered within the gray matter of patients with this dysgenetic disorder.

Bottom: At higher magnification, the glassy cytoplasm and nuclear pleomorphism of these cells suggest an astrocytic nature, although they are generally nonreactive for GFAP.

distant second. The majority of hemangioblastomas occur in the cerebellum. Many are multiple, either at initial presentation or over time as additional lesions appear. Other sites of predilection include the spinal cord and brain stem. Rare examples affect the supratentorial

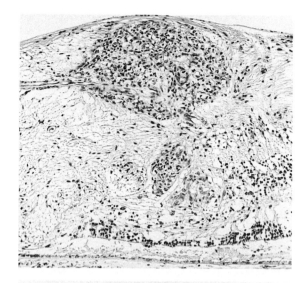

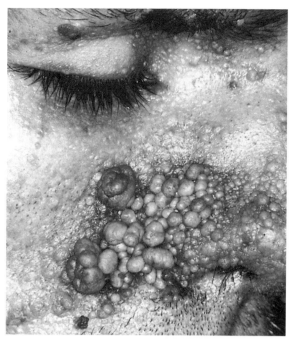

Figure 18-11
TUBEROUS SCLEROSIS
Adenoma sebaceum classically presents as multiple smooth excrescences. The nasal-labial fold is a favored site.

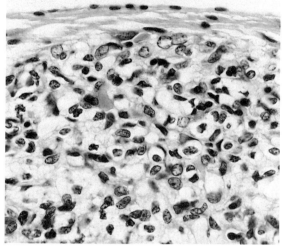

Figure 18-10
OCULAR HEMANGIOBLASTOMA IN
VON HIPPEL-LINDAU SYNDROME
This retinal hemangioblastoma, seen at low (top) and high (bottom) magnification, is analogous to its intracranial counterparts. It is discrete, highly vascular, and noted for interstitial or stromal cells. Such tumors may also affect the optic nerve. (Courtesy of Dr. Robert Folberg, Iowa City, IA.)

Tuberous Sclerosis

Also known as *Bourneville disease* or *epiloia*, this disorder is characterized clinically by the combination of cutaneous lesions, epilepsy, and associated mental deficiency (fig. 18-11) (34, 37,41). The responsible genes are on chromosomes 9 and 16 (33a). The three principal intracranial abnormalities include tubers, subependymal hamartomas, and subependymal giant cell astrocytomas. In histologic terms, the astrocytoma is essentially a large version of the hamartoma but one restricted to the region of the foramen of Monro. Cutaneous lesions include the adenoma sebaceum, subungual fibromas, the shagreen patch, fibrous forehead plaques, and patches of depigmentation. Café-au-lait spots similar to those of neurofibromatosis may also be seen. The term adenoma sebaceum is a misnomer since the raised lesion resembles an angiofibroma rather than a neoplasm of sebaceous glands. The ocular lesions consist of retinal astrocytic hamartomas and are histologically similar to subependymal nodules and giant cell astrocytomas. Visceral abnormalities include

leptomeninges (25). Brain stem lesions most often arise in the medulla and project into the fourth ventricle. Like the schwannomatosis of peripheral nerve roots in neurofibromatosis 2, multiple microscopic hemangioblastomas of the nerve root have been described (24).

The hemangioblastoma, the histogenesis of which is uncertain, is identical histologically at all sites including the retina.

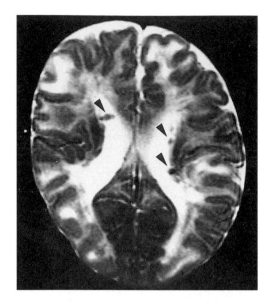

Figure 18-17
TUBEROUS SCLEROSIS
The calcified subependymal hamartomas appear as dark excrescences on the walls of the lateral ventricles (arrows) in this T2-weighted image. Multiple tubers are also present.

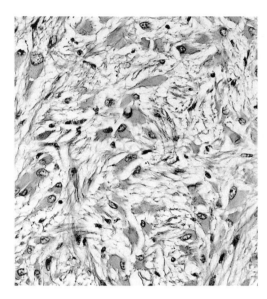

Figure 18-19
TUBEROUS SCLEROSIS
The fibrillated cells of the subependymal nodule are similar to those of symptomatic giant cell astrocytoma.

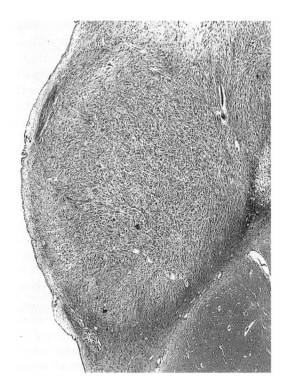

Figure 18-18
TUBEROUS SCLEROSIS
The subependymal nodule is a discrete subependymal mass of moderate cellularity. (Courtesy of Dr. H. Okazaki, Rochester, MN.)

normally populate the leptomeninges of the base of the brain and the ventral surface of the upper cervical spinal cord.

Clinical complications of the disease include hydrocephalus, seizures, and symptomatic infiltration of cranial or spinal nerves. Melanocytic lesions of the eye may be seen. Not all cases are inherited nor are cutaneous lesions always present. Rare forms of neurocutaneous melanosis have been associated with neurofibromatosis.

Radiologically, contrast enhancement of the leptomeninges has been reported. The intracranial lesions vary considerably, both in distribution and in the extent to which they form single or even multiple nodular masses. The proliferation, though often diffuse, usually does not appreciably thicken the leptomeninges. In other instances, the process diffusely expands the subarachnoid space without the formation of a distinct tumor. When mass lesions do arise, they are usually superimposed upon diffuse lesions.

Histologically, the lesions vary considerably from very well-differentiated melanocytic neoplasms to unequivocal malignant melanomas (see fig. 14-4) (44); in many instances, they are of intermediate grade. Solitary discrete melanocytomas have not been specifically identified as part of the syndrome.

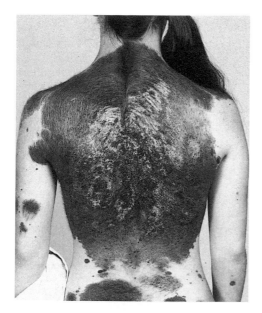

Figure 18-20
NEUROCUTANEOUS MELANOSIS
This large "bathing trunk" nevus in a 13-year-old is one expression of this syndrome. The ultimately lethal meningeal malignant melanoma is shown in figure 14-4. (Courtesy of Dr. E. Hsu, Ottawa, Canada.)

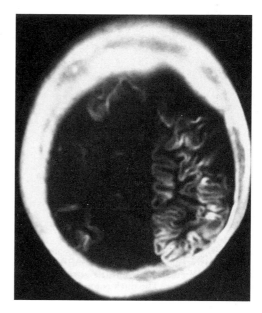

Figure 18-21
STURGE-WEBER DISEASE
As seen here by computerized tomography, the intracortical calcification produces a sinuous or gyriform pattern of radiographic density. As is often the case, the process is asymmetric.

Sturge-Weber Disease

Sturge-Weber disease is a sporadic rather than inherited disorder. Although included here among dysgenetic disorders, no clear genetic basis of the disease has been shown. It features both a cutaneous vascular nevus and a leptomeningeal angioma of the venous type (55). Independent involvement of the skin or leptomeninges may be a "forme fruste" expression.

The cutaneous capillary-venous lesions typically stain the face over a variable area which always includes a portion innervated by the ophthalmic division of the trigeminal nerve. Not only may mucosal, gingival, and orbital soft tissue be involved, but angiomas of the retina and choroid plexus are seen with some frequency. Concurrent involvement of the skin of the neck or upper body is less common. Associated brain lesions are usually ipsilateral to the facial abnormality and generally include the parieto-occipital region. Bilaterality is observed in some cases; cerebellar or brain stem involvement is less common. A spinal counterpart of the disorder, termed *Kippel-Trenaunay-Weber disease*, is associated with enlargement of the affected limb.

Radiologically, leptomeningeal angiomas produce thickening and contrast enhancement of the subarachnoid space in association with atrophy of the underlying brain (51,55). Cortical calcification, when present, produces a classic "tram track" pattern (fig. 18-21) (51,55).

Clinically, the intracranial lesions frequently induce seizures (50,54), whose control may require surgical resection of the calcified epileptogenic cortex (fig. 18-22) (52,53). With time, brain atrophy ensues on the side of the leptomeningeal angioma, with resultant contralateral motor deficits in some cases. In many instances, diminished intellect, if not frank dementia, is noted. Cognitive deficits are understandably more pronounced with bilateral cerebral involvement (50).

Macroscopically, the affected region is hypervascularized and red. The underlying brain may exhibit particulate calcification but is less affected. The dura is normal.

Microscopically, the abnormal vessels within the subarachnoid space are thin-walled channels largely devoid of smooth muscle (fig. 18-23). Calcospherites, although initially localized to perivascular regions, later become so abundant within the upper cortex as to escape precise localization.

Tuberous Sclerosis

33. Chou TM, Chou SM. Tuberous sclerosis in the premature infant: a report of a case with immunohistochemistry on the CNS. Clin Neuropathol 1989;8:45–52.

33a. European Chromosome 16 Tuberous Sclerosis Consortium. Identification and characterization of the tuberous sclerosis gene on chromosome 16. Cell 1993; 75:1305–15.

34. Gomez MR. Tuberous sclerosis. 2nd ed. New York: Raven Press, 1988.

35. Iwaki T, Wisniewski T, Iwaki A, et al. Accumulation of αB-crystallin in central nervous system glia and neurons in pathologic condition. Am J Pathol 1992;140:345–56.

36. Iwasaki S, Nakagawa H, Kichikawa K, et al. MR and CT of tuberous sclerosis: linear abnormalities in the cerebral white matter. AJNR Am J Neuroradiol 1990;11:1029–34.

37. Nagib MG, Haines SJ, Erickson DL, Mastri AR. Tuberous sclerosis: a review for the neurosurgeon. Neurosurgery 1984;14:93–8.

38. Nixon JR, Houser OW, Gomez MR, Okazaki H. Cerebral tuberous sclerosis: MR imaging. Radiology 1989;170:869–73.

39. _____, Miller GM, Okazaki H, Gomez MR. Cerebral tuberous sclerosis: postmortem magnetic resonance imaging and pathologic anatomy. Mayo Clin Proc 1989;64:305–11.

40. Scheithauer BW. The neuropathology of tuberous sclerosis. J Dermatol 1992;19:897–903.

41. Smirniotopoulos JG, Murphy FM. The phakomatoses. AJNR Am J Neuroradiol 1992;13:725–46.

42. Trombley IK, Mirra SS. Ultrastructure of tuberous sclerosis: cortical tuber and subependymal tumor. Ann Neurol 1981;9:174–81.

Neurocutaneous Melanosis

43. Faillace WJ, Okawara SH, McDonald JV. Neurocutaneous melanosis with extensive intracerebral and spinal cord involvement: report of two cases. J Neurosurg 1984;61:782–5.

44. Kaplan AM, Itabashi HH, Hanelin LG, Lu AT. Neurocutaneous melanosis with malignant leptomeningeal melanoma: a case with metastases outside the nervous system. Arch Neurol 1975;32:669–71.

45. Leaney BJ, Rowe PW, Klug GL. Neurocutaneous melanosis with hydrocephalus and syringomyelia. Case report. J Neurosurg 1985;62:148–52.

46. Reed WB, Becker SW Sr, Becker SW Jr, Nickel WR. Giant pigmented nevi, melanoma, and leptomeningeal melanocytosis. Arch Dermatol 1965;91:100–19.

47. Sagar HJ, Ilgren EB, Adams CB. Nevus of Ota associated with meningeal melanosis and intracranial melanoma: case report. J Neurosurg 1983;58:280–3.

48. Slaughter JC, Hardman JM, Kempe LG, Earle KM. Neurocutaneous melanosis and leptomeningeal melanomatosis in children. Arch Pathol 1969;88:298–304.

49. Smirniotopoulos JG, Murphy FM. The phakomatoses. AJNR Am J Neuroradiol 1992;13:725–46.

Sturge-Weber Disease

50. Bebin EM, Gomez MR. Prognosis in Sturge-Weber disease: comparison of unihemispheric and bihemispheric involvement. J Child Neurol 1988;3:181–4.

51. Benedikt RA, Brown Dc, Walker R, Gihaed VN, Mitchell M, Geyer CA. Sturge-Weber syndrome. Cranial MR imaging with Gd-DTPA. Am J Neuroradiol 1993;14:409–15.

52. Ito M, Sato K, Ohnuki A, Uto A. Sturge-Weber disease: operative indications and surgical results. Brain Dev 1990;12:473–7.

53. Ogunmekan AO, Hwang PA, Hoffman HJ. Sturge-Weber-Dimitri disease: role of hemispherectomy in prognosis. Can J Neurol Sci 1989;16:78–80.

54. Peterman AF, Hayles AB, Dockerty MB, Love JG. Encephalotrigeminal angiomatosis (Sturge-Weber disease): clinical study of thirty-five cases. JAMA 1958;167:2169–76.

55. Smirniotopoulos JG, Murphy FM. The phakomatoses. AJNR Am J Neuroradiol 1992;13:725–46.

Mesencephalo-Oculo-Facial Angiomatosis (Wyburn-Mason Disease)

56. Patel U, Gupta SC. Wyburn-Mason syndrome. A case report and review of the literature. Neuroradiology 1990;31:544–6.

57. Théron J, Newton TH, Hoyt WF. Unilateral retinocephalic vascular malformations. Neuroradiology 1974;7:185–96.

58. Wyburn-Mason R. Arteriovenous aneurysm of midbrain and retina, facial naevi and mental changes. Brain 1943;66:163–203.

Hereditary Hemorrhagic Telangiectasia (Rendu-Osler-Weber Disease)

59. Aesch B, Lioret E, de Toffel B, Jan M. Multiple cerebral angiomas and Rendu-Osler-Weber disease: case report. Neurosurgery 1991;29:599–602.

60. Sobel D, Norman D. CNS manifestations of hereditary hemorrhagic telangiectasia. Am J Neuroradiol 1984 ;569–73.

61. Willinsky RA, Lasjaunias P, Terbrugge K, Burrows P. Multiple cerebral arteriovenous malformations (AVMs). Review of our experience from 203 patients with cerebral vascular lesions. Neuroradiology 1990;32:207–10.

Cowden Syndrome

62. Albrecht S, Haber RM, Goodman JC, Duvic M. Cowden syndrome and Lhermitte-Duclos disease. Cancer 1992;70:869–76.

63. Padberg GW, Schot JD, Vielvoye GJ, Bots GT, de Beer FC. Lhermitte-Duclos disease and Cowden disease: a single phakomatosis. Ann Neurol 1991;29:517–23.

19

REACTIVE AND INFLAMMATORY MASSES SIMULATING NEOPLASIA

Demyelinating Disease

General Comments. In its classic form, a demyelinating disease such as *multiple sclerosis* is recognized on the basis of its clinical and radiographic presentation. Typically, a constellation of neurologic signs and symptoms arise in the face of multiple lesions which make their appearance over time. A biopsy is generally performed only if there is a solitary lesion suspected of being neoplastic (2,4). Such lesions may be accompanied by atypical radiologic features including significant mass effects. A rare form of multifocal demyelinating disease occurs during chemotherapy for colonic carcinoma (1). Metastases may be suspected in this setting.

Clinical and Radiographic Features. Demyelinating lesions, including those mimicking neoplasms, generally affect adolescents or young adults. Occasional examples are encountered in older patients, even the elderly. In accord with the known sex predilection of multiple sclerosis, most patients are women.

Demyelinating lesions are seen well on magnetic resonance images (MRIs) where they appear as bright (white) foci in T2-weighted images (figs. 19-1, 19-2). Classically, these foci, termed plaques, lie either adjacent to the lateral ventricles or beneath the cortex, or affect the spinal cord, brain stem, or visual pathways. The cerebellum is less frequently involved, particularly early in the disease. The plaques may be small, measuring a centimeter or less, but are occasionally large and accompanied by considerable mass effect (2a).

Microscopic Findings. The outpouring of macrophages that accompanies demyelination creates a hypercellular state that can closely resemble a neoplasm, particularly at low power or in frozen sections (figs. 19-3, 19-4). Scattered

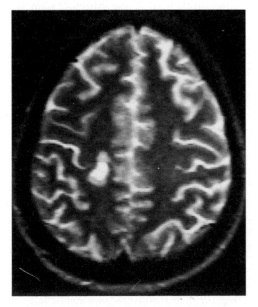 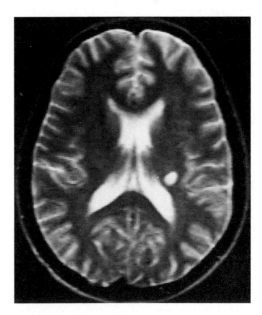

Figure 19-1
MULTIPLE SCLEROSIS

Left: A college student presented with hemiparesis due to the fronto-parietal lesion seen in a T2-weighted magnetic resonance image. Given the numerous reactive astrocytes and macrophages resembling oligodendrocytes, a diagnosis of mixed glioma was made. The patient improved considerably following steroid therapy alone.

Right: A follow-up scan 3 months later disclosed a second lesion in the contralateral hemisphere.

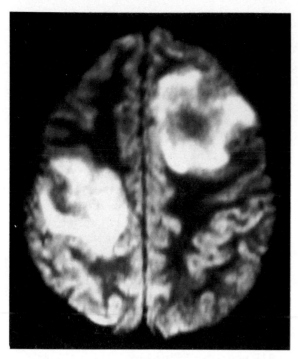

Figure 19-2
MULTIPLE SCLEROSIS
Because of their size and mass effect, large demyelinating lesions can clinically and radiographically mimic brain tumors.

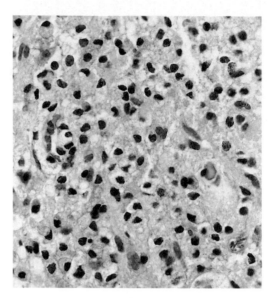

Figure 19-4
DEMYELINATING DISEASE
The hypercellularity of this plaque is due largely to macrophages whose cell borders may be only faintly visible.

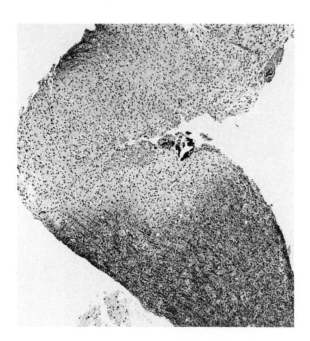

Figure 19-3
DEMYELINATING DISEASE
As seen in this needle biopsy specimen stained for myelin, demyelinating plaques are well circumscribed and moderately cellular. The sharp interface between the pale lesion and the normal darkly stained myelin (bottom) is well seen.

mitoses within macrophages further add to the confusion. Such cells are noted for their generally round uniform nuclei, vacuolated cytoplasm, and distinct cell borders (fig. 19-5). The recognition of demyelinating disease hinges upon identifying these cells. Once a few are identified as phagocytes, it usually becomes apparent that most of the remaining cells are similar. At that point, two differential diagnoses come to mind: demyelinating disease and infarction. Progressive multifocal leukoencephalopathy is another consideration.

As lipid-laden macrophages return to the vasculature, they appear to hesitate before reentering the blood stream. The distinctive perivascular huddle of monomorphous, vacuolated, periodic acid–Schiff (PAS)-positive cells is typical of both demyelinating and ischemic lesions, but is not generally a feature of neoplasia (fig. 19-6). Lying among the macrophages in affected brain parenchyma are reactive astrocytes with their prominent pink cytoplasm and stellate array of tapering processes. Although their nuclei are often large and may be somewhat polymorphous, there is not a notable increase in these cells over the number of normal astrocytes. Their luxurious symmetric array of processes, best appreciated on smear or glial fibrillary acidic protein (GFAP) preparations, readily excludes consideration of

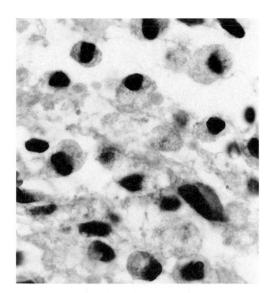

Figure 19-5
DEMYELINATING DISEASE
The sharp cell borders, granular cytoplasm, and nuclear uniformity of the macrophages are readily apparent at high magnification.

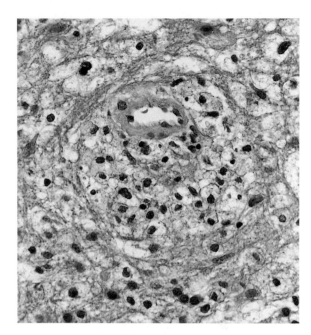

Figure 19-6
DEMYELINATING DISEASE
Macrophages often congregate around vessels. Such perivascular aggregations are unusual in brain tumors.

astrocytoma. Perivascular lymphocytic infiltrates are also a common and important diagnostic feature of demyelination. Commonly encountered are so-called "granular mitoses," a misnomer for the multiplicity of minute nuclei in large reactive astrocytes (fig. 19-7).

Stains for myelin highlight the remarkable discreteness of the lesion (fig. 19-3), which, particularly in large specimens, is often strikingly perivenous. Aside from poor-staining fragments of myelin within the cytoplasm of macrophages, the lesion is largely devoid of myelin. On balance, axis cylinders are spared although in active plaques some fragmentation and axonal loss is to be expected (fig. 19-8). Surviving axons may be less precisely aligned than those in the adjacent normal white matter and reactive swellings (spheroids) are commonly seen. In rapidly evolving plaques, or at sites where tissue is restrained from swelling (optic nerve or spinal cord), tissue necrosis may be observed.

Immunohistochemical Findings. The phagocytic elements are strongly immunoreactive for macrophage markers such as HAM-56, KP-1, or lysozyme (fig. 19-9) (1a). The cytoplasm and stellate processes of reactive astrocytes are impressively positive for GFAP. The lymphocytic infiltrate is polyclonal; most cells are T lymphocytes.

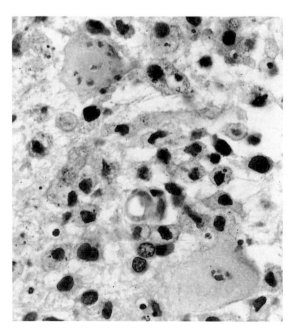

Figure 19-7
DEMYELINATING DISEASE
Astrocytes with dispersed but viable-appearing nuclear fragments are frequently seen in demyelinating disease. The misnomer "granular mitoses" has been applied to this finding. Such cells are seen less often in other reactive conditions and are only rarely observed in gliomas.

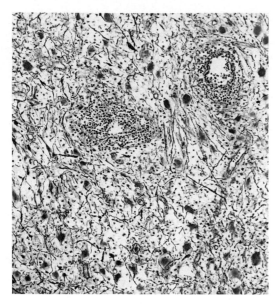

Figure 19-8
DEMYELINATING DISEASE
As seen in this Glees stained section for axis cylinders, considerable edema and chronic inflammation is evident in a demyelinating plaque, but there is relative sparing of the dark thread-like axons.

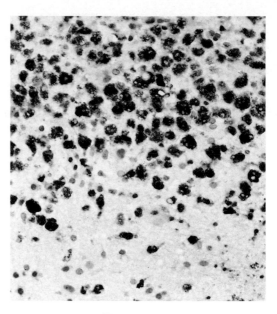

Figure 19-9
DEMYELINATING DISEASE
Immunostaining, as here in a HAM-56 preparation, is extremely useful in the diagnosis of macrophage-rich lesions. Note the sharp border of the plaque.

Ultrastructural Findings. Macrophages are identified by their sharp cell borders without junctional contact and the cytoplasmic content of phagocytized myelin debris. Oligodendrocytes are sparse. Remyelination may occur.

Differential Diagnosis. A demyelinating lesion should be considered when a cellular lesion with chronic perivascular inflammation is seen in a younger patient, especially a woman. In the absence of suggestive clinical or radiographic data, a demyelinating lesion can be misinterpreted as infarct, infection, or glioma (see Appendices A, C). In the immunosuppressed, the finding of macrophage-rich areas of demyelination should prompt consideration of the opportunistic papovavirus infection, progressive multifocal leukoencephalopathy (PML). Distinguishing features of this disease are oligodendroglia with "ground glass" nuclear inclusions and large viral-infected glial cells with dark nuclei, best seen at the edges of the demyelinated foci. As in the plaques of conventional demyelinating disease, the lesions of PML contain reactive astrocytes. Their often striking atypia in PML occasionally results in an erroneous diagnosis of malignant glioma.

Among gliomas, the oligodendroglioma enters into the differential diagnosis given the uniformity, nuclear roundness, and cytoplasmic vacuolization of the macrophages. In contrast to neoplastic oligodendrocytes, however, the macrophages have discrete cell borders, vacuolated rather than clear cytoplasm, uniform size, and normochromatic nuclei. When reactive astrocytes are particularly prominent, a diagnosis of mixed glioma or of astrocytoma may be entertained. In such instances, the application of macrophage markers is useful in confirming the histiocytic nature of the oligodendroglia-like cells. Given the configuration and uniform distribution of reactive astrocytes, a diagnosis of astrocytoma can usually be excluded.

Treatment and Prognosis. The classic demyelinating disease, multiple sclerosis, is noted for the appearance, often over a period of years, of plaques at a variety of sites. There is, however, great variability in the course of the disease and some demyelinating lesions remain unifocal. Rarely, a neoplasm develops in the setting of demyelinating disease, but it remains to be established whether the two processes are pathogenetically related (3).

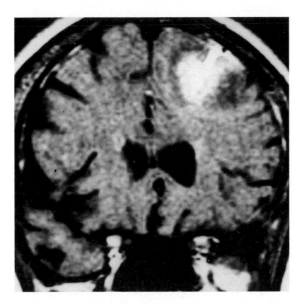

Figure 19-10
CEREBRAL INFARCT
Although this contrast-enhancing lesion involves the cerebral cortex as is typical of cerebral infarcts, an atypical clinical course prompted biopsy of this expansile lesion.

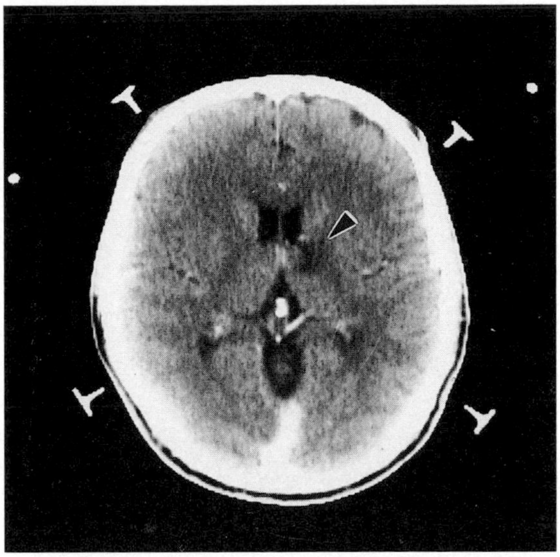

Figure 19-11
CEREBRAL INFARCT
Deep-seated small infarcts in the internal capsule (arrow) may produce neurologic signs and prompt a biopsy to rule out neoplasm.

Cerebral Infarct

With the exception of those rare situations in which decompressive surgery is undertaken knowingly with a cerebral infarct (5), ischemic lesions are generally biopsied only inadvertently. A radiographic low-density mass effect and the appearance of ring enhancement about 1 week into the course, places malignant glioma at the top of the list of differential diagnoses. Large infarcts may be approached by craniotomy (fig. 19-10), whereas small deep-seated lesions in the basal ganglia or thalamus are more often sampled by stereotactic biopsy (fig. 19-11). Although early infarcts may exhibit mass effects, with time they result in shrinkage of affected regions.

Macroscopic Findings. Acute arterial cerebral infarcts are soft expansile masses confined to the distribution of a single cerebral blood vessel. In contrast, large hemispheric lesions are characteristically wedge shaped and, in contrast to most fibrillary astrocytomas, extend to involve the cortex. Such classic lesions are less likely to be biopsied than are atypical infarcts that mimic glioma. Infarcts of the basal ganglia or thalamus are generally round and lack the wedge-shape configuration of large, more superficial lesions.

Venous infarcts are more superficial than arterial infarcts and are often hemorrhagic.

Microscopic Findings. By the time cerebral infarcts come to surgery, they have generally become macrophage rich and are, therefore, cellular lesions resembling either neoplasms or foci of demyelination (figs. 19-12, 19-13). When capillaries react, vascular cells become hypertrophic and atypical, with plump and mitotically active endothelial cells (fig. 19-14). Such vessels may closely resemble their proliferating counterparts in malignant gliomas. Early in infarction, large neurons become intensely eosinophilic ("red" neurons) as their nucleoplasm undergoes karyolysis (fig. 19-15).

In a well-established infarct, engorged macrophages known as gitter cells make their appearance. These have well-defined cell borders, uniform round nuclei, and cytoplasm filled with granular material (pl. XA). Occasional mitoses are noted. As in demyelinating lesions, these cells often crowd around blood vessels, an uncommon finding in settings other than infarct or demyelination. Well-defined cell borders are one of the most distinctive characteristics of macrophages and one which should be carefully sought. Their often granular and foamy appearance is due to

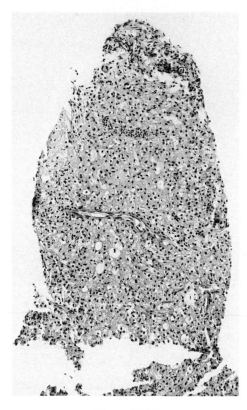

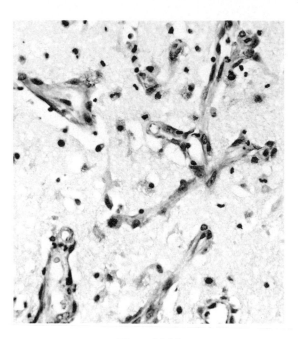

Figure 19-14
CEREBRAL INFARCT
The hypertrophy and hyperplasia of vascular elements should not be taken as evidence of neoplasia.

Figure 19-12
CEREBRAL INFARCT
As seen in this needle biopsy section, infarcts are moderately cellular masses with considerable nuclear uniformity.

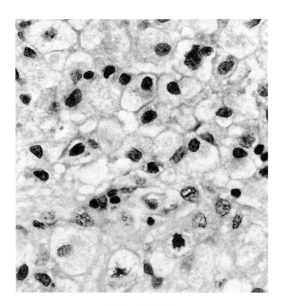

Figure 19-13
CEREBRAL INFARCT
When cellularity is high, the cell borders of macrophages may be less evident and an erroneous diagnosis of a glioma may be forthcoming. Note the mitoses within macrophages (bottom).

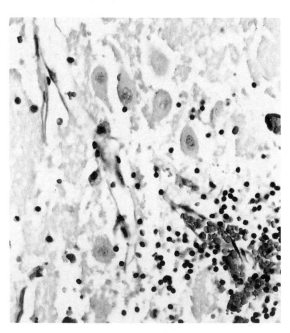

Figure 19-15
CEREBRAL INFARCT
As in this surgical specimen, ischemic or "red" neurons are a classic finding in recent cerebral infarction. The nuclei in various stages of dissolution are characteristic of such eosinophilic cells.

PLATE X

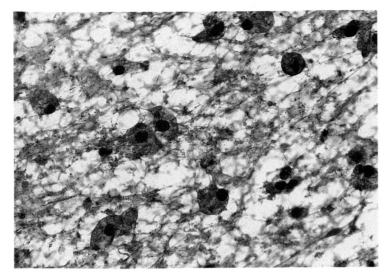

A. CEREBRAL INFARCT

Large, discrete, finely granular or foamy macrophages with uniform nuclei are well visualized in cytologic preparations. Such cells are unusual in brain neoplasms.

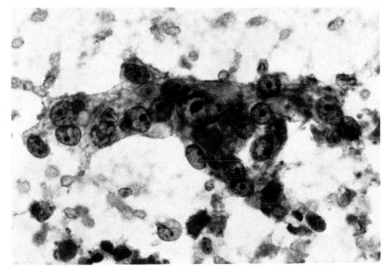

B. METASTATIC CARCINOMA

Cohesion as a tissue fragment; a "dirty" background; and, in this case of adenocarcinoma, prominent nucleoli, are typical cytologic findings.

C. METASTATIC CARCINOMA

The prominent cytoplasm of some carcinomas creates a resemblance to gliomas. In contrast, however, the metastatic cells are discrete isolated elements or aggregates in tissue fragments. Lacking is the fibrillar background typical of most gliomas.

phagocytized myelin fragments, the nature of which can be demonstrated with histochemical stains, particularly Luxol fast blue and PAS. The degree to which frankly necrotic tissue or cellular debris is apparent varies considerably. With time, infarcts are cleared of necrosis and evolve into rarefied or frankly cystic tissue wherein reactive astrocytes greatly outnumber phagocytes.

Immunohistochemical Findings. As in demyelinating disease, the macrophages are strongly positive for macrophage markers such as HAM-56 (fig. 19-16), KP-1, or lysozyme; the lymphocytes for T-cell and, to a lesser extent B-cell markers; and the reactive astrocytes to GFAP.

Differential Diagnosis. The hypercellularity and vascular changes that accompany early and organizing infarction may at first glance suggest a malignant glioma (see Appendices A, C). Given the round nuclei and generally pale cytoplasm of macrophages, oligodendroglioma comes to mind. The misdiagnosis is most likely when zones of subtotal necrosis are biopsied, areas in which gitter cells are intermixed with viable tissue. The cytoplasmic pallor of an infarct-associated macrophage is not an autolytic consequence of fluid imbibition, as in oligodendrogliomas, but rather the result of an accumulation of phagocytized myelin and cellular debris. On high magnification, the granular or foamy appearance is most readily apparent. Differential stains such as the Luxol fast blue or PAS are relatively inexpensive ways to confirm the macrophages' nature. Glioblastoma may also be considered, but is usually excluded on the basis of the uniformity of the macrophage nuclei and the discreteness of their cell borders. The telltale clustering of macrophages around blood vessels is another helpful feature. Immunostaining for macrophage markers and lack of GFAP reactivity within the monotonous cells easily confirms the diagnosis of infarction.

Infarcts may also resemble so-called granular cell gliomas (see fig. 3-54), most of which are glioblastomas. These rare tumors consist of neoplastic cells with features reminiscent of macrophages, including nuclear roundness, discrete cell borders, and granular cytoplasm. In large, sufficiently representative specimens, however, transition to obvious glioma is usually seen. Not only are some tumor cells positive for GFAP but most, if not all, are negative for macrophage markers.

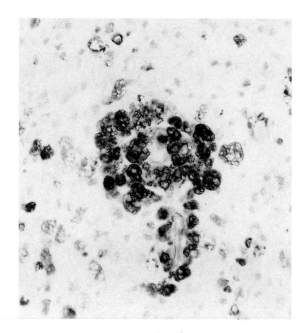

Figure 19-16
CEREBRAL INFARCT
Macrophages in cerebral infarcts are immunoreactive for HAM-56. Note the perivascular aggregation of the phagocytes.

Although most infarcts occur in the elderly, they still must be distinguished from demyelinating disease. In concept, this is not difficult since, in most cases, axons are preserved in demyelinating disease but are destroyed in infarcts. In practice, the distinction is not always straightforward since some axonal loss and fragmentation regularly occurs in demyelination. Indeed, rapidly progressive plaques may show frank central necrosis.

Treatment and Prognosis. Infarcts resolve within weeks to months. Depending upon their size, gliotic rarefied to grossly cystic foci may result. With advanced organization, infarcts become contracted foci readily distinguished from neoplasms by radiography.

Radionecrosis

For the purposes of this volume, the most relevant complication of craniospinal radiotherapy is late-delayed radionecrosis. Radiation leukoencephalopathy is an equally important, yet not fully characterized, complication of radiotherapy associated with decremental and potentially disabling loss of intellectual function. The

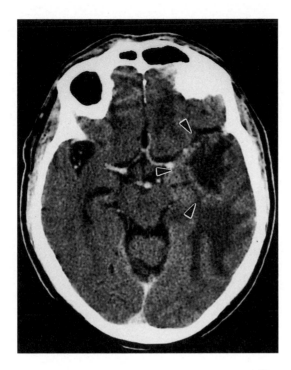 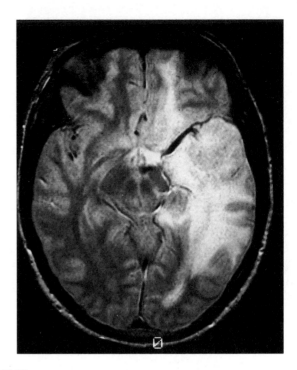

Figure 19-17
RADIONECROSIS

Radionecrosis may present as a contrast-enhancing lesion surrounded by considerable edema, as in this patient irradiated 2 years earlier for an orbital sarcoma.

Left: A malignant glioma was expected preoperatively in view of a ring configuration of the enhancement (arrows) and extensive perilesional edema.

Right: The latter is seen better in a proton density magnetic resonance image.

latter consists of a diffuse degeneration of the white matter with resultant hydrocephalus ex vacuo, rather than a mass requiring surgical intervention. On the other hand, radionecrosis is a rapidly evolving expansile lesion which may demand surgical decompression and histologic assessment to exclude a diagnosis of neoplasia (6–9). Radionecrosis is an especially common complication of interstitial radiation (9).

Clinical and Radiographic Features. Cerebral radionecrosis is generally encountered as a consequence of radiation therapy for malignant gliomas. Less commonly, it presents after treatment of well-differentiated brain tumors, non-neoplastic lesions, or extracranial malignancies of the head and neck. The occurrence of radionecrosis is radiation rate dependent, generally occurring with doses of 50 Gy or more. The effect is not immediate: a postradiation interval of 6 months to 2 years is observed in most cases. In extent, radionecrosis is limited to the treatment field.

As an expansile process, radionecrosis often exerts a neurologically evident mass effect. Imaging typically shows an aggressive-appearing lesion with contrast enhancement and surrounding edema (fig. 19-17) (6,8). This image is a misrepresentation since on positron emission tomography (PET) these lesions are hypometabolic or "cold," whereas recurrent neoplasm is hypermetabolic or "hot" (see fig. 3-43). Foci of radionecrosis frequently undergo dystrophic calcification with time and the dense deposits appear as either sizable plaque-like lesions in deep white matter or small foci along the gray-white junction. Surgery is rarely undertaken at such late stages since the affected region is contracting rather than expanding.

Macroscopic Findings. Externally, the mass effect of radionecrosis is reflected in swollen but otherwise intact gyri. On cut sections, the necrotic areas have a patchy, granular quality and are frequently yellow-gray and punctuated by multiple petechiae (fig. 19-18). With

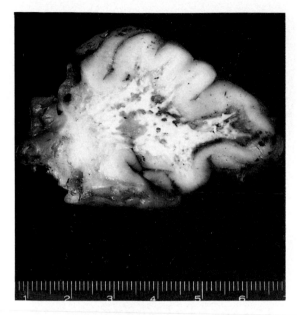

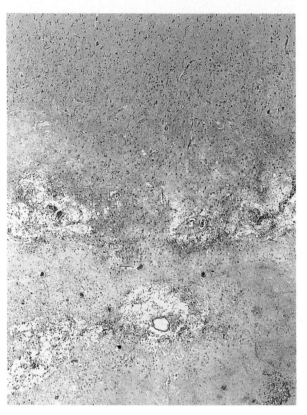

Figure 19-19
RADIONECROSIS
As is evident at low magnification, radionecrosis evolves by the confluence of multiple, often perivascular areas of necrosis which are most prominent in the white matter and in deeper layers of the cerebral cortex.

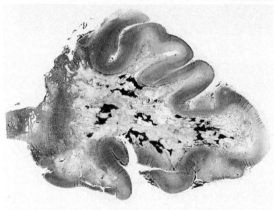

Figure 19-18
RADIONECROSIS
Top: Radionecrosis is characteristically a granular, somewhat yellow, petechiae-rich process largely confined to the white matter.

Bottom: As seen in a whole mount histologic section, the gray matter is largely spared. Note the characteristic darkly stained subcortical calcifications.

time, large chalky areas of calcification and cystic foci evolve. Although the process is largely a disorder of white matter, it does encroach upon deep cortical layers (7). In advanced lesions, cortical necrosis and atrophy may be seen.

Microscopic Findings. Radionecrosis is a distinctive form of coagulative necrosis which often appears as multiple discrete foci undergoing confluence at low magnification (fig. 19-19). It is also an unusual form of tissue reaction since

it does not elicit the degree of macrophage response so characteristic of ordinary ischemic infarcts and demyelinating disease. The relative paucity of histiocytes may relate to vascular injury which presumably retards their influx. In failing to undergo timely resolution, the lesions remain as granular areas of coagulative necrosis as much prone to dystrophic calcification as to cystic change. Deep layers of the overlying cortex often demonstrate a peculiar hypocellular state in which underlying tissue fades from view but reactive glia and neurons are relatively preserved.

Vascular damage is a prominent feature of radionecrosis and has led many to suggest an ischemic basis for chronic radiation injury. In active lesions, fibrinoid necrosis, as evidenced by amorphous thickening and eosinophilia of small blood vessels, is often widespread and accompanied by thrombosis. Pools of fibrin may be seen

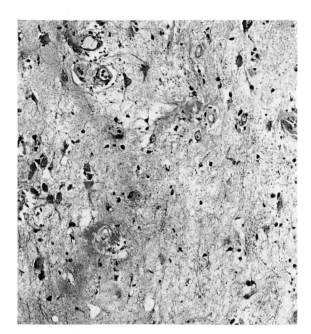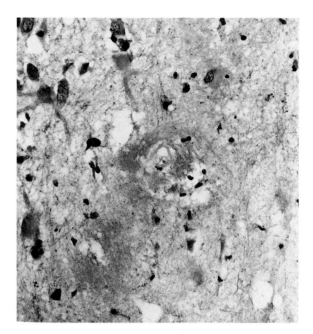

Figure 19-20
RADIONECROSIS

Left: As seen in this section of cerebral cortex, fibrinoid vascular necrosis is prominent. Also apparent is the characteristic hypocellularity and paucity of phagocytic elements.

Right: The typical vascular changes and perivascular pools of fibrin are seen at higher magnification.

surrounding vessels (figs. 19-20). Although not generally prominent, overt microvascular proliferation, such as the glomeruloid appearance seen in malignant gliomas, may ensue. Chronic changes include recanalization and mural hyalinization in addition to the formation of telangiectases. In more chronic lesions endothelial cells may be large, atypical, or even absent. Granulation tissue may be seen (fig. 19-21). Reactive astrocytes are often abundant, particularly surrounding areas of frank necrosis and may show irradiation atypia: nuclear and cytoplasmic enlargement as well as hyperchromasia (fig. 19-22).

Differential Diagnosis. In the setting of radiation for an extracranial lesion, neoplastic or not; a well-differentiated glioma such as pilocytic astrocytoma; or other benign intracranial neoplasms, radionecrosis is a distinctive and readily recognized process in which prominent and sometimes atypical astrocytes are quickly identified as reactive rather than neoplastic. This contrasts with a necrosis-prone malignant glioma in which two practical problems arise: distinguishing inherent necrosis from radiation-induced tumor necrosis and distinguishing the

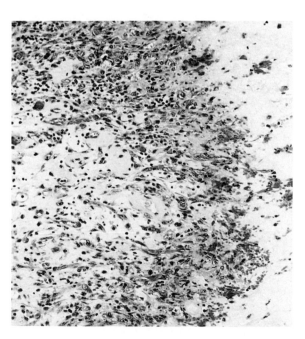

Figure 19-21
RADIONECROSIS

Late organization by granulation tissue formation is noted in some instances. The vascular component of this proliferation should not be interpreted as vascular proliferation indicative of a malignant glioma.

401

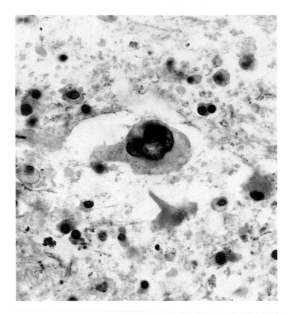

Figure 19-22
RADIATION-INDUCED ATYPIA
Considerable cytologic atypia may be noted in radiated tissues.

desired tumor necrosis (radiation effect) from injury to peritumoral brain substance (radionecrosis). This is discussed in the section on glioblastoma in chapter 3. In brief, all combinations of parenchymal radionecrosis, radiation effect upon the neoplasm, and recurrent actively growing necrotic tumor may be seen in specimens from the same patient. Without adequate tissue sampling, knowledge of the current radiographic images, and correlation with clinical as well as radiotherapeutic data, it may be impossible to determine which component of the lesion is responsible for a patient's clinical or radiographic deterioration. This is particularly true when only small specimens are provided.

Treatment and Prognosis. Delayed radionecrosis is generally a self-limited process which, in the absence of a life-threatening mass effect, evolves into a cystic or densely calcified focus.

Langerhans Cell Histiocytosis

Definition. A group of lesions consisting in part of a proliferation of Langerhans histiocytes.

General Comments. Historically, Langerhans cell histiocytosis (formerly histiocytosis X) was divided into three disorders: eosinophilic granuloma, Hand-Schüller-Christian disease, and Letterer-Siwe disease. In view of considerable clinical overlap, there is an effort now to dispense with such terms and refer to the disease on the basis of its extent: Langerhans histiocytosis of unifocal, multifocal, or disseminated type. The pathogenesis is unknown, but is generally assumed to be inflammatory rather than neoplastic, although the disseminated forms in the very young can be biologically malignant. The principal cells exhibit both immunohistochemical and ultrastructural features of Langerhans cells, thus supporting the unifying concept that these clinically dissimilar disorders are related proliferations of a unique cell common to many tissues.

The most commonly occurring and innocuous form of Langerhans cell histiocytosis is *solitary eosinophilic granuloma*. Its importance in the context of this volume relates to the frequency with which it affects the skull or spine. Only rarely does eosinophilic granuloma arise primarily within brain parenchyma. When the same process is multifocal and associated with signs and symptoms of hypothalamic disease, the complex is known as *Hand-Schüller-Christian disease*. *Letterer-Siwe disease* is a less secure entity but has been considered a systemic disease of skin, lymph nodes, and viscera, usually in young children.

Most cases of Langerhans cell histiocytosis that directly affect the central nervous system (CNS) do so by extension from one or more osseous foci. This is typically the case in multifocal eosinophilic granuloma involving the base of the skull (Hand-Schüller-Christian disease) in which interference with hypothalamic function results in endocrine deficiency states. Children and young adults are most often affected. Less commonly, unifocal or multifocal infiltrates appear to arise primarily within the hypothalamus (15), infundibulum (16,20), optic chiasm (18,19), choroid plexus (16a), or cerebral hemispheres (fig. 19-23) (11,13,14,17).

In the work-up of disturbances in hypothalamic or pituitary function, particularly diabetes insipidus, the sensitivity of MRI readily permits the visualization of small infundibular or hypothalamic lesions (16,20). In this setting, the necessarily small size of most biopsy specimens requires they be only sparingly assessed at frozen section and that optimally fixed tissue be reserved for immunohistochemistry and electron

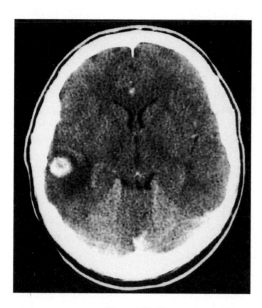

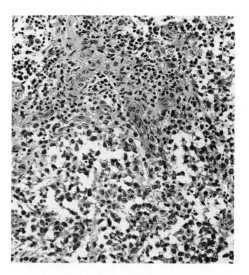

Figure 19-23
LANGERHANS CELL HISTIOCYTOSIS

Although Langerhans cell histiocytosis usually affects the cranial vault and basal structures, occasional lesions are intraparenchymal, thus suggesting a neoplasm. This brightly enhancing expansile lesion is surrounded by a dark zone of cerebral edema.

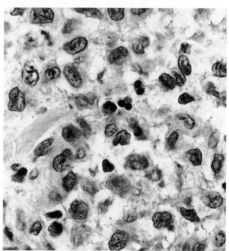

Figure 19-24
LANGERHANS CELL HISTIOCYTOSIS

Top: The lesion seen at low magnification is a typical example of Langerhans cell histiocytosis with the nodules of large cells surrounded by aggregates of small inflammatory cells including eosinophils.

Bottom: The complicated folded and clefted nuclear contours of the Langerhans cells are easily seen at higher magnification.

microscopy. Foci of Langerhans cell histiocytosis must be differentiated from inflammatory lesions such as sarcoidosis, infection, and neoplasms, both glial and germ cell.

Macroscopic Findings. The often yellow lesions vary from discrete nodules attached to the dura to granular intraparenchymal infiltrates. Those in the region of the hypothalamus may be either discrete or ill-defined lesions infiltrative of the meninges.

Microscopic Findings. Langerhans cell histiocytosis in its consummate form consists of a mixed infiltrate composed of Langerhans cells; chronic inflammatory cells, including plasma cells; and focal aggregates of eosinophils (fig. 19-24). Langerhans cells are noted for their large indented or convoluted nuclei (fig. 19-24, bottom). Lesions presenting primarily in the brain may exhibit a conspicuous xanthomatous reaction replete with foamy histiocytes and Touton giant cells (fig. 19-25) (14a). As in chronic osseous foci of Langerhans cell histiocytosis, abundant collagen and reticulin deposition is often seen. Striking and vigorous gliosis is elicited in areas of brain involvement. The presence of inflammatory cells within the cytoplasm of histiocytes is a common finding.

Immunohistochemical Findings. Langerhans cells are conspicuously positive for S-100 protein, vimentin, and certain histiocyte markers such as CD1a. Demonstration of CD1a requires fresh frozen tissue (10). Mac-387 has been suggested as a means of distinguishing immunonegative Langerhans cell histiocytosis from immunoreactive macrophage-derived lesions such as xanthogranulomas (12).

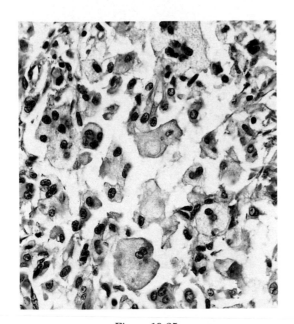

Figure 19-25
LANGERHANS CELL HISTIOCYTOSIS
Some lesions of Langerhans cell histiocytosis are noted for their cells with extensive foamy cytoplasm.

Ultrastructural Findings. At the ultrastructural level, multilobulation and complex folding of the nuclear membrane is seen in Langerhans cells. The diagnostic feature of Langerhans cell histiocytosis is a distinctive pentalaminar organelle with cross striations and frequent expansion. The appearance has been likened to a tennis racket. Langerhans cell granules appear to form from infoldings of the cell membrane and intracellular organelles.

Differential Diagnosis. Given the often minute nature of the specimen, particularly from parenchymal infiltrates in the hypothalamus, the precise nature of these lesions may not be apparent in routine histologic sections. Immunohistochemistry and electron microscopy aid in distinguishing Langerhans cell histiocytosis from lymphomas and nonspecific inflammatory reactions. The identification of S-100- and CD1a-positive Langerhans cells and the ultrastructural demonstration of the granules confirm the diagnosis.

The rather prominent gliosis elicited by parenchymal infiltrates of Langerhans cell histiocytosis must be recognized for what it is in order to avoid an erroneous diagnosis of either pilocytic or fibrillary astrocytoma.

The distinction between Langerhans cell histiocytosis and sinus histiocytosis with lymphadenopathy (Rosai-Dorfman disease) is discussed later in this chapter.

Treatment and Prognosis. Although common solitary and even multifocal Langerhans cell histiocytoses generally respond to low-dose radiotherapy, it is not clear whether this treatment is always necessary. Despite significant morbidity in multifocal examples, a fatal outcome is uncommon.

Xanthomatous Lesions

A disparate group of CNS lesions is noted for cells with abundant intracytoplasmic lipid. Some are diffuse and metabolic or degenerative in character, whereas others present as masses despite their non-neoplastic character. Occasionally, it is unclear whether a lesion is reactive or neoplastic. As a whole, the entities in this group warrant the nonspecific description "xanthomatous." Although tumors like pleomorphic xanthoastrocytoma and glioblastomas often contain varying numbers of xanthic cells, the present discussion focuses upon reactive or presumably reactive non-neoplastic processes. Langerhans cell histiocytosis is treated separately. The xanthomatous response to some colloid cysts of the third ventricle is discussed in chapter 16.

Xanthomas of the Choroid Plexus. The stroma and, to a far lesser extent, the epithelium of the choroid plexus may be sites of considerable xanthomatous change in normal individuals (fig. 19-26) (22,23,38,40). Unilateral or bilateral xanthogranulomatous enlargement of the plexus, especially its glomus in the trigone or atrium of the lateral ventricles, is a common radiographic or postmortem finding. Older patients are most affected. The nodular, yellow, and often partially cystic masses consist largely of xanthoma cells within the myxoid stroma of the choroid plexus. Extracellular release of the lipid results in the formation of cholesterol to which macrophage and giant cells respond. Xanthomatous enlargement of the choroid plexus is usually of no clinical significance and is only rarely symptomatic (23,26).

Xanthomas Associated with Hyperlipidemia. Xanthomatous change in congenital or acquired hyperlipidemia and hyperlipoproteinemia may manifest as intracranial masses affecting bone and dura. Histologically, the lesions are replete with

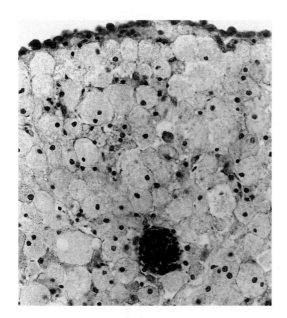

Figure 19-26
XANTHOMA OF THE CHOROID PLEXUS
Masses of xanthoma cells are common incidental postmortem findings.

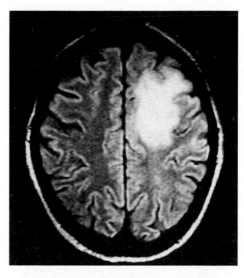

Figure 19-27
PROGRESSIVE MULTIFOCAL
LEUKOENCEPHALOPATHY
Although this process is classically multifocal, some patients, particularly those with acquired immunodeficiency syndrome, present with a solitary lesion requiring a biopsy to exclude a neoplasm.

foamy histiocytes and extracellular cholesterol clefts. Superficial cutaneous xanthomas are frequently an associated systemic finding (21,35).

Xanthomas in Systemic Xanthogranulomatosis. On rare occasion, intracranial or intraspinal masses appear as part of a systemic disorder characterized by multiple, usually cutaneous, xanthomas (25,27,32,34).

Xanthomatous Lesions Associated with Weber-Christian Disease. Rare dura-based xanthomatous foci may be seen in Weber-Christian disease, a relapsing panniculitis with a broad spectrum of clinical expressions. Histologically, these lesions consist in varying proportions of inflammatory infiltrates, fibrosis, and xanthomatous change (33,37).

Xanthomas, Fibroxanthomas, and Xanthogranulomas Not Associated with Systemic Disease. These rare processes consist of xanthomas or fibroxanthomas in the absence of a recognizable predisposing disorder. Heterogeneous in nature, some possibly neoplastic, these lesions share common histologic features including a variable content of xanthomatous cells, fibrous tissue, and chronic inflammation. Most are dura based (24,28–31,36,39).

Progressive Multifocal Leukoencephalopathy

Progressive multifocal leukoencephalopathy (PML) is a demyelinating disease seen in the immunosuppressed, usually with acquired immunodeficiency syndrome (AIDS). This multifocal or occasionally unifocal (fig. 19-27) process is in essence a papova virus infection of oligodendrocytes which produces discrete foci of demyelination. Numerous macrophages attracted by myelin debris and reactive atypical-appearing astrocytes combine to simulate a neoplasm (figs. 19-28, 19-29) (see Appendix A).

Distinguishing the process from a neoplasm is the abundance of macrophages and the presence of large hyperchromatic oligodendroglia, some with purple ground glass nuclei of the type seen in viral infections (fig. 19-30). Immunohistochemistry and in situ hybridization for JC virus confirm the diagnosis in minimally representative biopsies (41,42).

Sarcoidosis

As it affects the CNS, sarcoidosis is usually a diffuse or multicentric meningeal process with diffuse, plaque-like, or nodular thickening of the

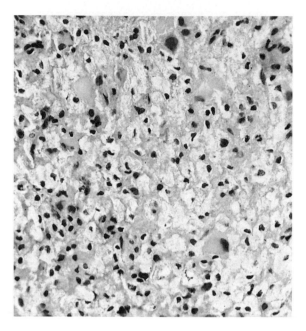

Figure 19-28
PROGRESSIVE MULTIFOCAL
LEUKOENCEPHALOPATHY
In addition to the considerable nuclear atypia of astrocytes and oligodendroglia, the hypercellularity imparted by macrophages contributes to the simulation of a neoplasm.

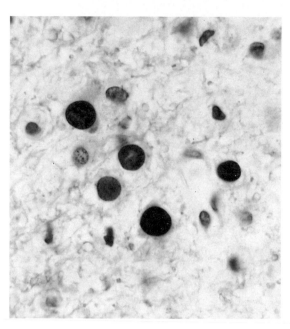

Figure 19-30
PROGRESSIVE MULTIFOCAL
LEUKOENCEPHALOPATHY
The diagnostic large, dark, round nuclei of infected oligodendroglia are best seen at the edge of the lesion.

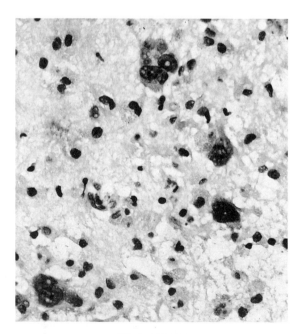

Figure 19-29
PROGRESSIVE MULTIFOCAL
LEUKOENCEPHALOPATHY
Marked nuclear hyperchromatism and pleomorphism of astrocytes are noted within the demyelinated regions.

meninges. The base of the brain is favored, as is the case in *parenchymal sarcoidosis* which typically affects the optic chiasm, infundibulum, and hypothalamus (45,47).

Relevant to this volume is the occurrence of *tumefactive sarcoidosis*. It usually presents as a dura-based meningioma-like mass (44) or as a small contrast-enhancing lesion in the suprasellar area. In the patients having no evidence of extracranial disease, the diagnosis of sarcoidosis is obviously problematic.

Histologically, the principal feature of sarcoidosis is multiple noncaseating granulomas with a tendency for gradual fibrosis (fig. 19-31). Geographic zones of necrosis are not expected, but small foci of fibrinoid necrosis within the granulomas are not uncommon. In the suprasellar region, the disease must be distinguished from the granulomatous inflammation that accompanies some germinomas (43) as well as from giant cell granuloma of the anterior pituitary, a process that may ascend from the sella and resembles sarcoidosis (46).

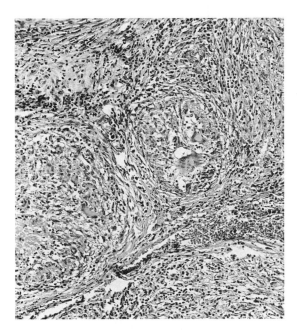

Figure 19-31
SARCOIDOSIS
As elsewhere in the body, meningeal sarcoidosis forms nodular masses of epithelioid histiocytes. Despite the association of necrosis with infectious disorders, such as tuberculosis, small foci of necrosis are not uncommon within the granulomatous nodules of sarcoidosis.

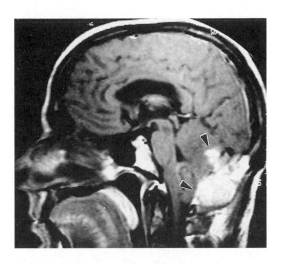

Figure 19-32
PLASMA CELL GRANULOMA
Intracranial plasma cell granulomas often present as dura-based masses (arrows).

Plasma Cell Granuloma

Dura-based meningioma-like masses with a prominent component of plasma cells occur at all levels of the neuraxis (fig. 19-32). Adults are primarily affected. Radiographically, these plasma cell granulomas are contrast enhancing (48–50,53–56).

Although plasma cell granulomas are discrete and are readily separable from underlying brain in most instances, penetration of the dura and involvement of adjacent bone may be noted. Most examples are adherent to the dura or are centered upon the arachnoid. Others are situated within the substance of the brain (51,52). The collagen of the lesions produces a firm texture. Depending upon the degree of collagenization, the color varies from white to gray.

Plasma cell granulomas are noted for their conspicuous content of mature plasma cells, often admixed with plasmacytoid and typical lymphocytes (fig. 19-33). Russell bodies are frequently encountered. Histiocytes, some lipid laden, may be noted. A fibroblastic reaction is typically seen and varies considerably in extent and degree. A storiform pattern is observed in some; in others bands of dense collagen lend a distinctive hyalinized appearance. In one reported case, designated "hyalinizing plasmacytic granulomatosis," the hyalinized fibers were surrounded by multinucleated giant cells (55).

Immunohistochemically, immunoglobulin production of the plasma cells is polyclonal.

Surgically, meningioma is the principal differential diagnosis. At the microscopic level, that diagnosis is entertained in cases in which proliferating histiocytes resemble nodules of meningothelial cells. Such lesions resemble plasma cell-rich or lymphoplasmacytoid meningiomas. Generally, plasma cell granulomas are overtly inflammatory in nature; the overrun meningothelial cells are a minimal component at best. If doubt remains regarding the presence of an underlying meningothelial lesion, further tissue sampling or immunohistochemistry for epithelial membrane antigen may be of assistance.

The distinction of plasma cell granuloma and plasmacytoma is usually apparent on hematoxylin and eosin (H&E) stained sections since the latter lesion is a cytologically monotonous plasma cell proliferation without the mixed inflammatory appearance of plasma cell granuloma.

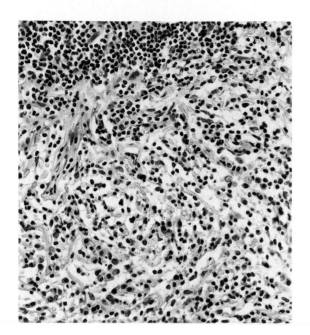 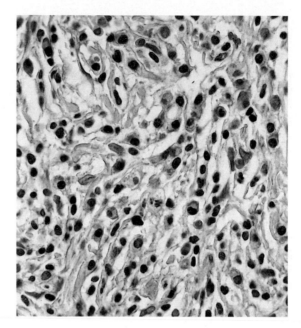

Figure 19-33
PLASMA CELL GRANULOMA
At low (left) and high (right) magnification, the lesion is a fibrotic mass with aggregated and dispersed populations of lymphocytes and plasma cells.

Immunohistochemical demonstration of polyclonality may be required in some cases, however.

The distinction between plasma cell granuloma and Castleman disease as well as sinus histiocytosis with massive lymphadenopathy (SHML, Rosai-Dorfman disease), is not as precise in the nervous system as at other sites. Indeed, it is possible that some reported cases of "plasma cell granuloma" belong to one of these other categories. Although rare, the lesion in Castleman syndrome is rather distinctive, featuring a more nodular pattern of lymphocytes associated with germinal center-like structures and hyperplastic vessels. Also rare, SHML exhibits a higher content of histiocytes, some showing emperipolesis.

An insufficient number of cases have been studied to permit generalization regarding the prognosis and optimum treatment of plasma cell granuloma. A number of patients have undergone postoperative radiation therapy with resolution of the lesion. On the other hand, many do well without lesion progression or recurrence after resection alone. The role of radiotherapy is thus debatable, particularly in cases in which total resection in gross or radiographic terms has been achieved (55).

Extranodal Sinus Histiocytosis with Massive Lymphadenopathy (Rosai-Dorfman Disease)

This uncommon non-neoplastic disorder usually presents as massive cervical lymphadenopathy with or without concurrent or subsequent involvement of other sites, either nodal or extranodal (59,62). An elevated erythrocyte sedimentation rate and polyclonal gammopathy are common. The process rarely affects the CNS, but may do so indirectly by pressure upon the brain or spinal cord from an epidural or intradural lesion (figs. 19-34, 19-35) (57,59,60,62a,63,64,). Clinically apparent nodal involvement may or may not accompany CNS symptoms. Intracranial, single or multiple, dura-based, meningioma-like lesions have been reported.

Histologically, extranodal lesions affecting the CNS are composed of sheets or nodules of vacuolated histiocytes interrupted by foci of chronic inflammatory cells containing lymphocytes and numerous plasma cells (figs. 19-36, 19-37). Emperipolesis may be seen but is often inconspicuous. The large histiocytes are S-100 positive (61).

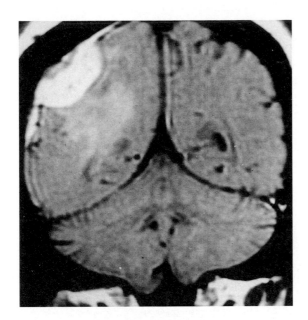

Figure 19-34
EXTRANODAL SINUS HISTIOCYTOSIS
WITH MASSIVE LYMPHADENOPATHY
(ROSAI-DORFMAN DISEASE)
Extranodal sinus histiocytosis with massive lymphadeno-
pathy is an uncommon cause of an intracranial mass. As here
over the parietal lobe, most lesions are dura based.

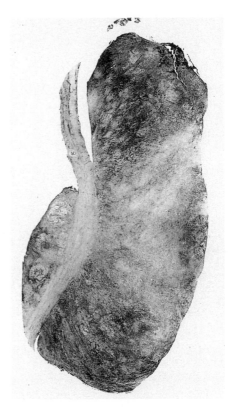

Figure 19-35
EXTRANODAL SINUS HISTIOCYTOSIS
WITH MASSIVE LYMPHADENOPATHY
(ROSAI-DORFMAN DISEASE)
The surgical specimen from the case illustrated in figure
19-34 shows both epidural and intradural involvement.

Although morphologic similarities exist between Langerhans cell histiocytosis and sinus
histiocytosis with massive lymphadenopathy
(SHML), the former exhibits more epithelioid-ap-
pearing histiocytes, a frequent eosinophil component, and less emperipolesis. Langerhans cell
granules are not found in SHML. SHML often
exhibits alpha-1-antitrypsin, alpha-1-anti-
chymotrypsin, and lysozyme whereas these are
lacking in Langerhans cell histiocytosis (58).

Although the meningeal lesions of SHML may
persist, and in some cases enlarge, the disorder
is rarely a cause of death.

Castleman Disease

Castleman disease is an uncommon reactive
lesion which may be systemic or limited to lymph
nodes, most often those of the mediastinum. Two
variants, the hyaline-vascular and plasma cell
types, are recognized. The former is noted for
germinal centers with hyalinization and prominent vessels whereas the latter may be accompanied by anemia, hypogammaglobulinemia,
and an elevated erythrocyte sedimentation rate.

Histologically, the latter is noted for the presence
of large numbers of plasma cells, often with
accompanying Russell bodies within interfollicu-
lar areas (66).

Intracranial or intraspinal involvement is
most unusual but the lesion has been reported
to form meningioma-like masses (65,67,68).

Too few cases are on record to permit conclusions concerning biologic behavior, although
most extracranial lesions are patently benign.

Syphilis (Gumma)

Neurosyphilis is usually a diffuse inflammatory
leptomeningeal process which in some cases involves traversing vessels (*meningovascular syphilis*). A stroke syndrome may result (74). Exceptionally, the process forms intracranial tumor-like
masses termed gummas (69,71–74a). Syphilis
may also affect patients with AIDS (70).

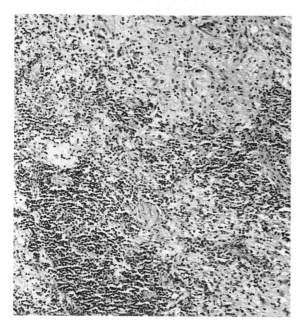

Figure 19-36
EXTRANODAL SINUS HISTIOCYTOSIS
WITH MASSIVE LYMPHADENOPATHY
(ROSAI-DORFMAN DISEASE)
A dense population of plasma cells and lymphocytes are
interrupted by aggregates of large histiocytes.

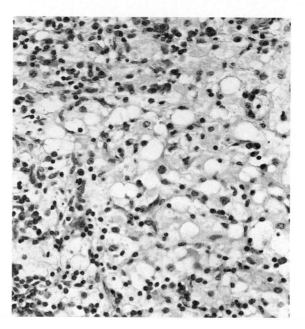

Figure 19-37
EXTRANODAL SINUS HISTIOCYTOSIS
WITH MASSIVE LYMPHADENOPATHY
(ROSAI-DORFMAN DISEASE)
Nodules of histiocytes abut zones of plasma cells and
lymphocytes. Emperipolesis is noted in some cases, but can
be inconspicuous.

Histologically, gummas consist of plasma cell–rich masses with or without foci of necrosis. Since attempts to differentially stain the organisms are usually unsuccessful, the diagnosis often rests on serologic studies.

Collagen-Vascular Diseases

Intracranial expressions of rheumatoid arthritis are rare. Most present as meningeal lesions, some of which are tumefactive (75,77,79). Histologically, the latter are fibroinflammatory in nature and exhibit necrosis centers surrounded by epithelial and scattered multinucleate cells. Such lesions look like classic rheumatoid nodules although radiating epithelioid cells may not be as prominent. Most lesions appear granulomatous, thus prompting consideration of infection, particularly tuberculosis.

Wegener granulomatosis rarely affects the CNS. It is more prone to form an inflammatory infiltrate within which regional vessels become occluded than a mass (78,80).

Cerebral symptoms are common in systemic lupus erythematosus but are rarely a consequence of vasculitis. Cerebral infarction, rather than an inflammatory mass, is the usual consequence.

Sjögren disease may occasionally be associated with a steroid-responsive dementia due to lymphocytic microperivasculitis (76).

Amyloidoma

On rare occasion, masses of amyloid present as extra- or intra-axial lesions and thus clinically and radiographically mimic a brain tumor in the absence of a plasma cell dyscrasia (82–85). Histologically, the amyloid may be deposited about vessels in concentric lamellae, or simply as scattered or cohesive spherical masses. A small number of lymphocytes and plasma cells may be seen. In one case, the plasma cells were apparently monoclonal (81,86). There is no association with systemic amyloidosis.

REFERENCES

Demyelinating Disease

1. Hook CC, Kimmel DW, Kvols LK, et al. Multifocal inflammatory leukoencephalopathy with 5-fluorouracil and levamisole. Ann Neurol 1992;31:262–7.
1a. Hulette CM, Downey BT, Burger PC. Macrophage markers in diagnostic neuropathology. Am J Surg Pathol 1992;16:493–9.
2. Hunter SB, Ballinger WE Jr, Rubin JJ. Multiple sclerosis mimicking primary brain tumor. Arch Pathol Lab Med 1987;111:464–8.
2a. Kepes JJ. Large focal tumor-like demyelinating lesions of the brain: intermediate entity between multiple sclerosis and acute disseminated encephalomyelitis? A study of 31 patients. Ann Neurol 1993;33:18–27.
3. Malmgren RM, Detels R, Verity MA. Co-occurrence of multiple sclerosis and glioma—case report and neuropathologic and epidemiologic review. Clin Neuropathol 1984;3:1–9.
4. Nesbit G, Forbes G, Scheithauer BW, et al. Multiple sclerosis: histopathologic and MR/CT correlation in 37 biopsied and three autopsied patients. Radiology 1991;80:467–74.

Cerebral Infarct

5. Kondziolka D, Fazl M. Functional recovery after decompressive craniectomy for cerebral infarction. Neurosurgery 1988;23:143–7.

Radionecrosis

6. Ball WS Jr, Prenger EC, Ballard ET. Neurotoxicity of radio/chemotherapy in children: pathologic and MR correlation. AJNR Am J Neuroradiol 1992;13:761–76.
7. Burger PC, Boyko OB. The pathology of central nervous system radiation injury. In: Gutin PH, Leibel SA, Sheline GE, eds. Radiation injury to the nervous system. New York: Raven Press, 1991:191–208.
8. Nelson DR, Yuh WT, Wen BC, Ryals TJ, Cornell SH. Cerebral necrosis simulating an intraparenchymal tumor. AJNR Am J Neuroradiol 1990;11:211–2.
9. Oppenheimer JH, Levy ML, Sinha U, et al. Radionecrosis secondary to interstitial brachytherapy: correlation of magnetic resonance imaging and histopathology. Neurosurgery 1992;31:336–43.

Langerhans Cell Histiocytosis

10. Ball WS Jr, Prenger EC, Ballard ET. Neurotoxicity of radio/chemotherapy in children: pathologic and MR correlation. AJNR Am J Neuroradiol 1992;13:761–76.
11. Eriksen B, Janinis J, Variakojis D, et al. Primary histiocytosis X of the parieto-occipital lobe. Hum Pathol 1988;19:611–4.
12. Fartasch M, Vigneswaran N, Diepgen TL, Hornstein OP. Immunohistochemical and ultrastructural study of histiocytosis X and non-X histiocytoses. J Am Acad Dermatol 1990;23:885–92.
13. Greenwood SM, Martin JS, Towfighi J. Unifocal eosinophilic granuloma of the temporal lobe. Surg Neurol 1982;17:441–4.
14. Itoh H, Waga S, Kojima T, Hoshino T. Solitary eosinophilic granuloma in the frontal lobe: case report. Neurosurgery 1992;30:295–8.
14a. Jamjoom ZA, Raina V, Al-Jamali A, Jamjoom AB, Yacub Y, Sharif HS. Intracranial xanthogranuloma of the dura in Hand-Schüller-Christian disease. Case report. J Neurosurg 1993;78:297–300.
15. Kepes JJ, Kepes M. Predominantly cerebral forms of histiocytosis-X. A reappraisal of "Gagel's hypothalamic granuloma," "granuloma infiltrans of the hypothalamus" and "Ayala's disease" with a report of four cases. Acta Neuropathol (Berl) 1969;14:77–98.
16. Maghnie M, Arico M, Villa A, Genovese E, Beluffi G, Severi F. MR of the hypothalamic-pituitary axis in Langerhans cell histiocytosis. AJNR Am J Neuroradiol 1992;13:1365–71.
16a. Morello A, Campesi G, Bettinazzi N, Albeggiani A. Neoplastiform xanthomatous granulomas of choroid plexus in a child affected by Hand-Schüller-Christian disease: case report. J Neurosurg 1967;26:536–41.
17. Moscinski LC, Kleinschmidt-DeMasters BK. Primary eosinophilic granuloma of frontal lobe. Diagnostic use of S-100 protein. Cancer 1985;56:284–8.
18. Smolik EA, Devecerski M, Nelson JS, Smith KR Jr. Histiocytosis X in the optic chiasm of an adult with hypopituitarism. Case report. J Neurosurg 1968;29:290–5.
19. Tabarin A, Corcuff JB, Dautheribes M, et al. Histiocytosis X of the hypothalamus. J Endocrinol Invest 1991;14:139–45.
20. Tien RD, Newton TH, McDermott MW, Dillon WP, Kucharczyk J. Thickened pituitary stalk on MR images in patient with diabetes insipidus and Langerhans cell histiocytosis. AJNR Am J Neuroradiol 1990;11:703–8.

Xanthomatous Lesions

21. Akazawa S, Ikeda Y, Toyama K, Miyake S, Takamori M, Nagataki S. Familial type IIa hyperlipoproteinemia associated with a huge intracranial xanthoma. Arch Neurol 1984;41:793–4.
22. Ayers WW, Haymaker W. Xanthoma and cholesterol granuloma of the choroid plexus. Report of the pathological aspects in 29 cases. J Neuropathol Exp Neurol 1960;19:280–95.

23. Brück W, Sander U, Blanckenberg P, Friede RL. Symptomatic xanthogranuloma of the choroid plexus with unilateral hydrocephalus. Case report. J Neurosurg 1991;75:324–7.

24. Carrillo R, Ricoy JR, Herrero-Vallejo J, Bravo G. Fibrous xanthomas of the brain. Report of two cases. Clin Neurol Neurosurg 1975;78:34–40.

25. Flach DB, Winkelmann RK. Juvenile xanthogranuloma with central nervous system lesions. J Am Acad Dermatol 1986;14:405–11.

26. Gaskill SJ, Saldivar V, Rutman J, Marlin AE. Giant bilateral xanthogranulomas in a child: case report. Neurosurgery 1992;31:114–7.

27. Giller RH, Folberg R, Keech RV, Piette WW, Sato Y. Xanthoma disseminatum. An unusual histiocytosis syndrome. Am J Pediatr Hematol Oncol 1988;10:252–7.

28. Kamiryo T, Abiko S, Orita T, Aoki H, Watanabe Y, Hiraoka K. Bilateral intracranial fibrous xanthoma. Surg Neurol 1988;29:27–31.

29. Kepes JJ. "Xanthomatous" lesions of the central nervous system: definition, classification and some recent observations. Progress Neuropathol 1979;4:179–213.

30. _____, Kepes M, Slowik F. Fibrous xanthomas and xanthosarcomas of the meninges and the brain. Acta Neuropathol (Berl) 1973;23:187–99.

31. Kimura H, Oka K, Nakayama Y, Tomonaga M. Xanthoma in Meckel's cave. A case report. Surg Neurol 1991;35:317–20.

32. Knobler RM, Neumann RA, Gebhart W, Radaskiewicz T, Ferenci P, Widhalm K. Xanthoma disseminatum with progressive involvement of the central nervous and hepatobiliary systems. J Am Acad Dermatol 1990;23:341–6.

33. Mangiardi JR, Rappaport ZH, Ransohoff J. Systemic Weber-Christian disease presenting as an intracranial mass lesion. Case report. J Neurosurg 1980;52:134–7.

34. Miyachi S, Kobayashi T, Takahashi T, Saito K, Hashizume Y, Sugita K. An intracranial mass lesion in systemic xanthogranulomatosis: case report. Neurosurgery 1990;27:822–6.

35. Okabe H, Ishizawa M, Matsumoto K, et al. Immunohistochemical analysis of spinal intradural xanthomatosis developed in a patient with phytosterolemia. Acta Neuropathol (Berl) 1992;83:554–8.

36. Paulus W, Kirchner T, Michaela M, et al. Histiocytic tumor of Meckel's cave. An intracranial equivalent of juvenile xanthogranuloma of the skin. Am J Surg Pathol 1992;16:76–83.

37. Pick P, Jean E, Horoupian D, Factor S. Xanthogranuloma of the dura in systemic Weber-Christian disease. Neurology 1983;33:1067–70.

38. Shuangshoti S, Netsky MG. Xanthogranuloma (xanthoma) of choroid plexus. The origin of foamy (xanthoma) cells. Am J Pathol 1966;48:503–33.

39. Vaquero J, Leunda G, Cabezudo JM, De Juan M, Herrero J, Bravo G. Posterior fossa xanthogranuloma. Case report. J Neurosurg 1979;51:718–22.

40. Wolf A, Cowen D, Graham S. Xanthomas of the choroid plexus in man. J Neuropathol Exp Neurol 1950;9:286–97.

Progressive Multifocal Leukoencephalopathy

41. Hulette CM, Downey BT, Burger PC. Progressive multifocal leukoencephalopathy. Diagnosis by in situ hybridization with a biotinylated JC virus DNA probe using an automated Histomatic Code-On slide stainer. Am J Surg Pathol 1991;15:791–7.

42. Schmidbauer M, Budka H, Shah KV. Progressive multifocal leukoencephalopathy (PML) in AIDS and in the pre-AIDS era. A neuropathological comparison using immunocytochemistry and in situ DNA hybridization for virus detection. Acta Neuropathol (Berl) 1990;80:375–80.

Sarcoidosis

43. Kraichoke S, Cosgrove M, Chandrasoma PT. Granulomatous inflammation in pineal germinoma. A cause of diagnostic failure at stereotaxic brain biopsy. Am J Surg Pathol 1988;12:655–60.

44. Ranoux D, Devaux B, Lamy C, Mear JY, Roux FX, Mas JL. Meningeal sarcoidosis, pseudo-meningioma, and pachymeningitis of the convexity. J Neurol Neurosurg Psychiatry 1992;55:300–3.

45. Sherman JL, Stern BJ. Sarcoidosis of the CNS: comparison of unenhanced and enhanced MR images. AJNR Am J Neuroradiol 1990;11:915–23.

46. Siqueira E, Tsung JS, Al-Kawi MZ, Woodhouse N. Case report: idiopathic giant cell granuloma of the hypophysis: an unusual cause of panhypopituitarism. Surg Neurol 1989;32:68–71.

47. Stern BJ, Krumholz A, Johns C, Scott P, Nissim J. Sarcoidosis and its neurological manifestations. Arch Neurol 1985;42:909–17.

Plasma Cell Granuloma

48. Cannella DM, Prezyna AP, Kapp JP. Primary intracranial plasma-cell granuloma. Case report. J Neurosurg 1988;69:785–8.

49. Eimoto T, Yanaka M, Kurosawa M, Ikeya F. Plasma cell granuloma (inflammatory pseudotumor) of the spinal cord meninges. Report of a case. Cancer 1978;41:1929–36.

50. Gangemi M, Maiuri F, Giamundo A, Donati P, De Chiara A. Intracranial plasma cell granuloma. Neurosurgery 1989;24:591–5.

51. Gochman GA, Duffy K, Crandall PH, Vinters HV. Plasma cell granuloma of the brain. Surg Neurol 1990;33:347–52.

52. Maeda Y, Tani E, Nakano M, Matsumoto T. Plasma-cell granuloma of the fourth ventricle. Case report. J Neurosurg 1984;60:1291–6.

53. Mirra SS, Tindall SC, Check IJ, Brynes RK, Moore WW. Inflammatory meningeal masses of unexplained origin. An ultrastructural and immunologic study. J Neuropathol Exp Neurol 1983;42:453–68.

54. Nakagawa K, Sakaki S, Fukui K, Sadamoto K. Intracranial nonspecific inflammatory granuloma. Surg Neurol 1990;33:221–5.

55. Nazek M, Mandybur TI, Sawaya R. Hyalinizing plasmacytic granulomatosis of the falx. Am J Surg Pathol 1988;12:308–13.

56. West SG, Pittman DL, Coggin JT. Intracranial plasma cell granuloma. Cancer 1980;46:330–5.

Extranodal Sinus Histocytosis with Massive Lymphadenopathy (Rosai-Dorfman Disease)

57. Carey MP, Case CP. Sinus histiocytosis with massive lymphadenopathy presenting as a meningioma. Neuropathol Appl Neurobiol 1987;13:391–8.
58. Eisen RN, Buckley PJ, Rosai J. Immunophenotypic characterization of sinus histiocytes with massive lymphadenopathy (Rosai-Dorfman disease). Semin Diagn Pathol 1990;7:74–82.
59. Foucar E, Rosai J, Dorfman RF. Sinus histiocytomas with massive lymphadenopathy (Rosai-Dorfman disease): review of the entity. Semin Diagn Pathol 1990;7:19–73.
60. Lopez P, Estes ML. Immunohistochemical characterization of the histiocytes in sinus histiocytosis with massive lymphadenopathy: analysis of an extranodal case. Hum Pathol 1989;20:711–5.

61. Montgomery EA, Meis JM, Frizzera G. Rosai-Dorfman disease of soft tissue. Am J Surg Pathol 1992;16:122–9.
62. Rosai J, Dorfman RF. Sinus histiocytosis with massive lymphadenopathy: a pseudolymphomatous benign disorder. Analysis of 34 cases. Cancer 1972;30:1174–88.
62a. Shaver EG, Rebsamen SL, Yachnis AT, Sutton LN. Isolated extranodal sinus histiocytosis in a 5-year-old boy. Case report. J Neurosurg 1993;79:769–73.
63. Song SK, Schwartz IS, Strauchen JA, et al. Meningeal nodules with features of extranodal sinus histiocytosis with massive lymphadenopathy. Am J Surg Pathol 1989;13:406–12.
64. Trudel M. Dural involvement in sinus histiocytosis with massive lymphadenopathy. Case report. J Neurosurg 1984;60:850–2.

Castleman Disease

65. Gianaris PG, Leestma JE, Cerullo LJ, Butler A. Castleman's disease manifesting in the central nervous system: case report with immunological studies. Neurosurgery 1989;24:608–13.
66. Keller AR, Hochholzer L, Castleman B. Hyaline-vascular and plasma-cell types of giant lymph node hyperplasia of the mediastinum and other locations. Cancer 1972;29:670–83.

67. Lacombe MJ, Poirier J, Caron JP. Intracranial lesion resembling giant lymph node hyperplasia. Am J Clin Pathol 1983;80:721–3.
68. Severson GS, Harrington DS, Weisenburger DD, et al. Castleman's disease of the leptomeninges. Report of three cases. J Neurosurg 1988;69:283–6.

Syphilis (Gumma)

69. Agrons GA, Han SS, Husson MA, Simeone F. MR imaging of cerebral gumma. AJNR Am J Neuroradiol 1991;12:80–1.
70. Berger JR, Waskin HA, Pall L, Hensley G, Ihmedian I, Post MJ. Syphilitic cerebral gumma with HIV infection. Neurology 1992;42:1282–7.
71. Fleet WS, Watson RT, Ballinger WE. Resolution of a gumma with steroid therapy. Neurology 1986;36:1104–7.
72. Ito M, Sato K, Tada H, Kuru Y. Neurosyphilis manifesting as a focal mass lesion: computed tomographic

and magnetic resonance imaging features. Case report. Neurol Med Chir (Tokyo) 1990;30:194–7.
73. Madsen FF, Pedersen KK, Stubbe-Teglbjaerg P. Cerebral gumma. Br J Neurosurg 1987;1:590–13.
74. Simon RP. Neurosyphilis. Arch Neurol 1985;42:606–13.
74a. Vogl T, Dresel S, Lochmüller H, Bergman, Reimers C, Lissner J. Third cranial nerve palsy caused by gummatous neurosyphilis: MR findings. AJNR Am J Neuroradiol 1993;14:1329–31.

Collagen-Vascular Diseases

75. Bathon JM, Moreland LW, DiBartolomeo AG. Inflammatory central nervous system involvement in rheumatoid arthritis. Semin Arthritis Rheum 1989;18:258–66.
76. Caselli RJ, Scheithauer BW, Bowles C, et al. The treatable dementia of Sjogrens syndrome: clinical, neuropsychologic, radiologic, and histopathologic correlations. Ann Neurol 1991;30:98–101.
77. Ouyang R, Mitchell DM, Rozdilsky B. Central nervous system involvement in rheumatoid disease. Report of a case. Neurology 1967;17:1099–105.

78. Satoh J, Miyasaka N, Yamada T, et al. Extensive cerebral infarction due to involvement of both anterior cerebral arteries by Wegener's granulomatosis. Ann Rheum Dis 1988;47:606–11.
79. Schachenmayr W, Friede RL. Dural involvement in rheumatoid arthritis. Acta Neuropathol (Berl) 1978;42:65–6.
80. Scully RE. Case records of the Massachusetts General Hospital. Case 12–1988. N Eng J Med 1988;318;760–8.

Amyloidoma

81. Cohen M, Lanska D, Roessmann U, et al. Amyloidoma of the CNS. I. Clinical and pathologic study. Neurology 1992;42:2019–23.
82. Ferreiro JA, Bhuta S, Nieberg RK, Verity MA. Amyloidoma of the skull base. Arch Pathol Lab Med 1990;114:974–6.
83. Spaar FW, Goebel HH, Volles E, Wickboldt J. Tumorlike amyloid formation (amyloidoma) in the brain. J Neurol 1981;224:171–82.

84. Townsend JJ, Tomiyasu U, MacKay A, Wilson CB. Central nervous system amyloid presenting as a mass lesion. Report of two cases. J Neurosurg 1982;56:439–42.
85. Ünal F, Hepgül K, Bayindir Ç, Bilge T, Imer M, Turantan I. Skull base amyloidoma. Case report. J Neurosurg 1992;76:303–6.
86. Vidal RG, Ghiso J, Gallo G, Cohen M, Gambetti PL, Frangione B. Amyloidoma of the CNS. II. Immunohistochemical and biochemical study. Neurology 1992;42:2024–8.

20

METASTATIC AND SECONDARY NEOPLASMS

Metastatic Carcinoma and Sarcoma

Definition. Neoplasms affecting the central nervous system (CNS) by local extension or by blood borne dissemination from a distant site.

General Comments. Metastatic carcinomas are common intracranial masses encountered both at surgery and autopsy. Selected references give clinical accounts of metastases from carcinomas of lung (18,37), breast (38), bladder (12), prostate (7,36), ovary (10,33), and placenta (2,20), and malignant melanoma (5,11,28). Metastatic sarcomas are much less common. All major sarcomas have been represented (22,30).

Clinical and Radiographic Features. *Metastatic Tumors of the Skull and Dura.* Most cranial metastases are irregular lytic lesions which, given time, enlarge and compress the underlying brain. Less common are globular, dura-based, meningioma-like masses with little, if any, detectable calvarial component. Extensive osteoblastic metastases, particularly at the skull base, are classically from carcinomas of the prostate, whereas metastatic lesions in and about the sella turcica frequently originate in the breast (24) and less often the lung. Prostatic carcinoma may affect the dura but only rarely involves brain parenchyma.

Carcinomas of the head and neck may extend in a seemingly discontinuous fashion along neurovascular structures to present intracranially. Such perineural extension, occasionally as far as the cavernous sinus, is typical of adenoid cystic carcinoma (figs. 20-1, 20-2) (14,27) and, to a lesser extent, basal cell carcinoma of the face or neck. The primary tumor is sometimes sufficiently small as to be undetected at the time the intracranial component becomes symptomatic.

Metastases to the Spinal Column and Epidural Space. Metastases to the vertebral column and epidural space are a common cause of spinal cord compression (fig. 20-3). Neoplasms of the breast, lung, and prostate are the common primary sources (6,32). Particularly with lung cancer, the primary may be unsuspected at the time the metastasis is discovered. Metastases of prostate carcinoma, usually osteoblastic, typically "creep" rostrally and laterally from lumbosacral levels to simultaneously involve the base of the skull, the lateral bony pelvis, and the ribs. This tumor, unlike some lytic lesions, does not generally produce vertebral collapse or symptomatic compression of the spinal cord. Back pain is the principal symptom.

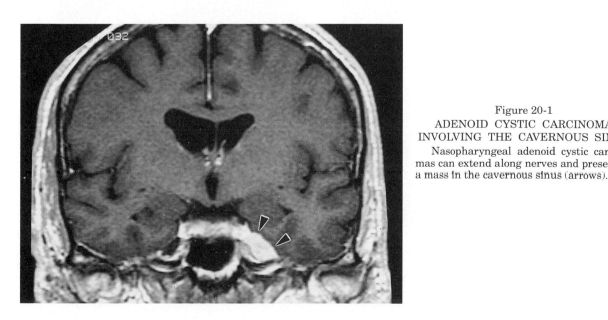

Figure 20-1
ADENOID CYSTIC CARCINOMA INVOLVING THE CAVERNOUS SINUS
Nasopharyngeal adenoid cystic carcinomas can extend along nerves and present as a mass in the cavernous sinus (arrows).

415

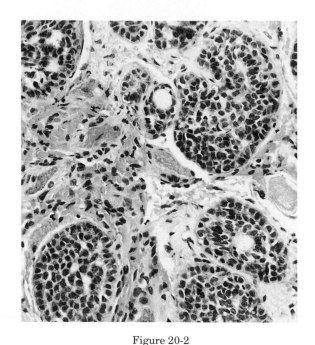

Figure 20-2
ADENOID CYSTIC CARCINOMA
INVOLVING THE GASSERIAN GANGLION
Individual cells and small glands are seen among nerve
fibers and ganglion of the trigeminal nerve.

Metastatic Tumors of the Meninges and Sub-arachnoid Space. Metastases to the leptomeninges are a frequent consequence of CNS metastases, both cranial and spinal (26,39). A special variant of meningeal carcinoma is a diffuse proliferation known as *carcinomatosis meningitis,* or *meningeal carcinomatosis* in the semantically correct form (see fig. 20-11) (3,17,21,34). By definition, the process is limited largely to the subarachnoid space, though access may be attained from the spine or skull (17,21). In practice, small parenchymal foci of metastatic carcinomas are sometimes encountered (26). Meningeal carcinomatosis typically occurs with adenocarcinoma of the stomach, lung, or breast. As a source, carcinoma of the stomach, once the classic primary, has now been largely supplanted by mammary carcinoma (3). Mental "clouding," headaches, and progressive cranial nerve deficits are common symptoms. The disorder is suggested when neuroimaging studies show thickening and contrast enhancement of the leptomeninges (34). Cytologic examination of cerebrospinal fluid is often

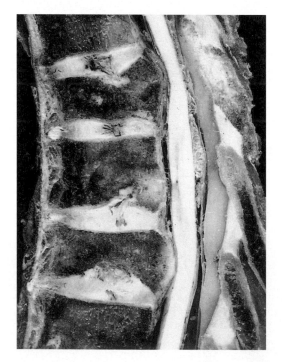

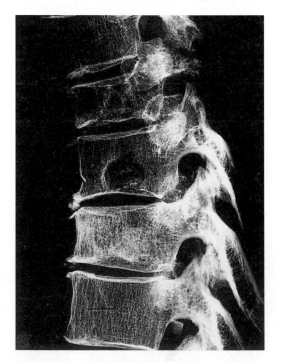

Figure 20-3
METASTATIC CARCINOMA
Left: As in this patient with breast carcinoma, vertebral collapse and spinal cord compression are common consequences of spinal metastases.
Right: The osteolytic nature of the lesions is apparent in a radiograph of the same specimen.

confirmatory (16). A meningeal biopsy must include a generous sample of leptomeninges; dural samples are typically nondiagnostic.

Metastases to the Parenchyma of the Brain and Spinal Cord. Metastases to CNS parenchyma are either solitary or multiple, and are almost always contrast enhancing (fig. 20-4, left). They characteristically incite a large zone of peritumoral cerebral edema commensurate with a rapidly growing mass (fig. 20-4, right). Such tumors originate at any of a number of primary sites. Neoplasms with a propensity to disseminate to the CNS, like malignant melanoma, often produce multiple metastases, whereas solitary deposits generally occur with tumors not prone to CNS metastasis, such as adenocarcinoma of the gastrointestinal tract. Symptoms of a brain metastasis as the first evidence of the disease are especially likely in carcinoma of the lung (37). Late and often solitary metastases are classically associated with a primary in the kidney or eye (melanoma). Abundant mucus in some metastatic gastrointestinal neoplasms can be observed by a dark signal in T2-weighted images (T2 shortening) (15).

Metastatic carcinoma to the brain usually affects either or both the cerebral hemispheres and cerebellum (figs. 20-5, 20-6). While any cerebral lobe or portion thereof may be involved, the distribution of metastases is not random. As a presumed consequence of circulatory dynamics, watershed areas between the anterior, middle, and posterior cerebral arteries are favored (13). Rarely are such locations as the pineal gland or tuber cinereum selectively affected (40). Brain stem lesions are also uncommon (41).

Metastases to spinal cord parenchyma are rare and generally found in the terminal stages of widely metastatic carcinoma from the bronchus or skin (melanoma) (fig. 20-7). It is highly unusual for patients to present with symptoms referable to an intramedullary metastasis (9).

Macroscopic Findings. Metastases to the parenchyma are well-circumscribed; firm; granular, mucoid, or necrotic in texture; and vary in color, with most gray-tan. Their epicenter is typically in gray matter and in the cortex near the gray-white junction (figs. 20-5, 20-6). Metastatic melanomas are variably pigmented due to melanin deposition or associated hemorrhage.

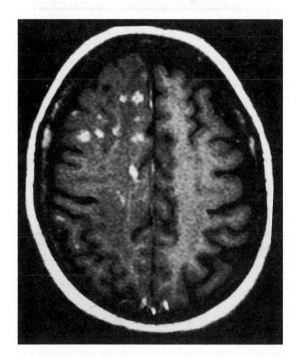 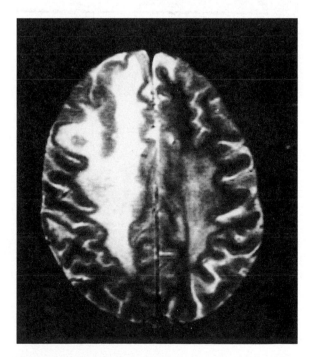

Figure 20-4
METASTATIC CARCINOMA
Multiplicity and contrast enhancement (left), and also considerable peritumoral edema (right), are cardinal radiographic features of metastatic carcinoma.

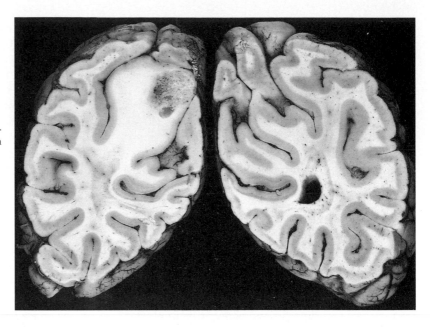

Figure 20-5
METASTATIC CARCINOMA
Metastatic carcinomas are usually superficially situated and associated with considerable surrounding edema.

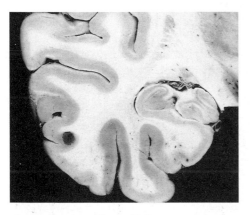

Figure 20-6
METASTATIC CARCINOMA
The typical location of metastases in gray matter is apparent in this small lesion in the temporal lobe.

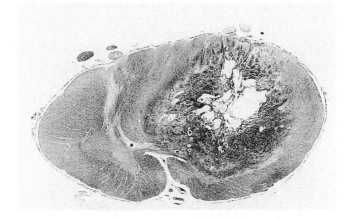

Figure 20-7
METASTATIC CARCINOMA
Although involvement of spinal meninges and nerve roots is common, intraparenchymal metastases to the spinal cord are rare.

Metastases are typically surrounded by a considerable rim of yellow, soft, edematous white matter (fig. 20-5). Extensive hemorrhage most often accompanies metastatic melanoma, choriocarcinoma, and, due primarily to its high incidence, bronchogenic carcinoma (23). Dystrophic calcification of metastases is unusual, occurs primarily in breast or carcinoid tumors, and is rarely evident on radiographs (35). Metastatic sarcomas, like osteosarcoma or malignant fibrous histiocytoma, are relatively infrequent and usually occur late in the course of the disease.

Microscopic Findings. Metastatic carcinomas affecting the CNS are similar histologically to those at other body sites and do not require detailed description, other than to stress the features that distinguish them from lesions with which they might be confused.

Parenchymal metastases are discrete lesions that largely displace rather than infiltrate adjacent tissues (fig. 20-8). Thus, although small tongues of tumor may extend into the brain, carcinoma cells do not extensively permeate parenchyma in an isolated manner as with gliomas

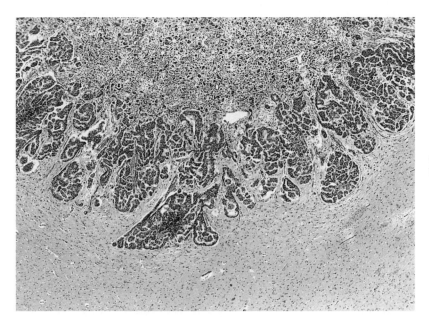

Figure 20-8
METASTATIC CARCINOMA
Metastases are generally well-circumscribed masses which displace, more
than permeate, parenchyma.

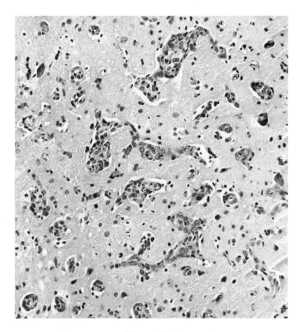

Figure 20-9
METASTATIC CARCINOMA
Occasional metastatic carcinomas track along small ves-
sels, creating a diffuse zone of infiltration.

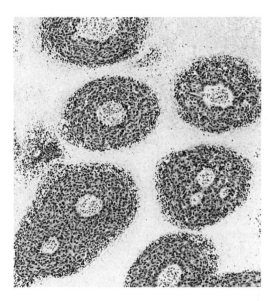

Figure 20-10
METASTATIC CARCINOMA
Sparing of an isometric zone of viable neoplastic cells is
common in necrotizing metastases.

and lymphomas. Metastatic small cell carcinomas
and occasional melanomas are an exception since,
to a limited extent, they may infiltrate both brain
tissue and perivascular zones (fig. 20-9) (31).

Metastases often undergo extensive necrosis
with viable tissue limited to a narrow rim of tumor

at the periphery of the lesion or to well-circumscribed perivascular cuffs (fig. 20-10). While uniform perivascular collars are occasionally seen
in malignant gliomas, this pattern of tumor sparing is more characteristic of metastases.

Vascular proliferation, typical of glioblastoma,
is infrequent in carcinoma metastases and is
spatially confined to occasional vessels in the

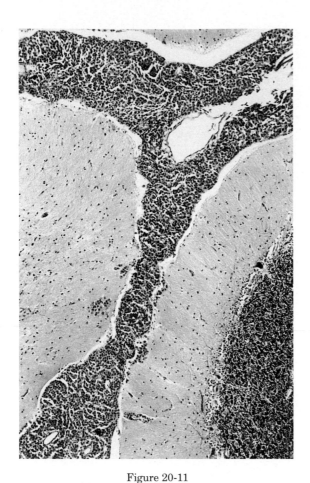

Figure 20-11
MENINGEAL CARCINOMATOSIS
Meningeal carcinomatosis is the diffuse proliferation of neoplastic cells without the formation of a tumorous mass.

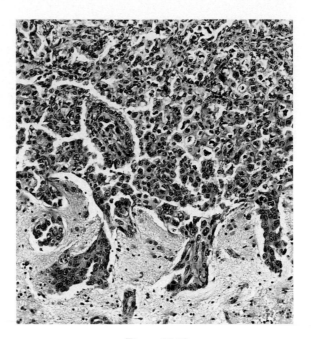

Figure 20-12
METASTATIC CARCINOMA TO THE MENINGES
Carcinomas metastatic to the meninges often follow the perivascular, or Virchow-Robin, spaces into the cerebral cortex.

immediate environs of the lesion. In contrast, vascular proliferation in glioblastomas may occur in peritumoral brain tissue or at remote sites such as in leptomeninges, but is also prominent within the tumor. Considerable vascular reaction may accompany some metastases, especially those of renal cell carcinoma.

The neoplastic cells in meningeal carcinomatosis proliferate freely within the subarachnoid space, opacify the leptomeninges, extend inwardly along perivascular (Virchow-Robin) spaces, and produce either diffuse or nodular enlargement of cranial and spinal nerves (figs. 20-11, 20-12). In most instances, the neoplasms are anaplastic or attain differentiation limited to mucus production by signet ring cells. Epithelial growth patterns and squamous differentiation are less often encountered.

Immunohistochemical Findings. Metastatic lesions share the immunoreactivity of the parent neoplasm so that positivity for cytokeratins and epithelial membrane antigen is expected in most nonmelanocytic neoplasms (fig. 20-13) (see Appendix H). The utility of cytokeratin staining is compromised by the frequent occurrence of cross reactivity, presumably with glial fibrillary acidic protein (GFAP), in some astrocytes. As a result, keratin staining should be done in concert with preparations for GFAP. Although the stain is not specific, malignant melanomas are often reactive with S-100 protein. They also stain positively with HMB-45 and other melanoma-specific antibodies.

Although the cells of metastatic tumors are GFAP negative, metastases do engender impressive reactive astrocytosis in their surroundings. Unlike primary malignant neoplasms such as gliomas and lymphomas, however, only rarely are significant numbers of reactive astrocytes found deep within metastatic tumors.

Ultrastructural Findings. Squamous cell carcinomas are noted for their intercellular connection by true desmosomes, many of which

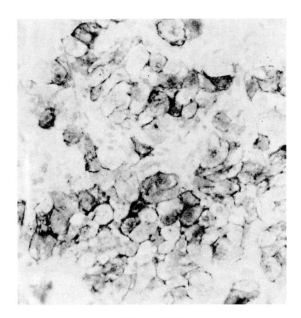

Figure 20-13
METASTATIC CARCINOMA
Immunoreactivity for epithelial membrane antigen is present in many carcinomas.

include bundles of tonofilaments which fan out into surrounding cytoplasm. Tonofilament bundles may also lie free in cytoplasm, not only in squamous cell carcinomas but also in adenocarcinomas. The latter typically have intracellular or intercellular microvillous-lined acinar spaces. Cytoplasmic and intraluminal mucus may be seen in some lesions. Some small cell (oat cell) carcinomas contain occasional neurosecretory granules. Metastatic melanoma features melanosomes in various stages of development and lack intercellular junctions.

The cells of lymphomas, most of which are of large cell type, vary considerably in terms of nuclear morphology. As a whole, nuclei are irregular and exhibit coarse chromatin and nucleolar prominence. At the ultrastructural level, they tend to be uncomplicated cells lacking junctions, pigments, granules, or specific cytoplasmic organelles. Nuclear "pockets" may be a common feature.

With the exception of ependymal tumors, which exhibit arrays of well-formed junctions, acinar spaces, and microvilli, most malignant gliomas show only intermediate filament formation and the presence of rudimentary (intermediate) junctions. The features of specific glioma variants are more completely discussed in their respective sections of this book.

Cytology. Metastatic carcinoma cells are known for their cohesion, the basis of cell aggregation into tissue fragments which in smears represent microbiopsies. Discrete cell borders, nuclear molding, large nuclei, prominent nucleoli (particularly in adenocarcinoma), and generally high nuclear-cytoplasmic ratios complete the picture (pl. XB, C, p. 397). Mucous vacuoles may also be apparent and, when large, displace the nucleus to produce the classic signet ring cells. Squamous cell carcinomas often exhibit at least some cells with peripherally situated, eosinophilic, somewhat refractile skeins of fibrils. Unlike malignant gliomas, intercellular spaces do not contain elongated cellular processes.

Frozen Section and Needle Biopsy Findings. The general architectural features of cell cohesion, microscopic circumscription, lobularity, and frequent fibrous septa withstand freezing and remain the diagnostic cornerstones of metastases. Attention only to high magnification microscopic features can, because of artifactual distortion, divert the pathologist's thinking toward gliomas.

Given the firm texture of some metastases, flexible biopsy needles may be deflected from the surface of the mass into the surrounding brain, resulting in sections of only gliotic tissue superficially resembling glioma. In such instances, smear preparations are useful since they highlight the typical cytologic features of reactive gliosis. On correlation of these cytologic and histologic findings with radiographic images, it quickly becomes apparent that the specimen has not been obtained from a targeted contrast-enhancing mass.

Differential Diagnosis. Little differential diagnostic consideration is necessary for overtly malignant, circumscribed neoplasms with glandular, squamous, or melanocytic differentiation. If only focal epithelial differentiation in a neoplasm of otherwise uncertain nature is seen, however, the uncommon occurrence of epithelial differentiation, either squamous or glandular, in glioblastomas and gliosarcomas should be considered (see fig. 3-33J, K). The finding of more typical glioblastoma features or GFAP positivity resolves this issue.

Papillary carcinomas related to the ventricular system, usually the fourth ventricle in adults,

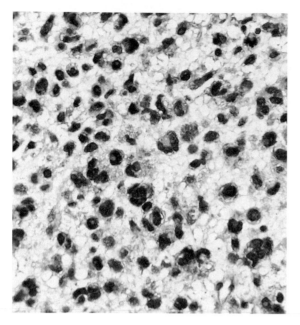

Figure 20-14
METASTATIC CARCINOMA
Metastases with a fibrillar background and considerable variation in nuclear size can closely resemble a malignant glioma.

prompts consideration of choroid plexus papilloma or carcinoma. Choroid plexus carcinomas are rare in adults. Unlike most carcinomas, choroid plexus tumors are vimentin and S-100 protein positive (1). They are also usually negative for epithelial membrane antigen (EMA). Although some choroid plexus carcinomas are reactive for carcinoembryonic antigen and most exhibit transthyretin staining, neither feature is diagnostic.

For metastatic carcinomas of the small cell type or those that are pleomorphic without obvious epithelial features, the possibility of a malignant glioma, particularly glioblastoma, cannot always be dismissed without supplementary studies (fig. 20-14). The same is sometimes true for metastatic renal cell carcinoma, which can closely resemble hemangioblastoma (fig. 20-15). In such cases, the remarkable degree of histologic circumscription that characterizes metastases is a helpful feature. Glioblastomas are not always diffusely infiltrative nor are hemangioblastomas always discrete masses. Immunohistochemistry then becomes exceedingly important. The presence of cytokeratins in association with EMA is conclusive evidence of

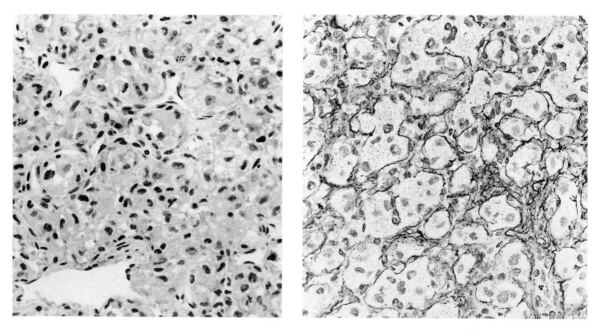

Figure 20-15
METASTATIC CARCINOMA
In sections stained for both hematoxylin and eosin (left) and reticulin (right), the lobular architecture suggests the possibility of a hemangioblastoma in this patient with von Hippel-Lindau syndrome. Immunoreactivity for epithelial membrane antigen (shown in figure 20-13) was definitive evidence for the diagnosis of carcinoma.

carcinoma although reactivity of gliomas for cytokeratins (8,25,29), and even EMA (19,29), is recognized. Sections prepared with such antibodies must be interpreted with caution and in conjunction with a reaction for GFAP. Despite the rare occurrence of GFAP-positive carcinomas (4), GFAP immunoreactivity must remain a diagnostic mainstay and strong evidence of a neoplasm's glial nature.

For obvious reasons, metastatic carcinoma must be distinguished from primary CNS lymphoma. In contrast to most metastases, lymphomas are deep-seated and distinctive for their angiocentricity. Necrosis in lymphomas is more likely to be of the single cell type, rather than widespread with confluent zones sparing perivascular cuffs. With immunosuppression, particularly in acquired immunodeficiency syndrome (AIDS), necrosis may be extensive. In small specimens, large cell lymphomas may mimic metastatic carcinoma. Smear preparations are most helpful because the distinctive cytologic characteristics of lymphoma are apparent in most cases. Even in small specimens it is obvious that lymphomas, unlike metastatic carcinoma, are infiltrative tumors that overrun rather than displace brain parenchyma. Lymphomas engender a considerable response in astrocytes, histiocytes, and even benign-reactive T lymphocytes. Lingering diagnostic uncertainty may be relieved by immunostaining for leukocyte common antigen (LCA), B- or T-cell markers, or immunoglobulin light or heavy chains. A special variant of large cell lymphoma, designated Ki-1, is immunoreactive for EMA, as are reactive and neoplastic plasma cells.

Treatment and Prognosis. Many clinical variables determine the outlook for patients with metastatic disease. Aside from patients with the occasional solitary metastasis, as from renal cell carcinoma, or with early osseous lesions in prostate cancer, most patients die within several months.

Leukemia

Secondary involvement of the CNS in leukemia occurs in three forms: 1) meningeal involvement; 2) intraparenchymal hemorrhagic foci containing intravascular and perivascular aggregates of immature or blast forms; and 3) the rare granulocytic sarcoma or chloroma.

Meningeal leukemia most often occurs in the setting of acute leukemia, particularly lymphoblastic leukemia. Headaches and cranial nerve dysfunction result from obstruction of flow of cerebrospinal fluid and from infiltration of cranial nerves (fig. 20-16) (43,44,47,48). The pathway by which these cells gain access to the meninges remains to be determined, but the frequent prominence of dural involvement suggests that meningeal relapse results from extension of tumor in the bone marrow. Although the infiltrate is confined to subarachnoid and Virchow-Robin spaces early in its course, with progression it can broach the pia-glial membrane and gain access to brain parenchyma (42). As is the case with primary lymphoma, neoplastic cells sometimes infiltrate the wall of vessels and become entwined in a lamellar network of reticulin.

In cases associated with markedly elevated leukocyte counts, as in blast crisis, cerebral vessels may become occluded by neoplastic cells (leukostasis) which proliferate locally to form sizable masses. Superimposed hemorrhage may enlarge such foci abruptly and often fatally (45). Macroscopically, such hemorrhages contain a distinctive central gray core of neoplastic cells.

Tumor masses termed chloroma of granulocytic sarcoma rarely occur with acute myelogenous leukemia (46,49). Intracranial as well as intraspinal examples have been reported. These usually arise in the epidural or subdural spaces.

Secondary Malignant Lymphoma

Secondary involvement of intradural structures by malignant lymphomas is generally confined to the leptomeninges and to cranial and spinal nerve roots. CNS involvement typically occurs late in the course of diffuse high-grade lymphomas, usually at a time when extranodal sites, such as bone marrow, become affected. As in meningeal carcinomatosis, symptoms of increased intracranial pressure and cranial nerve dysfunction are common.

Macroscopically, little may be seen other than hypertrophy of cranial and spinal nerve roots. Microscopically, the neoplastic cells proliferate within the leptomeninges, extend into the Virchow-Robin spaces, and permeate nerves (50–54). Cytologic examination of the cerebrospinal fluid is a worthwhile diagnostic procedure.

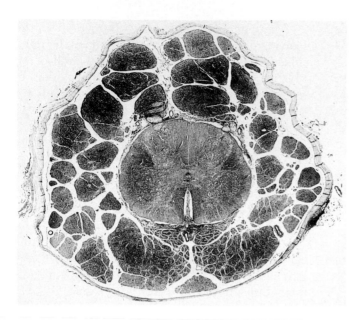

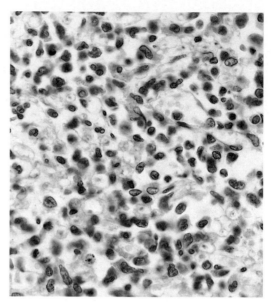

Figure 20-16
SECONDARY INVOLVEMENT BY LEUKEMIA
Leukemic involvement of the central nervous system frequently involves both the leptomeninges and nerve roots. The roots are thickened (left) by the darkly stained infiltrate of neoplastic cells (right).

Spinal Epidural Lymphoma

Occasional lymphomas, either of non-Hodgkin or less often of Hodgkin type, involve the spinal epidural space and compress the spinal cord. In some cases, particularly with Hodgkin disease, the underlying disease process has previously been recognized at other body sites (56); in other patients the neoplasm makes its first appearance in the intraspinal space (55,57). In some instances no extraspinal focus is ever found. It remains unclear whether such ostensibly isolated lymphomas are truly primary in the epidural space or represent spread from occult visceral or lymphoreticular primary foci (58).

Spinal epidural lymphomas are noted for their lack of osseous involvement, a feature in contrast to the frequent osteolytic or osteoblastic involvement of bone in spinal metastatic carcinoma.

Intravascular Lymphoma

Definition. An angiotropic, largely intravascular malignant lymphoma potentially affecting any number of nonlymphoreticular organs; the lymph nodes and spleen are usually excluded. The process exhibits a particular affinity for the vasculature of the skin, brain, and spinal cord.

Clinical and Radiographic Features. This curious disorder usually presents in adulthood. The diffuse or focal neurologic signs are the consequence of ischemia, produced by "sludging" or vascular occlusion of cerebrospinal vessels (60,62). Infarcts of the brain or spinal cord are therefore common. An associated rash is a common consequence of cutaneous involvement. Renal and adrenal infiltrates are also frequent.

Macroscopic Findings. Although prominent engorged vessels may be noted in some cases, macroscopic findings are generally limited to those of secondary infarction.

Microscopic Findings. The lesion consists of a striking intravascular proliferation of cytologically malignant lymphocytes, generally of large or mixed cell type (fig. 20-17, left). Vesicular nuclei and prominent nucleoli are therefore regular features, as is entrapment of cells in fibrin. Large, medium, and small vessels are all affected. As in the case of primary CNS lymphoma, the neoplastic cells may in some cases be found beneath endothelium or within vessel walls where they can incite a fibrous reaction. At first glance such vessels resemble those in chronic reaction or inflammation. Perivascular parenchymal infiltration is uncommon.

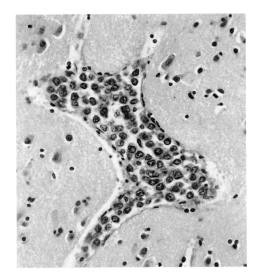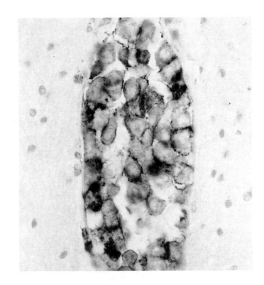

Figure 20-17
DIFFUSE INTRAVASCULAR LYMPHOMA
Left: Atypical lymphoid cells pack the vessels in this systemic form of lymphoma which frequents the central nervous system.
Right: The neoplastic cells are immunoreactive for leukocyte common antigen.

Immunohistochemical Findings. Although this tumor was originally considered a proliferation of endothelial cells, hence the term angioendotheliomatosis, it exhibits no endothelial markers such as *Ulex europaeus* agglutinin-I (UEA-I) or von Willebrand factor (factor VIII) (61,62). In contrast, immunoreactivity is noted for lymphoid hematopoietic markers such as leukocyte common antigen (fig. 20-17, right). As would be expected of an angiocentric lymphoma, a B-cell phenotype has been reported (60) although in one case a T-cell nature was demonstrated (59).

Differential Diagnosis. This uncommon lesion must be distinguished from the far more common primary CNS lymphoma which, in contrast to the angiotropic lesion, is a largely parenchymal neoplasm. Angiotropic lymphomas are essentially restricted to the vasculature. On rare occasion, metastatic carcinomas exhibit a striking intravascular pattern of growth; appropriate immunomarker studies readily distinguish such neoplasms from lymphoma.

Treatment and Prognosis. Although steroid therapy has a beneficial short-term effect, producing dramatic clinical improvements, most patients survive less than 1 year from the onset of symptoms. At autopsy, many systemic sites are affected, particularly skin, kidney, heart, lung, prostate, and adrenals and other endocrine organs.

Lymphomatoid Granulomatosis

Lymphomatoid granulomatosis is a controversial lesion since it is not always clear whether it represents an atypical inflammatory response or an angiocentric lymphoma. Most observers consider it a malignant lymphoma of the T-cell type or an atypical lymphoid lesion in evolution to a lymphoma.

The CNS is symptomatically involved in approximately 25 percent of cases (64). Sometimes, the disease appears to be limited to the CNS at the time of presentation (65,66). Because this is the exception, the disorder is discussed under Metastatic and Secondary Neoplasms. CNS symptoms may result in either case. The CNS lesions are typically multifocal when assessed by neuroradiologic methods. Lymphomatoid granulomatosis has been reported with AIDS (63).

Macroscopically, the lesions are frequently hemorrhagic and necrotic. Microscopically, they consist of a mixed inflammatory infiltrate associated with atypical lymphocytes, plasmacytoid lymphocytes, occasional bizarre mononuclear cells, and macrophages. Immunohistochemically, the process consists of a polyclonal population of plasma cells and lymphocytes as well as a predominant population of T lymphocytes. The infiltrate is characteristically angiocentric and is accompanied by multiple concentric laminae of perivascular reticulin, a feature also typical of malignant lymphomas. Perivascular infarction and hemorrhage are common. Areas of associated malignant lymphoma have been noted in some cases occurring in AIDS (63).

The differential diagnosis focuses primarily on distinguishing malignant lymphoma from reactive lymphoplasmacytic proliferations. Distinguishing features include the mixed cellular infiltrate of lymphomatoid granulomatosis which contrasts with the more monomorphic and generally atypical elements comprising malignant lymphomas. Some AIDS patients develop atypical lymphoid proliferations of uncertain nature and etiology, as well as inflammatory masses due to *Treponema pallidum* infection. Both these lesions are generally richer in plasma cells than is lymphomatoid granulomatosis.

The appropriate therapy for lymphomatoid granulomatosis remains to be established. Some patients have responded to chemotherapy and radiotherapy whereas steroids have successfully, if temporarily, arrested the disease in others.

REFERENCES

Metastatic Carcinoma and Sarcoma

1. Ang LC, Taylor AR, Bergin D, Kaufmann JCE. An immunohistochemical study of papillary tumors in the central nervous system. Cancer 1990;65:2712–9.
2. Athanassiou A, Begent RH, Newlands ES, Parker D, Rustin GJ, Bagshawe KD. Central nervous system metastases of choriocarcinoma. 23 years' experience at Charing Cross Hospital. Cancer 1983;52:1728–35.
3. Boogerd W, Hart AA, van der Sande JJ, Engelsman E. Meningeal carcinomatosis in breast cancer. Prognostic factors and influence of treatment. Cancer 1991; 67:1685–95.
4. Budka H. Non-glial specificities of immunocytochemistry for the glial fibrillary acidic protein (GFAP). Triple expression of GFAP, vimentin and cytokeratin in papillary meningiomas and metastasizing renal carcinoma. Acta Neuropathol (Berl) 1986;72:43–54.
5. Bullard DE, Cox EB, Seigler HF. Central nervous system metastases in malignant melanoma. Neurosurgery 1981;8:26–30.
6. Byrne TN. Spinal cord and compression from epidural metastases. N Eng J Med 1992;327:614–9.
7. Castaldo JE, Bernat JL, Meier FA, Schned AR. Intracranial metastases due to prostatic carcinoma. Cancer 1983;52:1739–47.
8. Cosgrove M, Fitzgibbons PL, Sherrod A, Chandrasoma PT, Martin SE. Intermediate filament expression in astrocytic neoplasms. Am J Surg Pathol 1989;13:141–5.
9. Costigan DA, Winkelman MD. Intramedullary spinal cord metastasis. A clinicopathological study of 13 cases. J Neurosurg 1985;62:227–33.
10. Dauplat J, Nieberg RK, Hacker NF. Central nervous system metastases in epithelial ovarian carcinoma. Cancer 1987;60:2259–62.
11. Davey P, O'Brien P. Disposition of cerebral metastases from malignant melanoma: implications for radiosurgery. Neurosurgery 1991;29:8–15.
12. Davis RP, Spigelman MK, Zappulla RA, Sacher M, Strauchen JA. Isolated central nervous system metastasis from transitional cell carcinoma of the bladder: report of a case and review of the literature. Neurosurgery 1986;18:622–4.
13. Delattre JY, Krol G, Thaler HT, Posner JB. Distribution of brain metastases. Arch Neurol 1988;45:741–4.
14. Dolan EJ, Schwartz ML, Lewis AJ, Kassel EE, Cooper PW. Adenoid cystic carcinoma: an unusual neurosurgical entity. Can J Neurol Sci 1985;12:65–8.
15. Engelhoff JC, Ross JS, Modic MT, Masaryk TJ, Estes M. MR imaging of metastatic GI adenocarcinoma in brain. AJNR Am J Neuroradiol 1992;13:1221–4.
16. Gasecki AP, Bashir RM, Foley J. Leptomeningeal carcinomatosis: a report of 3 cases and review of the literature. Eur Neurol 1992;32:74–8.
17. Gonzalez-Vitale JC, Garcia-Bunuel R. Meningeal carcinomatosis. Cancer 1976;37:2906–11.
18. Hirsch FR, Paulson OB, Hansen HH, Vraa-Jensen J. Intracranial metastases in small cell carcinoma of the lung. Correlation of clinical and autopsy findings. Cancer 1982;50:2433–7.
19. Hitchcock E, Morris CS. Cross reactivity of anti-epithelial membrane antigen monoclonal for reactive and neoplastic glial cells. J Neurooncol 1987;4:345–52.
20. Ishizuka T, Tomoda Y, Kaseki S, Goto S, Hara T, Kobayashi T. Intracranial metastasis of choriocarcinoma. A clinicopathologic study. Cancer 1983;52:1896–903.
21. Kokkoris CP. Leptomeningeal carcinomatosis. How does cancer reach the pia-arachnoid? Cancer 1983;51:154–60.
22. Lewis AJ. Sarcoma metastatic to the brain. Cancer 1988;61:593–601.
23. Mandybur TI. Intracranial hemorrhage caused by metastatic tumors. Neurology 1977;27:650–5.
24. Marin F, Kovacs K, Scheithauer, BW, Young Jr WF. The pituitary gland in patients with breast carcinoma: a histologic and immunocytochemical study of 125 cases. Mayo Clinic Proc 1992;67:949–56.
25. Ng HK, Lo ST. Cytokeratin immunoreactivity in gliomas. Histopathology 1989;14:359–68.
26. Olson ME, Chernik NL, Posner JB. Infiltration of the leptomeninges by systemic cancer. A clinical and pathologic study. Arch Neurol 1974;30:122–37.
27. Piepmeier JM, Virapongse C, Kier EL, Kim J, Greenberg A. Intracranial adenocystic carcinoma presenting as a primary brain tumor. Neurosurgery 1983;12:348–52.
28. Retsas S, Gershuny AR. Central nervous system involvement in malignant melanoma. Cancer 1988;61:1926–34.

29. Rosenblum MK, Erlandson RA, Budzilovich GN. The lipid-rich epithelioid glioblastoma. Am J Surg Pathol 1991;10:925–34.
30. Sarno JB, Wiener L, Waxman M, Kwee J. Sarcoma metastatic to the central nervous system parenchyma: a review of the literature. Med Pediatr Oncol 1985; 13:280–92.
31. Scully RE. Case Records of the Massachusetts General Hospital Case 28–1992. N Eng J Med 1992;327:107–16.
32. Stark RJ, Henson RA, Evans SJ. Spinal metastases. A retrospective survey from a general hospital. Brain 1982;105(Pt 1):189–213.
33. Stein M, Steiner M, Klein B, et al. Involvement of the central nervous system by ovarian carcinoma. Cancer 1986;58:2066–9.
34. Sze G, Soletsky S, Bronen R, Krol G. MR imaging of the cranial meninges with emphasis on contrast enhancement and meningeal carcinomatosis. AJNR Am J Neuroradiol 1989;10:965–75.

35. Tashiro Y, Kondo A, Aoyama I, et al. Calcified metastatic brain tumor. Neurosurgery 1990;26:1065–70.
36. Taylor HG, Lefkowitz M, Skoog SJ, Miles BJ, McLeod DG, Coggin JT. Intracranial metastases in prostate cancer. Cancer 1984;53:2728–30.
37. Trillet V, Catajar JF, Croisile B, et al. Cerebral metastases as first symptom of bronchogenic carcinoma. A prospective study of 37 cases. Cancer 1991;67:2935–40.
38. Tsukada Y, Fouad A, Pickren JW, Lane WW. Central nervous system metastasis from breast carcinoma. Autopsy study. Cancer 1983;52:2349–54.
39. Wasserstrom WR, Glass JP, Posner JB. Diagnosis and treatment of leptomeningeal metastases from solid tumors: experience with 90 patients. Cancer 1982;49:759–72.
40. Weber P, Shepard KV, Vijayakumar S. Metastases to pineal gland. Cancer 1989;63:164–5.
41. Weiss HD, Richardson EP Jr. Solitary brainstem metastasis. Neurology 1978;28:562–6.

Leukemia

42. Azzarelli B, Roessmann U. Pathogenesis of central nervous system infiltration in acute leukemia. Arch Pathol Lab Med 1977;101:203–5.
43. Bleyer WA. Biology and pathogenesis of CNS leukemia. Am J Pediatr Hematol Oncol 1989;11:57–63.
44. Bojsen-Møller M, Nielsen JL. CNS involvement in leukaemia. An autopsy study of 100 consecutive patients. Acta Pathol Microbiol Immunol Scand [A] 1983;91:209–16.
45. Freireich EJ, Thomas LB, Frei E III, Fritz RD, Forkner CE Jr. A distinctive type of intracerebral hemorrhage associated with "blastic crisis" in patients with leukemia. Cancer 1960;13:146–54.

46. Llena JF, Kawamoto K, Hirano A, Feiring EH. Granulocytic sarcoma of the central nervous system: initial presentation of leukemia. Acta Neuropathol (Berl) 1978;42:145–7.
47. Moore EW, Thomas LB, Shaw RK, Freireich EJ. The central nervous system in acute leukemia. Arch Intern Med 1960;105:451–68.
48. Price RA, Johnson WW. The central nervous system in childhood leukemia: I. The arachnoid. Cancer 1973;31:520–33.
49. van Veen S, Kluin PM, de Keizer RJ, Kluin-Nelemans HC. Granulocytic sarcoma (chloroma). Presentation of an unusual case. Am J Clin Pathol 1991;95:567–71.

Secondary Malignant Lymphoma

50. Griffin JW, Thompson RW, Mitchinson MJ, De Kiewiet JC, Welland FH. Lymphomatous leptomeningitis. Am J Med 1971;51:200–8.
51. Jellinger K, Radaszkiewicz. Involvement of the central nervous system in malignant lymphomas. Virchow Arch [A] 1976;370:345–62.
52. Liang R, Chiu E, Loke SL. Secondary central nervous system involvement by non-Hodgkin's lymphoma: the risk factors. Hematol Oncol 1990;8:141–5.

53. MacKintosh FR, Colby TV, Podolsky WJ, et al. Central nervous system involvement in non-Hodgkin's lymphoma: an analysis of 105 cases. Cancer 1982;49:586–95.
54. Young RC, Howser DM, Anderson T, Fisher RI, Jaffe E, DeVita VT Jr. Central nervous system complications of non-Hodgkin's lymphoma. The potential role for prophylactic therapy. Am J Med 1979;66:435–43.

Spinal Epidural Lymphoma

55. Epelbaum R, Haim N, Ben-Shahar M, Ben-Arie Y, Feinsod M, Cohen Y. Non-Hodgkin's lymphoma presenting with spinal epidural involvement. Cancer 1986;58:2120–4.
56. Friedman M, Kim TH, Panahon AM. Spinal cord compression in malignant lymphoma. Treatment and results. Cancer 1976;37:1485–91.

57. Grant JW, Kaech D, Jones DB. Spinal cord compression as the first presentation of lymphoma—a review of 15 cases. Histopathology 1986;30:1191–202.
58. Lyons MK, O'Neill BP, Marsh WR, Kurtin PJ. Primary spinal epidural non-Hodgkin's lymphoma: report of eight patients and review of the literature. Neurosurgery 1992;675–80.

Intravascular Lymphoma

59. Abe S, Shimbo Y, Saito T, Kohno M, Nishiyama A, Kumanishi T. An immunohistochemical study on "neoplastic angioendotheliosis": demonstration of B lymphocyte markers in the neoplastic cells. Acta Neuropathol (Berl) 1988;75:313–6.
60. Clark WC, Dohan FC Jr, Moss T, Schweitzer JB. Immunocytochemical evidence of lymphocytic derivation of neoplastic cells in malignant angioendotheliomatosis. J Neurosurg 1991;74:757–62.

61. Wick MR, Mills SE, Scheithauer BW, Cooper PH, Davitz MA, Parkinson K. Reassessment of malignant "angioendotheliomatosis": evidence in favor of its reclassification as "intravascular lymphomatosis." Am J Surg Pathol 1986;10:112–23.
62. Wrotnowski U, Mills SE, Cooper PH. Malignant angioendotheliomatosis. An angiotropic lymphoma? Am J Clin Pathol 1985;83:244–8.

Lymphomatoid Granulomatosis

63. Anders KH, Latta H, Chang BS, Tomiyasu U, Quddusi AS, Vinters HV. Lymphomatoid granulomatosis and malignant lymphoma of the central nervous system in the acquired immunodeficiency syndrome. Hum Pathol 1989;20:326–34.

64. Katzenstein AL, Carrington CB, Liebow AA. Lymphomatoid granulomatosis. A clinicopathologic study of 152 cases. Cancer 1979;43:360–73.

65. Kleinschmidt-DeMasters BK, Filley CM, Bitter MA. Central nervous system angiocentric, angiodestructive T-cell lymphoma (lymphomatoid granulomatosis). Surg Neurol 1992;37:130–7.

66. Schmidt BJ, Meagher-Villemure K, Del Carpio J. Lymphomatoid granulomatosis with isolated involvement of the brain. Ann Neurol 1984;15:478–81.

21

DIAGNOSTIC METHODS IN NEURO-ONCOLOGY

Frozen Section

Frozen sections of lesions from the central nervous system (CNS) are usually requested to determine the specific histologic diagnosis, to ensure that appropriate procedures for special tissue processing are set in motion, and to receive assurance that diagnostically adequate tissue has been obtained. The assessment of resection margins is less often an issue than it is for tumors at other body sites.

It is essential that interpretation of frozen sections be done in conjunction with an adequate clinical history since the latter aids in sorting possible diagnoses into the likely and the unlikely. As is emphasized throughout this volume, it is also very important for the pathologist to be acquainted with the radiographic anatomy of the lesion in question. Neuroimages provide resolution equivalent to that of gross or even low-power microscopic examination. The combination of clinical and radiographic findings is, therefore, diagnostically important, increasing the likelihood of, or virtually excluding, certain entities. Imaging studies are useful also in determining whether a specimen has been taken from the most abnormal area.

Because of the considerable variation in physical facilities available at medical institutions, no one procedure for frozen section preparation can be prescribed, although a visit by the pathologist to the operating room is highly recommended. Either there or in the frozen section suite, clinical data and radiographic findings can be reviewed in direct contact with the surgeon. This personal interaction is invaluable in any setting, but is especially important when frozen section findings are negative or equivocal and a decision must be made about what to do next.

The quality of frozen sections is greatly affected by technical artifacts. For instance, edematous brain tissue submitted to freezing is prone to the formation of ice crystals, artifactual distortion, and condensation of nuclei. Such changes are enhanced by the relatively slow freezing that occurs when refrigerants are dribbled over the specimen, but are minimized by the rapid freezing possible when small specimens are quenched in cryogens such as liquid nitrogen. Nuclear details are preserved and the processes of reactive and neoplastic glial cells are clearly seen, often better than in formalin-fixed, paraffin-embedded sections. Although rapid freezing minimizes the artifacts evident on paraffin-embedded permanent sections, it remains important to reserve the bulk of the specimen for processing without freezing.

Unlike sections of many other tissues which need to be warmed on glass slides to prevent detachment during staining, those of the CNS not only do not require such a procedure but in fact suffer from it. The dried, artifactually spread, hypodense nuclei complicate the process of diagnosis which can be difficult even under optimal circumstances.

Techniques for staining frozen sections vary. We stain one section with an aqueous method such as toluidine blue and another with hematoxylin and eosin (H&E). Sections stained by the aqueous method exhibit superior nuclear detail and retain tissue lipids since they never pass through alcohols and xylenes.

Stereotactic Biopsy

Since cores of tissue can be taken at predetermined depths along a prescribed projectory of the needle, magnetic resonance imaging (MRI)- or computerized tomography (CT)-directed biopsies sample predetermined targets with remarkable precision. Multiple cores can be taken at any one target point simply by rotating the needle or trochar between sampling. The stereotactic technique was originally advocated for inaccessible lesions or for use in patients in whom general anesthesia was considered hazardous. At present, it is widely employed in cases in which open biopsy could be performed readily and safely. It is debated whether this expanded role of stereotaxy is always appropriate.

The needle retrieving the specimen is either a large bore cutting needle or trochar which delivers a core of tissue, or a fine needle capable of aspirating cells and microscopic tissue fragments suitable for cytologic study but not for frozen sections. Most surgeons use the former. It is our practice to excise a small fragment of each core in order to obtain cytologic preparations. When necessary, a 1-mm segment of core may also be taken for ultrastructural study. We use the remainder for frozen or permanent sections. As much tissue as possible is reserved for routine processing.

Interpretation of small specimens can obviously be challenging. As a result, it is absolutely essential that all relevant information is gathered before histologic and cytologic findings are reviewed and reported. Radiographic findings, clinical history, and the surgeon's intraoperative observations are key to an accurate diagnosis. It is also important for the surgeon to consider the use of frozen section controls in determining the adequacy of the specimen. Although stereotactic biopsy has great theoretical precision, it is not uncommon for the needle to miss the lesion. Even with a massive glioblastoma, the procedure may obtain near normal or reactive brain tissue as the needle passes the target point by a millimeter or two. Metastatic carcinomas are usually sufficiently rich in collagen that a large, blunt-tipped needle may slide off the firm surface and into surrounding edematous brain. By comparing histologic to radiographic findings, the pathologist faced with a sample of gliotic or only mildly abnormal tissue can quickly determine whether the most radiographically abnormal area was sampled or not.

Needle biopsy specimens of paucicellular lesions such as low-grade gliomas are especially difficult to interpret. In such cases, it is important to reserve unfrozen tissue for optimal processing since the process of freezing obscures cytologic features, particularly those of oligodendroglia. Sampling problems also confound tumor grading. It is not surprising, therefore, that the ratio of anaplastic astrocytoma to glioblastoma is higher in needle biopsy cores than in large specimens obtained by open biopsy (20).

Cytology

Cytologic preparations are invaluable adjuncts to histologic study, particularly frozen sections, since they reveal fine nuclear and cytoplasmic detail. For "touch" preparations, the slide is gently applied to a freshly cut surface of the tissue, lifted, and immediately immersed in fixative. Even the slightest drying induces artifacts, particularly nuclear pallor and enlarge-

ment. This technique is ideal for pituitary adenomas and malignant lesions such as lymphomas and metastatic carcinomas, but more forceful methods are necessary in order to obtain cells from most lesions of the CNS. Thus, the "squash" or the "smear" technique is generally used for gliomas. Squash preparations involve immersion of a small tissue fragment in polychrome stain, followed by the application of a coverslip and compression of the fragment. The smear technique involves compression of tissue followed by gentle drawing apart of the two opposing glass slides. Prompt alcohol fixation is recommended prior to staining by any one of a number of methods.

In the above noted preparations, nuclear details are best captured following fixation in 95 percent alcohol and staining with the Papanicolaou method which, with some modifications, can be done with the time allotted to a frozen section. A satisfactory alternative, which is perhaps a better method for studies of cytoplasm, is fixation in 95 percent alcohol followed immediately by staining with H&E. The hemalum phloxine method (14) is particularly well suited to CNS cytology.

Immunohistochemistry

Immunohistochemistry has become an indispensable tool in the diagnosis and classification of CNS tumors (see Appendix H for a summary), but must be thoughtfully applied since 1) many antibodies are less cell specific than was originally, or is widely, thought (10); 2) negative staining may be artifactual and does not exclude the presence of the antigen in question; and 3) it can be difficult to determine whether an immunoreactive cell is neoplastic. The results must always be interpreted in the context of the findings in classically stained histologic sections. Details of immunohistochemical staining are provided throughout the volume under the discussion of specific entities.

Special Stains

Part of the appeal of neuropathology stems from its use of specialized, visually elegant histochemical stains for glial cells, neurons, and other CNS elements. These techniques, much to the relief of laboratories that found them difficult to perform, have been largely supplanted by the more sensitive and specific immunohistochemical methods described above. The Cajal gold chloride sublimate method has thus been replaced with the glial fibrillary acidic protein (GFAP) technique and the Bielschowsky method by antibodies to synaptophysin, neurofilament protein, and microtubular protein. The Rio Hortego silver carbonate technique for microglia has given way to staining by the lectin Ricinus communis agglutinin-1 or by various antibodies including HAM-56 for the cells in an activated state. Use of the phosphotungstic acid hematoxylin (PTAH) technique for glial processes, though still retained in some centers for other uses, is rapidly disappearing. The GFAP immunostaining method has taken its place. Many of the classic special stains remain, however, including some methods that do not need detailed review here. Of these, variations of the reticulin stain are in common use as are various stains for myelin, the best known being the Luxol fast blue method, usually combined with the H&E or periodic acid–Schiff (PAS) counterstain.

Cytologic Examination of Cerebrospinal Fluid

Cytologic examination of cerebrospinal fluid (CSF) is valuable in the diagnosis of metastatic, and to a lesser extent, primary CNS neoplasms that have gained access to the subarachnoid space (6,8). The method is particularly likely to detect neoplastic cells of leptomeningeal metastases from systemic primaries. In contrast, the cells of gliomas are more cohesive and less likely to appear in detached or floating form. Since leukemias and lymphomas metastasize to the nervous system and often involve the leptomeninges, screening of CSF in cases of suspected disease relapse is a common practice. In approximately 10 percent of primary and in even higher percentages of recurrent medulloblastomas, malignant cells are present in CSF. The same immunohistochemical methods used in tissue sections can be used in CSF specimens, especially cytospin preparations. Thus, gliomas may demonstrate reactivity for GFAP, lymphoid neoplasms for leukocyte common antigen (LCA) or other hemopoietic markers, carcinomas for keratin, etc.

Proliferation Markers

In this rapidly evolving field, a number of markers have been used, with varying success, to measure cell turnover and to predict the tempo of tumor recurrence. Others are under study, and new, more innovative ones no doubt await development. As is the case for any grading method, the regional variation in proliferative rates must be recognized (13a).

One time-tested technique relies upon the use of a monoclonal antibody to bromodeoxyuridine (BrdU) (28,32,36,37). The halogenated pyrimidine is a thymidine analogue and, after intravenous injection, is incorporated into the tumor's newly synthesized DNA. Its presence in a nucleus, revealed by immunostaining of paraffin-embedded tissue sections, indicates the S-phase of the cell cycle. This technique has been widely applied to gliomas and meningiomas and its clinical utility is specifically discussed in sections dealing with those entities.

A second antibody, Ki-67, is directed toward an antigen within the nuclei of cells in all phases of the cell cycle except G0. It is, therefore, a marker of cycling cells (11,35a,36,41,47). The technique is advantageous since it requires no preoperative or intraoperative injections of a compound, and can be applied to paraffin-embedded tissue (29a). Staining in many cells is nuclear, with prominent or exclusive localization to nucleolar organizing regions and nucleoli (49). As is the case for BrdU studies, a general correlation exists between histologically determined tumor grade and the Ki-67 staining index.

The number and area of nucleolar organizing regions have also been used as indicators of cell proliferation. These structures can be demonstrated readily in paraffin-embedded tissue using a silver nitrate stain (11a,30a,30b,42,49). Since they represent sites of transcription of DNA coding for ribosomal RNA, their number and prominence are indirect indicators of cell proliferative activity. Despite initial optimism, considerable disagreement exists regarding the prognostic value of the so-called nucleolar organizer region (AgNOR) technique (35). A number of studies have found a correlation between histologically determined tumor grade and AgNOR counts, especially in meningiomas (12,23,24,35, 38,40,44). One other study suggested that the

AgNOR number might aid in the distinction of gliosis from low-grade glioma (34).

Staining for proliferating cell nuclear antigen (PCNA) or cyclin may be of prognostic utility but considerable disagreement surrounds this issue (3,11a,30–30b,33). The antibody intensely stains the nuclei of cells in the S-phase, but also stains, with less intensity, a variable percentage of cells in other phases of the cell cycle (48). As a consequence, a large number of immunoreactive nuclei may be seen even in low-grade tumors such as schwannomas (33). Unlike Ki-67 and BrdU preparations, considerable variability of nuclear staining is seen, from faint to intense. As a result, it is difficult to determine at what point a nucleus is sufficiently stained to be considered in S-phase. It is of course also difficult to identify all faintly staining nuclei (33).

Other antibodies of use in determining the cellular proliferative index include ones directed toward DNA polymerase alpha (4) and P105 (31).

DNA Cytofluorometry

Cytofluorometric measurement of DNA can be performed upon either cell suspensions obtained from fresh tissue or upon nuclei from deparaffinized blocks (26,50). As is described in the prognosis sections of specific tumor entities, the presence of aneuploidy as measured by this method or even an increase in proliferative antibody labeling in some lesions such as infiltrating fibrillary astrocytic neoplasms, has been associated with a higher histologic grade and a poorer prognosis (13,27,17,55). In other situations, however, such as in medulloblastoma, aneuploidy is correlated with a more favorable prognosis (43,54). Sometimes, cytofluorometry provides no prognostically significant data.

Molecular Techniques

Previously, the grading of CNS tumors was based upon morphologic findings. There is now a tendency to augment histologic grading, not only with proliferation indices but with data regarding specific chromosomal or genomic abnormalities. Since the latter may identify milestones in tumor progression, it seems likely that they have prognostic use, particularly in small specimens in which pathologic examination is more often cytologic than histologic. Amplification of the epidermal growth factor receptor gene (1,7,29,53), p53 mutations (9,19,25,45), loss of heterozygosity (51,52), and others that await discovery, are changes that may be utilized diagnostically. Initial evidence suggests that immunohistochemical detection of p53 in fibrillary astrocytic neoplasms provides little prognostic information. Analyses to detect these changes would be most appropriate in otherwise lower-grade lesions, in effect detecting tumor progression at an early stage.

Neuroimaging

As is emphasized throughout this volume, neuroimaging has undergone remarkable evolution, resulting in sophisticated procedures that resolve small anatomic details, define cerebral blood flow, and localize as well as measure the concentration of brain metabolites. The images produced are extremely relevant to the pathologic evaluation of lesions affecting the CNS.

Computerized tomography (CT) scanning is a conventional radiologic method that relies upon regional anatomic differences in cellular and extracellular density and the absorbance of X-ray photons in generating an image. By employing tomographic exposures and computerized analysis, CT produces images that are "shadows" in the true sense of the word. In such radiographs, gray matter has attenuation (absorption) properties that give an intermediate light gray density (hyperattenuation), whereas white matter produces a considerably darker density (hypoattenuation). Calcified structures, such as bone and the concretions of normal choroid plexus and pineal gland, are highly absorbent and appear white (pronounced hyperattenuation). Freshly clotted blood is also hyperattenuating.

For routine diagnostic purposes, CT may be performed both with and without contrast enhancement. Enhanced CT studies are obtained following the intravenous administration of an iodinated contrast medium such as is used in systemic angiography. CT readily detects the hyperattenuating contrast medium passing through the cerebral vasculature and that which enters the interstitial space as a consequence of a defective blood-brain barrier. The presence, absence, and distribution of such contrast enhancement are important characteristics of various brain tumors, and widely used in formulation of preoperative differential diagnoses. Among diffuse or fibrillary astrocytic neoplasms, for example, enhancement is usually seen only in the more malignant tumors. Enhancement is not an indicator of anaplasia since it is commonly observed in pilocytic astrocytomas and in non-neoplastic conditions such as demyelinating disease, radionecrosis, and subacute cerebral infarction.

Magnetic resonance imaging (MRI) uses a magnetic field and delivers pulses of radiofrequency (RF) waves to the target tissue. During intervals between pulses, the tissue relaxes and emits a RF "echo" which can be detected by surface coils, the scanner's receiving antennae. The detected echo is then transformed, reconstructed, and presented as an image. The instrument thus is tuned to listen to the RF emissions from excited and then relaxed tissue slices, and does not produce images in the usual radiographic manner by recording regional differences in the absorbance of photons. Current MRI scanners are tuned to receive the RF largely from hydrogen protons, which are most numerous in water but are also present in proteins and lipids. In the most common form of imaging, spin-echo, two RF pulses are intermittently directed at the tissues at a 90° and then 180° angle.

The length of the interval following a RF pulse, during which the tissue is allowed to relax before recording, can be varied. In images described as T1-weighted, there is a shorter interval between cessation of the pulse and recording the "time to echo," or TE. Twenty milliseconds is typical. The entire "time for repetition" of the 90É and 180É pulse, or TR, is generally 500 m/s. In practice, T1-weighted images are generally used to define fine details of normal or pathologic anatomy, and is the procedure used after injection of gadolinium contrast agent for enhancement, a process discussed below. On T1-weighted images, the cortex has an intermediate gray signal intensity whereas white matter is somewhat more hyperintense (lighter) due to the presence of protons in the cholesterol of myelin. Bone and calcified structures are dark or nearly black and are therefore not well seen, while fat in both bone marrow and free adipose tissue has an extremely hyperintense white signal. Protein-rich cyst contents, such as those of the colloid cyst or Rathke cleft cyst, are often markedly hyperintense, requiring no contrast enhancement.

Proton density images have a longer TR than T1-weighted acquisitions (usually 2000 to 2500 m/s) and a short TE (commonly 30 m/s) much like that of the T1-weighted acquisition. The true T2-weighted image is sometimes referred to as the second echo. For this image, the TE is commonly 80 m/s or longer. Both first (proton density) and second echoes produce images that are especially sensitive to edema or increased water concentration. Only on T2 imaging does CSF appear hyperintense or white.

T2-weighted imaging detects increased water in tumors, in other expansile lesions such as infarcts, and in the peritumoral vasogenic edema that accompanies many intracranial lesions. An additional application of T2-weighted images is the detection of iron, such as in hemosiderin, which produces a dark signal described as T2 shortening. Iron deposition is found within brain tissue surrounding longstanding vascular malformations such as cavernous angiomas. Other causes of a dark signal in T2-weighted images are calcium, dense fibrous connective tissue, melanin, and deoxyhemoglobin as in subacute hemorrhage. Flowing blood is dark ("flow void") in both T1 and T2 images. Replacement of normal lipid-rich and water-poor white matter by a demyelinating plaque makes the water-containing focus readily apparent on proton density or T2-weighted images, where it appears as a hyperintense signal. The normal white matter in T2-weighted images has a dark signal intensity due to the T2-shortening effect of myelin.

Like CT images, those produced by MRI may be enhanced by the intravenous injection of a contrast compound, such as the paramagnetic rare-earth metal gadolinium which is chelated to diethylenetriaminepentacetic acid (DTPA). This technique can be employed either as a form of angiography or as tumoral contrast enhancement as is used in CT scanning to define the permeability of vessels.

MRI technology is used in magnetic resonance angiography and spectroscopy. At present, limited information exists regarding the diagnostic specificity of various magnetic resonance spectra in the identification of different tumor types and grades, but the technique appears to have promise since it uses the same basic equipment as conventional MRI (5,46).

Although it requires a cyclotron to prepare the necessary isotopes, *positron emission tomography (PET)* is increasingly used. With the isotope [^{18}F] fluorodeoxyglucose (FDG), it is possible to map the metabolic activity of intracranial neoplasms. Appropriately, cellular mitotically active lesions, such as glioblastomas and lymphomas, are metabolically hyperactive or "hot," whereas low-grade tumors are hypometabolic or "cold." Thus, PET scanning may provide useful data regarding tumor grade (2,39) and may permit visualization of anaplastic transformation in lower-grade tumors (18). Furthermore, it may be helpful in distinguishing recurrent, often high-grade tumors from necrosis (see fig. 3-44) (15,16,21). PET scanning can also aid in the selection of a precise biopsy site by identifying the most highly metabolic (malignant) areas of primary brain tumors (22).

REFERENCES

1. Agosti RM, Leuthold M, Gullick WJ, Yasargil MG, Wiestler OD. Expression of the epidermal growth factor receptor in astrocytic tumors is specifically associated with glioblastoma multiforme. Virchows Arch [A] 1992;420:321–5.

2. Alavi JB, Alavi A, Chawluk J, et al. Positron emission tomography in patients with gliomas: a predictor of prognosis. Cancer 1988;62:1074–8.

3. Allegranza A, Girlando S, Arrigoni GL, et al. Proliferating cell nuclear antigen expression in central nervous system neoplasms. Virchows Arch [A] 1991;419:417–23.

4. Appley AJ, Fitzgibbons PL, Chandrasoma PT, Hinton DR, Apuzzo ML. Multiparameter flow cytometric analysis of neoplasms of the central nervous system: correlation of nuclear antigen p105 and DNA content with clinical behavior. Neurosurgery 1990;27:83–96.

5. Arnold DL, Emrich JF, Shoubridge EA, Villemure JG, Feindel W. Characterizations of astrocytomas, meningiomas and pituitary adenomas by phosphorus magnetic resonance spectroscopy. J Neurosurg 1991;74:447–53.

6. Bigner SH. Cerebrospinal fluid (CSF) cytology: current status and diagnostic implications. J Neuropathol Exp Neurol 1992;51:235–45.

7. _____, Burger PC, Wong AJ, et al. Gene amplification in malignant human gliomas: clinical and histopathologic aspects. J Neuropathol Exp Neurol 1988;47:191–205.

8. _____, Johnston WW. Cytopathology of the central nervous system. New York: Masson, 1983.

9. Bruner JM, Saya H, Moser RP. Immunocytochemical detection of p53 in human gliomas. Mod Pathol 1991;4:671–4.

10. Budka H. Non-glial specificities of immunocytochemistry for the glial fibrillary acidic protein (GFAP). Triple expression of GFAP, vimentin and cytokeratins in papillary meningioma and metastasizing renal carcinoma. Acta Neuropathol (Berl) 1986;72:43–54.

11. Burger PC, Shibata T, Kleihues P. The use of the monoclonal antibody Ki-67 in the identification of proliferating cells: application to surgical neuropathology. Am J Surg Pathol 1986;10:611–7.

11a. Centeno BA, Louis DN, Kupsky WJ, Preffer FI, Sobel RA. The AgNOR technique, PCNA immunohistochemistry, and DNA ploidy in the evaluation of choroid plexus biopsy specimens. Am J Clin Pathol 1993;100:690–6.

12. Chin LS, Hinton DR. The standardized assessment of argyrophilic nucleolar organizer regions in meningeal tumors. J Neurosurg 1991;74:590–6.

13. Coons SW, Davis JR, Way DL. Correlation of DNA content and histology in prognosis of astrocytomas. Am J Clin Pathol 1988;90:289–93.

13a. _____, Johnson PC. Regional heterogeneity in the proliferative activity of human gliomas as measured by the Ki-67 labeling index. J Neuropathol Exp Neurol 1993;52:609–18.

14. Daumas-Duport C, Scheithauer BW, Kelly PJ. A histologic and cytologic method for the spatial definition of gliomas. Mayo Clin Proc 1987;62:435–49.

15. Di Chiro G, Oldfield EH, Wright DC, et al. Cerebral necrosis after radiotherapy and/or intraarterial chemotherapy for brain tumors: PET and neuropathologic studies. AJR Am J Roentgenol 1988;150:189–97.

16. _____, Patronas NJ, Oldfield EH, Wright DC, Katz DA. PET, CT and NMR of cerebral necrosis following radiotherapy or intraarterial chemotherapy for cerebral tumors [Abstract]. Am J Neuroradiol 1985;6:473–4.

17. Fitzgibbons PL, Turner RR, Appley AJ, et al. Flow cytometric DNA and nuclear antigen content in astrocytic neoplasms. Am J Clin Pathol 1988;89:640–4.

18. Francavilla TL, Miletich RS, Di Chiro G, Patronas NJ, Rizzoli HV, Wright DC. Positron emission tomography in the detection of malignant degeneration of low-grade gliomas. Neurosurgery 1989;24:1–5.

19. Fults D, Brockmeyer D, Tullous MW, Pedcone CA, Cawthon RM. p53 mutation and loss of heterozygosity on chromosomes 17 and 10 during human astrocytoma progression. Cancer Res 1992;52:674–9.

20. Glantz MJ, Burger PC, Herndon JE II, et al. Influence of the type of surgery on the histologic diagnosis in patients with anaplastic gliomas. Neurology 1991; 41:1741–4.

21. _____, Hoffman JM, Coleman RE, et al. Identification of early recurrence of primary central nervous system tumors by [^{18}F] fluorodeoxyglucose positron emission tomography. Ann Neurol 1991;29:347–55.

22. Hanson MW, Glantz MJ, Hoffman JM, et al. FDG-PET in the selection of brain lesions for biopsy. J Comput Assist Tomogr 1991;15:796–801.

23. Hara A, Hirayama H, Sakai N, Yamada H, Tanaka T, Mori H. Correlation between nucleolar organizer region staining and Ki-67 immunostaining in human gliomas. Surg Neurol 1990;33:320–4.

24. _____, Sakai N, Yamada H, Hirayama H, Tanaka T, Mori H. Nucleolar organizer regions in vascular and neoplastic cells of human gliomas. Neurosurgery 1991; 29:211–5.

25. Hayashi Y, Yamashita J, Yamaguchi K. Timing and role of p53 gene mutation in the recurrence of glioma. Biochem Biophy Res Commun 1991;180:1145–50.

26. Hedley DW, Freidlander ML, Taylor IW, Rugg CA, Musgrove EA. Method for analysis of cellular DNA content of paraffin-embedded pathological material using flow cytometry. J Histochem Cytochem 1983;31:1333–5.

27. Hirakawa K, Suzuki K, Ueda S, et al. Multivariate analysis of factors affecting postoperative survival in malignant astrocytoma. Importance of DNA quantification. J Neurooncol 1984;2:331–40.

28. Hoshino T, Nagashima T, Murovic JA, et al. In situ cell kinetics studies on human neuroectodermal tumors with bromodeoxyuridine labeling. J Neurosurg 1986;64:453–9.

29. Hurtt MR, Moossy J, Donovan-Peluso M, Locker J. Amplification of epidermal growth factor receptor gene in gliomas: histopathology and prognosis. J Neuropathol Exp Neurol 1992;51:84–90.

29a. Karamitopoulou E, Perentes, Diamantis I, Maraziotis T. Ki-67 immunoreactivity in human central nervous system tumors: a study with MIB 1 monoclonal antibody on archival material. Acta Neuropathol 1994;87:47–54.

30. _____, Perentes E, Melachrinou M, Mariziotis T. Proliferating cell nuclear antigen immunoreactivity in human central nervous system neoplasms. Acta Neuropathol (Berl) 1993;85:316–22.

30a. Khoshyomn S, Maier H, Morimura T, Kitz K, Budka H. Immunostaining for proliferating cell nuclear antigen: its role in determination of proliferation in routinely processed human brain tumor specimens. Acta Neuropathol 1993;86:582–9.

30a. Korkolopoulou P, Christodoulo P, Papanikolaou A, Thomas-Tsagli E. Proliferating cell nuclear antigen and nucleolar organizer regions in CNS tumors: correlation with histological type and tumor grade. Am J Surg Pathol 1993;17:912–9.

31. Kunishio K, Mishima N, Matsuhisa T, et al. Immunohistochemical demonstration of DNA polymerase α in human brain-tumor cells. J Neurosurg 1990;72:268–72.

32. Labrousse F, Daumas-Duport C, Batorski L, Hoshino T. Histological grading and bromodeoxyuridine labeling index of astrocytomas. Comparative study in a series of 60 cases. J Neurosurg 1991;75:202–5.

33. Louis DN, Edgerton S, Thor AD, Hedley-Whyte ET. Proliferating cell nuclear antigen and Ki-67 immunohistochemistry in brain tumors: a comparative study. Acta Neuropathol (Berl) 1991;81:675–9.

34. _____, Meehan SM, Ferrante RJ, Hedley-Whyte ET. Use of the silver nucleolar organizer region (AgNOR) technique in the differential diagnosis of central nervous system neoplasia. J Neuropathol Exp Neurol 1992;51:150–7.

35. Maier H, Morimura T, Öfner D, Hallbrucker C, Kitz K, Budka H. Argyrophilic nucleolar organizer region proteins (Ag-NORs) in human brain tumors: relations with grade of malignancy and proliferation indices. Acta Neuropathol (Berl) 1990;80:156–62.

35a. Montine TJ, Vandersteenhoven JJ, Aguzzi A, et al. Prognostic significance of Ki-67 proliferation index in supratentorial fibrillary astrocytic neoplasms. Neurosurgery. In press.

36. Morimura T, Kitz K, Stein H, Budka H. Determination of proliferative activities in human brain tumor specimens: a comparison of three methods. J Neurooncol 1991;10:1–11.

37. Nishizaki T, Orita T, Kajiwara K, et al. Correlation of in vitro bromodeoxyuridine labeling index and DNA aneuploidy with survival or recurrence in brain-tumor patients. J Neurosurg 1990;73:396–400.

38. Orita T, Kajiwara K, Nishizaki T, Ikeda N, Kamiryo T, Aoki H. Nucleolar organizer regions in meningioma. Neurosurgery 1990;26:43–6.

39. Patronas NJ, Di Chiro G, Kufta C, et al. Prediction of survival in glioma patients by means of positron emission tomography. J Neurosurg 1985;62:816–22.

40. Plate KH, Rüschoff J, Behnke J, Mennel HD. Proliferative potential of human brain tumours as assessed by nucleolar organizer regions (AgNORs) and Ki-67-immunoreactivity. Acta Neurochir (Wien) 1990;104:103–9.

41. Raghavan R, Steart PV, Weller RO. Cell proliferation patterns in the diagnosis of astrocytomas, anaplastic astrocytomas and glioblastoma multiforme: a Ki-67 study. Neuropathol Appl Neurobiol 1990;16:123–33.

42. Rüschoff J, Plate K, Bittinger A, Thomas C. Nucleolar organizer regions (NORs). Basic concepts and practical application in tumor pathology. Pathol Res Pract 1989;185:878–85.

43. Schofield DE, Yunis EJ, Geyer JR, Albright AL, Berger MS, Taylor SR. DNA content and other prognostic features in childhood medulloblastoma. Proposal of a scoring system. Cancer 1992;69:1307–14.

44. Shiraishi T, Tabuchi K, Mineta T, Momozaki N, Takagi M. Nucleolar organizing regions in various human brain tumors. J Neurosurg 1991;74:979–84.

45. Sidransky D, Mikkelsen T, Schwechheimer K, Rosenblum ML, Cavanee W, Vogelstein B. Clonal expansion of p53 mutant cells is associated with brain tumour progression. Nature 1992;335:846–7.

46. Sutton LN, Wang Z, Gusnard D, et al. Proton magnetic resonance spectroscopy of pediatric brain tumors. Neurosurgery 1992;31:195–202.

47. Tsanaclis AM, Robert F, Michaud J, Brem S. The cycling pool of cells within human brain tumors: in situ cytokinetics using the monoclonal antibody Ki-67. Can J Neurol Sci 1991;18:12–7.

48. van Dierendonck JH, Wijsman JH, Keijzer R, van de Velde CJ, Cornelisse CJ. Cell-cycle-related staining patterns of anti-proliferating cell nuclear antigen monoclonal antibodies. Comparison with BrdU labeling and Ki-67 staining. Am J Pathol 1991;138:1165–72.

49. Verheijen R, Kuijpers HJ, Schlingemann RO, et al. Ki-67 detects a nuclear matrix-associated proliferation-related antigen. I. Intracellular localization during interphase. J Cell Sci 1989;92(Pt 1):123–30.

50. Vindeløv LL, Christensen IJ, Nessen NI. A detergent-trypsin method for the preparation of nuclei for flow cytometric DNA analysis. Cytometry 1983;3:323–7.

51. von Deimling A, Eibl RH, Ohgaki H, et al. p53 mutations all associated with 17p allelic loss in grade II and grade III astrocytoma. Cancer Res 1992;52:2987–90.

52. _____, Louis DN, von Ammon K, Wiestler OD, Seizinger BR. Evidence for a tumor suppressor gene on chromosome 19q associated with human astrocytomas, oligodendrogliomas, and mixed gliomas. Cancer Res 1992;52:4277–9.

53. _____, Louis DN, von Ammon K, et al. Association of epidermal growth factor receptor gene amplification with loss of chromosome 10 in human glioblastoma multiforme. J Neurosurg 1992;77:295–301.

54. Yasue M, Tomita T, Engelhard H, Gonzalez-Crussi F, McLone DG, Bauer KD. Prognostic importance of DNA ploidy in medulloblastoma of childhood. J Neurosurg 1989;70:385–91.

55. Zaprianov Z, Christov K. Histological grading, DNA content, cell proliferation and survival of patients with astroglial tumors. Cytometry 1988;9:380–6.

APPENDIX A

NON-NEOPLASTIC LESIONS POTENTIALLY MISINTERPRETED AS NEOPLASMS

Reactive Gliosis

May be misinterpreted as a glioma if attention is focused only on the cytoplasmic features and not on cell density and distribution. Well-differentiated astrocytomas are hypercellular and the cells are irregularly distributed. Unlike glioma cells, those of reactive gliosis are stellate in configuration with long, tapering, radiating processes; they are hypertrophic but not notably increased in number.

Demyelinating Disease

May be misinterpreted as glioma because of the high cellularity produced by the influx of macrophages. The large reactive, albeit "atypical-appearing" astrocytes, lend additional overtones of neoplasia. The diagnosis of demyelinating disease is based upon heightened suspicion in a young patient with one or more white matter lesions, especially when paraventricular or subcortical, but any central nervous system lesion rich in macrophages should be suspect. The presence of perivascular inflammation, although sometimes seen in gliomas, alerts the pathologist to the possibility of demyelinating disease. Smear preparations greatly facilitate the recognition of macrophages and reactive astrocytes. Either PAS or one of several immunohistochemical stains for macrophages are appropriate if the presence of these phagocytes is suspected.

Cerebral Infarct

May be interpreted as a glioma, particularly a malignant variety, because of the high cellularity, necrosis, and hypertrophic vascular changes. The radiographic findings of a contrast-enhancing mass makes this misinterpretation even more likely. As in the case of demyelinating disease, macrophages are the principal constituent cells.

Pineal Cyst

May be mistaken for either a) a glioma if, out of context of the radiographic features, attention is focused on the gliotic wall surrounding the cyst cavity or b) a pineocytoma if attention is directed toward the residual gland. Correct identification of the pineal cyst is aided by the radiographic finding of a largely thin-walled pineal cyst and by cognizance of the normal histologic appearance of the pineal gland, which may suggest a neoplasm.

Meningioangiomatosis

May be interpreted as a meningioma if meningothelial cells are prominent, a glioma because of the overall hypercellularity, or a ganglion cell neoplasm due to entrapment of preexisting neurons. A correct diagnosis depends largely on the recognition of the entity as an intracortical perivascular proliferation of meningothelial cells and fibroblasts.

Hypothalamic Hamartoma

May be misinterpreted as a ganglion cell tumor if attention is focused only on the neurons. Correct identification follows the recognition of its hypocellularity, similarity to normal grey matter, and relative degree of organization of mature neurons and glia.

Progressive Multifocal Leukoencephalopathy

May be misconstrued as a malignant glioma because of the often considerable pleomorphism and hyperchromasia of oligodendroglia and astrocytes within this demyelinating lesion. Identification depends on recognizing the macrophage-rich background and virus-infected oligodendroglia which are most abundant at the edge of the lesion.

Dysplastic Gangliocytoma (Lhermitte-Duclos Disease)

May be misinterpreted as a glioma or a ganglion cell tumor because of the abnormal, large, closely packed cells. The lesion is recognized by its radiographic features as well as the neuronal character of its constituent cells. The latter are topographically restricted to the internal granular cell layer.

Syrinx (Spinal Cord)

The gliotic non-neoplastic cyst wall of a spontaneous or tumor-associated intramedullary cavity can closely resemble a well-differentiated astrocytoma of the spinal cord. The frequent presence of Rosenthal fibers makes the pilocytic astrocytoma a frequent, and potentially difficult, differential diagnostic problem as is discussed above under Reactive Gliosis.

APPENDIX B

CNS TUMORS POTENTIALLY OVERGRADED AS AGGRESSIVE OR ANAPLASTIC NEOPLASMS

Pilocytic Astrocytoma

Is overgraded when mistaken for a fibrillary or "diffuse" astrocytoma of any grade. This error is especially likely to occur with lesions in the cerebral hemispheres and spinal cord where pilocytic astrocytomas are incorrectly assumed to be rare. A diagnosis of pilocytic astrocytoma should always be suspected in the face of a discrete, contrast-enhancing cystic lesion.

Ganglion Cell Tumors

May be overgraded as fibrillary or diffuse astrocytoma if attention is focused only on the glial component. The pleomorphism of both neurons and glia can, particularly at the time of frozen section, be misinterpreted as evidence of histologic malignancy.

Pleomorphic Xanthoastrocytoma (PXA)

May, given its pleomorphism, be mistaken for a malignant glioma. This error is avoided by awareness of the clinical and radiographic features of classic PXA, and by noting the disparity between extensive cytologic atypia and the absence of mitotic figures and necrosis.

Hemangioblastoma

The neoplasm proper may closely resemble a glioma, particularly in frozen sections. In addition, the non-neoplastic cyst wall resembles a pilocytic astrocytoma. Awareness of the tumor's radiographic features and occurrence at sites other than the cerebellum (e.g. medulla and spinal cord) minimizes the likelihood of diagnostic confusion.

Central Neurocytoma

From a therapeutic point of view, this uncommon neoplasm is overgraded if mistaken for oligodendroglioma, ependymoma, or neuroblastoma. The lesion is readily recognized in the context of its clinical and radiographic features: a large intraventricular, often calcified, midline mass with little or no apparent intraparenchymal component.

Dysembryoplastic Neuroepithelial Tumor (DNT)

May appear similar, if not identical, to oligodendroglia, particularly in small, nonrepresentative fragments. The presence of occasional abnormal ganglion cells may alternatively suggest a ganglion cell tumor. Recognition of the lesion is aided by awareness of its stereotypic and radiographic features, as well as by its intracortical loose-textured nodules.

Desmoplastic Infantile Ganglioglioma (DIG)

May be misinterpreted as a meningeal sarcoma, malignant glioma, or embryonal tumor because of the cellular component in some examples. The lesion is recognized by the radiographic features, cyst with superficial tumor mass, and histologic findings which include a prominent desmoplastic component.

APPENDIX C

SUSPECT DIAGNOSES IN SURGICAL NEUROPATHOLOGY

- Malignant tumor (especially in young adults) with either a long clinical history (usually seizures), or with associated scalloping of the inner table of the skull.

- Well-differentiated fibrillary astrocytoma in the face of a radiographically contrast-enhancing lesion.

- Infiltrating glioma, of any grade, for a cystic lesion, especially one with a mural nodule.

- Malignant neoplasm in the absence of neuroradiologic evidence of peritumoral edema.

- Glioma in the setting of a macrophage-rich lesion, especially one that is multifocal.

- Infiltrating glioma, especially high grade, for a tumor with Rosenthal fibers or eosinophilic granular bodies.

- Glioma or pineocytoma in the face of a cystic lesion in the pineal gland.

APPENDIX D

FREQUENTLY CYSTIC LESIONS

Pilocytic astrocytoma

Ganglion cell tumors

Desmoplastic infantile ganglioglioma

Ependymoma (supratentorial and spinal)

Hemangioblastoma

Pleomorphic xanthoastrocytoma

Craniopharyngioma

Cysts
  Colloid
  Rathke cleft
  Endodermal
  Ependymal (glioependymal)
  Choroid plexus
  Epidermoid and dermoid
  Arachnoid
  Pineal
  Nerve root
  Spinal synovial

Intramedullary spinal cord neoplasm with a syrinx

Syringomyelia

Meningioma (occasional)

Schwannoma (usually larger examples)

APPENDIX E

FREQUENTLY CALCIFIED TUMORS

Oligodendroglioma

Pilocytic astrocytoma

Subependymal giant cell astrocytoma (tuberous sclerosis)

Ependymoma

Subependymoma

Choroid plexus papilloma (fourth ventricular)

Ganglion cell tumors

Central neurocytoma

Pineal cyst (residual pineal)

Meningioma

Vascular malformations

Craniopharyngioma (adamantinomatous type)

Meningioangiomatosis

Retinoblastoma

APPENDIX F

INTRAVENTRICULAR TUMORS

Ependymoma (lateral, third, and fourth)

Subependymoma (lateral and fourth)

Subependymal giant cell astrocytoma (tuberous sclerosis) (lateral)

Choroid plexus tumors (lateral and third in children; fourth in adults)

Pilocytic astrocytoma (third, fourth, and lateral)

Central neurocytoma (lateral and rarely, third)

Pineal parenchymal and germ cell tumors (posterior third)

Papillary craniopharyngioma (third)

Colloid cyst (third)

Meningioma (uncommon in lateral, third, or fourth)

APPENDIX G

DIFFERENTIAL DIAGNOSES OF INTRASPINAL LESIONS BY ANATOMIC LOCATION

EXTRADURAL

    Herniated nucleus pulposus

    Metastatic carcinoma

    Lymphoma

    Myeloma

    Abscess

    Tuberculosis

    Primary spine and soft tissue tumors

    Neuroblastoma/ganglioneuroblastoma

INTRADURAL

    Extramedullary

        Schwannoma

        Meningioma

        Non-neoplastic cysts (endodermal, meningeal, Tarlov)

        Meningeal carcinomatosis (subarachnoid)

        Drop metastasis (subarachnoid)

        Inflammatory lesions, e.g., tuberculosis, sarcoid (subarachnoid)

    Intramedullary

        Astrocytoma

            Pilocytic

            Fibrillary

        Oligodendroglioma

        Ependymoma

            Cellular

            Myxopapillary (filum terminale)

        Subependymoma

        Ganglion cell tumor

        Hemangioblastoma

        Paraganglioma (filum terminale)

        Schwannoma (uncommon)

        Demyelinating disease

        Syringomyelia

APPENDIX H

IMMUNOREACTIVITY OF SELECTED CNS TUMORS

	Epithelial Membrane Antigen (EMA)	Cyto-keratin (CK)	S-100 Protein	Chromo-granin	HMB-45	Synapto-physin
Metastatic carcinoma	+	+	±	±	±	−
Lymphoma	−[3]	−	−	−	−	−
Plasmacytoma/myeloma	+	−	−	−	−	−
Germinoma	−	10%+	−	−	−	−
Chordoma	+	+	+	−	−	−
Meningioma	+	±[1]	±	−	−	−
Hemangiopericytoma	−	−	−	−	−	−
Esthesioneuroblastoma	−	±[2]	±[2]	±	−	+
Melanoma	−	−	+	−	+	−
Glioma	−[4]	+[6]	+	−	−	−
Medulloblastoma	−	−	±[8]	−	−	+
Central neurocytoma	−	−	−	−	−	+
Choroid plexus tumors	±	±	+	−	−	−
Schwannoma	±[5]	−	+	−	±[7]	−
Paraganglioma	−	−	±[9]	+	−	+

[1] Secretory variant of meningioma contains PAS-positive pseudopsammoma bodies; surrounding cells are CEA- and CK-reactive.

[2] Tumors with olfactory rosettes may be reactive for CK. Sustentacular cells, present in some tumors, are S-100 reactive.

[3] Ki-1 lymphoma is commonly LCA negative and EMA positive. CD 30 reactivity distinguishes this tumor.

[4] EMA reactivity may be seen rarely in astrocytoma and gliosis. Epithelial surfaces may be positive in ependymomas.

[5] Schwannoma may exhibit cytoplasmic EMA reactivity.

[6] Reactivity is common with commercial antisera.

[7] Melanotic schwannomas are positive.

[8] Positive in medulloblastomas with glial differentiation.

[9] Sustentacular cells are positive, chief cells are variably stained.

[10] Sustentacular cells are positive, chief cells are negatively stained.

IMMUNOREACTIVITY OF SELECTED CNS TUMORS

	Carcino-embryonic Antigen (CEA)	Placental Alkaline Phosphatase (PLAP)	Leukocyte Common Antigen (LCA)	Vimentin	Glial Fibrillary Acidic Protein (GFAP)
Metastatic carcinoma	±	±	−	±	−
Lymphoma	−	−	+	±	−
Plasmacytoma/myeloma	−	−	±	+	−
Germinoma	−	+	−	±	−
Chordoma	10%+	−	−	+	−
Meningioma	±[1]	−	−	+	−
Hemangiopericytoma	−	−	−	+	−
Esthesioneuroblastoma	−	−	−	−	−
Melanoma	−	−	−	+	−
Glioma	−	−	−	+	+
Medulloblastoma	−	−	−	±[8]	±[8]
Central neurocytoma	−	−	−	−	−
Choroid plexus tumors	±	−	−	+	±
Schwannoma	−	−	−	+	±
Paraganglioma	−	−	−	±[10]	±[10]

APPENDIX I

IMMUNOCYTOLOGY OF PRIMARY INTRACRANIAL GERM CELL TUMORS*

	Placental Alkaline Phosphatase	Alpha Feto-protein	Human Chorionic Gonado-tropin	Human Placental Lactogen	Preg-nancy-Specific Protein	Keratin	Epithelial Membrane Antigen
Germinoma**	+	−	±[†]	−	−	10%	−
Teratoma	+	±	−	−	−	±	±
Embryonal carcinoma	+	−	−	−	−	+	−
Yolk sac carcinoma	±	+	−	−	−	+	±
Choriocarcinoma	±	−	+	+	+	+	+

* Modified from Scheithauer BW: Neuropathology of pineal region tumors. Clin Neurosurg 1985;32:351–83.

**Germinomas have been reported to show immunoreactivity for vimentin (15 percent) as well as neuron-specific enolase (90 percent).

[†] Isolated syncytiotrophoblastic cells are present in 50 percent of germinomas.

Index*

---

*Numbers in boldface indicate table and figure pages.

❖❖❖